Advanced Practice Nursing:
Emphasizing Common Roles

Advanced Practice Nursing: Emphasizing Common Roles

Christine M. Sheehy, PhD, RN
Associate Professor
Arizona State University
Tempe, Arizona

Marianne McCarthy, PhD, RN, CS
Assistant Professor
Arizona State University
Tempe, Arizona

F. A. DAVIS COMPANY ● **Philadelphia**

F. A. Davis Company
1915 Arch Street
Philadelphia, PA 19103

Printed in the United States of America

Last digit indicates print number: 10 9 8 7 6 5 4

Acquisitions Editor: Joanne P. DaCunha, RN, MSN
Production Editors: Michael Schnee, Jessica Howie Martin
Cover Designer: Louis J. Forgione

As new scientific information becomes available through basic and clinical research, recommended treatments and drug therapies undergo changes. The authors and publisher have done everything possible to make this book accurate, up to date, and in accord with accepted standards at the time of publication. The authors, editors, and publisher are not responsible for errors or omissions or for consequences from application of the book, and make no warranty, expressed or implied, in regard to the contents of the book. Any practice described in this book should be applied by the reader in accordance with professional standards of care used in regard to the unique circumstances that may apply in each situation. The reader is advised always to check product information (package inserts) for changes and new information regarding dose and contraindications before administering any drug. Caution is especially urged when using new or infrequently ordered drugs.

Library of Congress Cataloging in Publication Data
Advanced practice nursing : emphasizing common roles / [edited by]
   Christine M. Sheehy, Marianne McCarthy.
      p.   cm.
   Includes bibliographical references and index.
   ISBN 0-8036-0234-0 (alk. paper)
   1. Nurse practitioners.   2. Midwives.   3. Nurse anesthetists.
I. Sheehy, Christine M., 1948–   . II. McCarthy, Marianne, 1953–
   [DNLM: 1. Nurse Clinicians.   2. Nurse Practitioners.   3. Nurse
Midwives.   WY   128   A2445   1998]
RT82.8.A37   1998
610.73'06'92—dc21
DNLM/DLC
for Library of Congress   97-34612
                                                               CIP

Foreword

The publication of this book, *Advanced Practice Nursing: Emphasizing Common Roles*, is timely and the title illustrates a major change in the conceptualization of advanced nursing practice that is underway in the United States today. For many years, emphasis has been placed on seeking ways to identify and validate differences in the practice and education of all levels of nurses, with the most emphasis on entry-level nurses. However, since health-care reform has spotlighted all advanced practice roles as being capable of providing safe and cost-effective care, these efforts to identify differences in practice have given way to identifying commonalties in advanced practice nursing. The terms *nurse practitioner* and *nurse midwife* have almost become household words. This public recognition of advanced practice roles and the need for cost control have become driving forces, helping to describe and define the roles through standardization of advanced practice curricula, professional and accreditation standards, and regulation. Thus, a book that combines the major issues and concepts related to the four advanced practice roles of nurse practitioner, certified nurse midwife, certified registered nurse anesthetist, and clinical nurse specialist is long overdue, and should reflect the current and future trends of advanced practice nursing. Speaking with one voice dissolves much of the confusion over what constitutes advanced nursing in both nursing education and practice.

The efforts of the contributing authors demonstrate the common body of knowledge specific to advanced nursing practice roles. At the same time, the authors have acknowledged the unique contribution each advanced nursing role brings to health care. This is absolutely critical today because the nursing, medical, and health-care paradigms we have known for the past 30 years are rapidly changing. The history of the development and legitimization of advanced practice differs for each role, but there are also experiences common to all. Nurse practitioner, certified nurse midwife, and certified registered nurse anesthetist roles were all developed in collaboration and/or in competition with medicine. The inclusion of specific, delegated medical acts as part of advanced practice nursing prompted many studies in the 1960s, '70s, and '80s to determine the safety, effectiveness, and cost of substituting advanced practice nursing roles for medicine in certain settings. Consequently, NPs, CNMs, and CRNAs were most often compared to other health professionals, such as physicians and physician assistants, rather than to each other. Less of an attempt was made to determine the similarities of each nursing role, and in many cases, the nature of the practice was described relative to medicine rather than nursing. This led to an emphasis in the health-care literature on the medical aspects of the role rather than furthering the development of advanced nursing roles. For this reason, acceptance of the roles in nursing education has not been readily forthcoming. In contrast to these three roles, CNSs were not compared to other professional groups, including medicine. However, if the role of the CNS was more palatable for nursing education, few studies were conducted to support and define the safety, effectiveness, and cost-benefit of the role. In general, although this comparison process may have been necessary developmentally, it truly inhibited the promotion of the concept of advanced practice nursing into the health-care arena.

The authors of *Advanced Practice Nursing* have adroitly moved beyond this past and truly captured the present trends. Efforts to identify and develop common standards for all advanced practice can also be seen in the standardization of core content and specialty curricula for master's programs that prepare advanced practice nurses, in the publications of professional and advanced practice nursing organizations, and in regulation. The American College of Nurse Midwives and the American Association of Nurse Anesthetists have had uniform educational standards for nurse midwifery and nurse anesthetist programs for many years. The lack of standards and guidelines for programs has been addressed by the National Organization of Nurse Practitioner Faculty in its recently published *Curriculum Guidelines and Program Standards for Nurse Practitioner Programs.* The publication of the American Association of Colleges of Nursing document, *Essentials of Master's Education for Advanced Practice Nursing,* represents the first national attempt to identify common core content for all master's programs that prepare graduates in the four advanced practice roles, and emphasizes standardization of nursing curricula for advanced practice.

The expectation of a master's degree as the entry requirement for advanced practice is becoming a reality and most likely will be universal sometime after the turn of the century. State nursing regulatory boards are moving toward setting a date after which a master's degree will be required for recognition as an advanced practice nurse; all current nurses in advanced practice roles will be "grandfathered" after that date. All of these parallel and joint efforts have contributed to the conceptualization of advanced practice nursing so that future graduate students, faculty, employers, advanced practice nurses, and consumers of health care may all share the same understanding and expectations of an advanced practice nurse.

I would like to applaud the editors, Dr. Christine Sheehy and Dr. Marianne McCarthy, and all contributors for their foresight and vision to produce a book that lays the groundwork for nursing to truly join forces for the next century.

Mary V. Fenton, DrPH, RN

Acknowledgments

This edited book has been made possible by the combined expertise and commitment of many friends, students, and colleagues, all of whom I cherish and hold in the highest regard. During the course of the project, personal circumstances often competed with writing efforts for many of the authors. I am extremely grateful to all of them for their willingness to see their chapters through to completion.

For a variety of reasons, the authorship of several chapters changed mid-production, requiring a new search for talent. Although, admittedly, it was difficult to deny my pleas, those who "jumped aboard" did so with graciousness and enthusiasm because they valued the product. These include Pauline Komnenich, Suzanne Hall Johnson, Marla Weston, and Vicki Buchda. Working under the pressure of an abbreviated timeline is not for the faint of heart. I am very grateful that you allowed me to lean on you.

Several people were particularly helpful in providing information and wisdom. Judith Berman provided much insight in the initial stages of production, and ultimately coauthored a chapter. Debra Bergstrom was instrumental in the early conceptualization of the chapter "Creating Excellence in Practice." The historical description in the chapter "The Evolution of Advanced Practice in Nursing," was greatly enhanced and made more meaningful by input from Joyce Roberts, PhD, CNMW, FAAN, FACNM; Betty Bear, PhD, CNMW, FAAN, FACNM; John Garde, CRNA, MS, FAAN; Pamela Minarik, MS, FAAN; Irene Riddle, PhD, MSN; and Loretta C. Ford, EdD, MS, FAAN. They generously gave of their time to describe the "lived experience," went out of their way to arrange times to be interviewed, to make supporting materials available, and to edit.

I am most indebted to my coeditor, Marianne McCarthy, for her collaboration. I thank our editor, Joanne DaCunha, who bore with me through many phases in learning and text production, and from whom I must now suffer gradual separation in my daily routine.

C.M.S.

This book is dedicated to my two beautiful boys, Zachary and Alec, who provided joyful distraction when I needed it most, and to Judith, my most cherished friend and ardent critic, who offered her kind support and expert advice during a rewarding but arduous endeavor. The hard work of Judith A. Berman is acknowledged and greatly appreciated.

M.C.M.

Contributors

Jeanne Pichette Bair, MSN, RN, CNM
Senior Instructor
University of Colorado Health
   Sciences Center
Denver, Colorado

Geraldine "Polly" Bednash, PhD, RN, FAAN
Executive Director
American Association of Colleges of
   Nursing
Washington, D.C.

Debra Bergstrom, MS, RN, CCRN, FNP
Nurse Practitioner
Mercy Integrated Health
Phoenix, Arizona

Judith A. Berman, JD, RN
Attorney
Doyle, Winthrop, & West
Phoenix, Arizona

Linda A. Bernhard, PhD, RN
Associate Professor
Nursing and Women's Studies
The Ohio State University
College of Nursing
Columbus, Ohio

Vicki L. Buchda, MS, RN
Director, Patient Care Resources
Mayo Arizona
Scottsdale, Arizona

Christine E. Burke, PhD, CNM
Faculty
University of Colorado Health
   Sciences Center
Denver, Colorado

Linda Callahan, PhD, CRNA
Assistant Director
Kaiser Permanente School of Nurse
   Anesthesia
California State University
Long Beach, California

Linda Lindsey Davis, PhD, RN, ANP
Professor, School of Nursing
Senior Scientist, Center for Aging
University of Alabama at Birmingham
Birmingham, Alabama

Linda Maria Dominguez, PhD, RN
Clinical Researcher
Maricopa Medical Center
Phoenix, Arizona

Julie Reed Erickson, PhD, RN, FAAN
Assistant Professor
University of Arizona College of
   Nursing
Tucson, Arizona

Margaret Faut-Callahan, DNSc, CRNA, FAAN
Professor and Program Director,
   Nurse Anesthesia Program
Rush University College of Nursing
Chicago, Illinois

Mary V. Fenton, DrPH, RN
Dean and Professor
The University of Texas Medical
   Branch School of Nursing at
   Galveston
Galveston, Texas

Catherine L. Gilliss, DNSc, RN, CS, FAAN
Professor
Department of Family Health Care
  Nursing
University of California
San Francisco, California

Senior Fellow
University of California at San
  Francisco Center for the Health
  Professions
San Francisco, California

Lucille A. Joel, EdD, RN, FAAN
Professor
Rutgers—The State University of New
  Jersey, College of Nursing
Newark, New Jersey

Suzanne Hall Johnson, MN, RNC, CNS
Director, Hall Johnson
  Communications, Inc.
Editor, *Dimensions of Critical Care
  Nursing; Recruitment, Retention &
  Restructuring Report;* and *Nurse
  Author & Editor*
Lakewood, Colorado

Pauline Komnenich, PhD, RN
Associate Professor
Arizona State University College of
  Nursing
Tempe, Arizona

Michael J. Kremer, DNSc, CRNA
Faculty Preceptor
Nurse Anesthesia Program
Rush University College of Nursing
Chicago, Illinois

Mary Jeanette Mannino, JD, CRNA
Director, Anesthesia and Ambulatory
  Surgery
The Mannino Group
Washington, D.C.

Joan M. Stanley, PhD, CRNP
Director of Education Policy
American Association of Colleges of
  Nursing
Washington, D.C.

Sara Torres, PhD, RN, FAAN
Associate Professor and Chair
Department of Psychiatric,
  Community Health, and Adult
  Primary Care
University of Maryland at Baltimore
School of Nursing
Baltimore, Maryland

Michelle Walsh, PhD, RN, CPNP
Pediatric Nurse Practitioner
Child Care Consultants, Inc.
Columbus, Ohio

Marla J. Weston, MS, RN
Acute Care Administrator
Columbia Paradise Valley Hospital
Phoenix, Arizona

Reviewers

Dorothy J. Brundage, PhD, RN, FAAN
Associate Professor of Nursing
Duke University School of Nursing
Durham, North Carolina

Mary B. Dressler, EdD, RN
Associate Professor, Graduate
    Nursing
Gwynedd Mercy College
Gwynedd Valley, Pennsylvania

Kelly A. Goudreau, M. Nurs., RN, CS, APRN
Assistant Professor
University of Maine
College of Nursing
Fort Kent, Maine

Lynne M. Hektor, PhD, ARNP, CS
Associate Professor
Florida Atlantic University
Boca Raton, Florida

Margaret McAllister, PhD(c), MA, SpCl N, FNP
Lecturer and Family Nurse
    Practitioner
Northeastern University
Boston, Massachusetts

Ann M. McGinn, EdD, RN
Associate Professor, Graduate
    Nursing
Gwynedd Mercy College
Gwynedd Valley, Pennsylvania

Geralyn R. Spollet, APRN, CDE
Assistant Professor
Adult Nurse Practitioner Program
Adult Health Division
Yale University
New Haven, Connecticut

Lois Van Cleve, PhD, MS, RN
Professor and Associate Dean
Loma Linda University, Graduate
    Program in Nursing
Loma Linda, California

Contents

CHAPTER 9

**Collaborative Practice: How We Get from Coordination to the
Integration of Skills and Knowledge** 217

Sara Torres, PhD, RN, FAAN
Linda Marie Dominguez, PhD, RN

CHAPTER 10

Clinical Research in the Advanced Practice Role 241

Julie Reed Erickson, PhD, RN, FAAN
Christine M. Sheehy, PhD, RN

CHAPTER 11

Publishing Scholarly Works 264

Suzanne Hall Johnson, MN, RNC, CNS

CHAPTER 12

Legal Aspects of Advanced Nursing Practice 280

Linda Callahan, PhD, CRNA
Mary Jeanette Mannino, JD, CRNA

CHAPTER 13

Marla J. Weston, MS, RN
Vickie L Buchda, MS, RN
Debra Bergstrom, MS, RN, CCRN, FNP

Introduction: Complement, Diversity, and Clarification

CHRISTINE M. SHEEHY, PhD, RN
MARIANNE McCARTHY, PhD, RNCS

Christine Sheehy, PhD, RN, has a doctoral degree in public policy and administration from Virginia Commonwealth University. Between 1989 and 1990, she taught in the master's and doctoral programs and was project director for the master's-level geriatric–nurse practitioner option at the University of Arizona College of Nursing. After a 2-year period as director of health services research for the Maricopa Health System, she returned to the academic setting at Arizona State University in Tempe. Dr. Sheehy's substantive expertise is in the area of health-policy analysis, quality-of-care and health-outcome measurement, and chronic illness and aging.

Marianne McCarthy, PhD, RNCS, is an assistant professor of nursing at Arizona State University. Dr. McCarthy is prepared as both a geriatric nurse practitioner and as a gerontological clinical nurse specialist and has completed a multidisciplinary Geriatric Fellowship Program at the San Francisco Institute of Aging. Dr. McCarthy has practiced extensively in a variety of settings as an advanced practice nurse for almost 20 years. Currently, she is involved in clinical practice in long-term care and coordinates and teaches theory and practicum courses in the Adult Advanced Practice Nursing Program at Arizona State University.

CHAPTER OUTLINE

THE BROADEST USE OF THE TERM
  CRITICAL THINKING
THE APPLICATION OF CRITICAL THINKING
  IN A COMPLEX AND UNCERTAIN
  NURSING-CARE ENVIRONMENT
SUMMARY

The impetus for this text was both immediate and gradual. The need was related directly to course development for graduate nurses enrolled in a geri-
atric-nurse practitioner option. No composite source could be found on
which to structure content considered essential to role development of the advanced practice nurse (APN). Because the nurse practitioner role is one of four
advanced practice nursing areas, it seemed meaningful to explore many aspects
of the nurse practitioner role with a view toward other APN roles. Although
each has distinctive practice features, there is increasing recognition of many
shared role components. As a practical matter, there are at least as many issues
that concern the four role areas as there are issues idiosyncratic to the respective
roles. Clarification of roles appeared best accomplished by comparing one to another, that is, by reflecting perspectives of each APN group on such matters as
historical development, credentialing, legal considerations, and reimbursement.
The four groups of professional nurses recognized as advanced practitioners are:

1. Nurse practitioners (NPs)
2. Clinical nurse specialists (CNSs)
3. Certified nurse midwives (CNMWs)
4. Certified registered nurse anesthetists (CRNAs)[1]

Paralleling this line of thinking, we were sensitive to the climate beyond the
university. Throughout our respective careers in nursing, we had mutually ob-
served that in practice settings, many health-care professionals were confused
about the various APN roles. At least some of the opportunities for APNs are
contingent on "others' " understanding about the potential contribution of
APNs. Role expansion arising from changes in the health-care environment
hinges not only on the clear articulation of role by APNs but also on appreciation
by interdisciplinary colleagues and, in turn, consumers. Therefore, we speculated that a book such as this could also serve as a reference for a wide variety of
clinicians and managers of organizations in which APNs are employed. These
include physicians and professionals in operations, such as chief executives, vice
presidents, and clinical service directors. Further, the book should be a valuable
document to State Boards of Nursing with regard to the APN regulatory interface. The information provided in the chapters and exercises are grounded in
real-world scenarios and challenges frequently encountered in health-care institutions and settings.

The purpose of the book is to put forth, within their historical and contemporary context, major themes crucial to the successful development and implementation of *all* APN roles. The text of each chapter describes *key* concepts of
particular relevance to advanced role development and practice. It is not intended to cover the universe of practice concerns for two reasons. First, this
would be a herculean task, which would delay publishing of vital information
and result in an encyclopedic product. Second, many generic topics would likely
be suitably addressed in other courses in a curriculum. The goal of the book is to
emphasize those issues *common* to the four professional groups that operational-
ize the APN role, thereby joining forces on issues critical to:

- Promoting favorable penetration of the health-care market, and
- Optimizing effective utilization in the health-care system.

Chapter 1 describes the evolution of the four advanced practice nursing
areas and highlights significant trends. In addition to the documented history,

APN leaders were interviewed and asked to reflect on their "lived experiences." This approach provides greater meaning and a richer understanding of the four roles than typical historical accounts. Chapter 2 addresses the broad overlay of the U.S. sociopolitical environment, and Chapter 3 focuses directly on the topic of managed care, which is presented in a contemporary perspective, illustrating trends in both corporate and managed competition. Chapter 4 encompasses numerous conceptual and theoretical models that are closely involved with practice, including leadership and change. Chapter 5 provides a framework for primary care in its most generic application. Chapter 6 covers, in depth, the critically important practice requirements of credentialing and clinical privileges.

Chapter 7 incorporates knowledge about the economics of medical care and implications for reimbursement. Chapter 8 describes the ways in which the roles can be successfully marketed, and strategies for negotiating position descriptions and benefits. It also explains the importance of mentors in accomplishing these activities. Chapter 9 addresses collaboration in terms of integration of skills and knowledge. In Chapter 10, the roles of APNs as consumers of research and as researchers are explored, and are consistent with expectations defined in standards of practice. Trends in the type and nature of research, barriers, and areas of continued need are highlighted for the practice areas. Chapter 11 focuses on the publication of scholarly works, Chapter 12 concerns the legal considerations surrounding role implementation, and Chapter 13 concludes the themes by emphasizing how excellence promotes all professional pursuits.

The chapter objectives build on Bloom's[2] taxonomy of application and analysis and are constructed at the higher end of that continuum of *synthesis* and *evaluation*. The Suggested Exercises at the end of each chapter focus on formation of *critical-thinking* ability. We committed to this approach:

- In the broadest use of the term, and

- As one that provides the greatest utility in comprehending a very complex and uncertain environment.

The Broadest Use of the Term
Critical Thinking

Nursing research has found no consistent relationship between critical thinking and either clinical judgment or achievement in nursing education.[3,4] Differences in study methods and design and the suspicion that critical thinking is a more complicated construct than that which is commonly measured are possible explanations.[3] Tanner[5,6] suggested that critical thinking has been conceptualized to be something that it is not, such as problem solving or the nursing process. Support for this proposition was demonstrated in a survey of nursing deans and faculty.[7] Their interpretation of critical thinking was often narrowly defined and contradictory, operationalized as a rational linear process, a problem-solving activity similar to the nursing process that uses principles of objectivity, prediction, and control. Findings such as these may result partly from reliance on logic-driven paradigms for critical thinking. Perhaps the most well-known example is that proposed by Watson and Glaser,[8] which outlines development of *attitudes* (viewing issues and problems), *knowledge acquisition* (e.g., evaluating the accuracy and logic of evidence, differentiating valid and invalid assumptions), and *skills* (deriving abstractions and generalizations, formulating conclusions, and selecting courses of action).

A more recent and broader impression of critical thinking, and the one that guided development of the exercises contained in this book, is that of Facione.[9] Using a panel of experts and the Delphi technique, he conceptualized critical thinking as having two dimensions:

1. Cognitive skills, and

2. Affective dispositions.

Cognitive skills include interpretation, analysis, evaluation, inference, explanation, and self-regulation (i.e., self-examination and self-correction). *Affective dispositions* that characterize good critical thinkers are inquisitiveness, precision, persistence, diligence in seeking relevant information, flexibility, honesty, and reasonableness among others.[9] The reader is referred to the last reference of the Introduction for the complete list of attributes.

However, even if one subscribes to this expanded perspective of critical thinking, there are many impediments to the application of critical thinking. Among them are:

- *Beliefs* that knowledge necessarily produces critical thinking, that mistakes are always bad, that there is a correct way, and that what is right is most valued[10–12]

- *The educational system,* which often emphasizes primarily factual knowledge[13] and remains largely examination driven[14]

- *Teaching practices,* such as the use of lecture when it is unsuitable to the content and/or learning styles of students[10]

Tanner[6] asserted there *is* recognition that some nursing pedagogy not only fails to enhance, but may actually impede, development of critical-thinking abilities in students. Critical-thinking modes such as questioning assumptions and recognizing historical context are often ignored,[15] and learning by discovery may be uncomfortable for some students, because pursuit of creative solutions threatens their security and desire to be correct.[10]

In a phenomenologic study of nurses, Brookfield[16] presented a self-description by nurses of the process of learning critical thinking. They explained it as

> a rhythm of learning that might be called "incremental fluctuation" . . . in a series of fluctuations marked by an overall movement forward . . . distinguished by an increased ability to take alternative perspectives on familiar situations, a developing readiness to challenge assumptions, and a growing tolerance for ambiguity. (p. 204)

Our aim in the Suggested Exercises is to support such a dynamic approach to learning.

The process of critical thinking also highlights the connectiveness of events and the human experience[13] and supports the searching out, recognizing, and explaining of patterns.[14,17] In most Suggested Exercises, there are no single or best answers, there are no test questions per se. The exercises can be used for classroom activities and/or assignments. Faculty can further individualize the exercises by attributing criteria and weighting in evaluating them for grading purposes. The exercises do not use exemplars, because we preferred to leave illustrations to those interpreting the chapter. In our experience, professional nurses are rich with their own exemplars.

Critical thinking then is fundamental to the advanced practice role because:

- It is indispensable in anticipating and responding to forces affecting professional practice.[13,18]
- Those who think critically can be expected to be effective change agents.[13]
- Critical thinking is essential to understanding personal relationships and evaluating perspectives, and to envisioning alternative ways to organize information.[19]
- Critical thinking is fundamental to productive participation in quality-assurance activities, shared governance, consultation, research, and peer review.[17]

Critical thinking has "emancipatory potential."[19] As Brookfield stated[16]:

> If we think critically, . . . we will make good clinical decisions that are grounded in an accurate understanding of our contexts for practice. (p.197)

According to Miller and Malcom[10]:

> While clinical judgement and critical thinking are not synonymous terms, they are related concepts. Critical thinking is inherent in making sound clinical judgements. (pp. 68–69)

The Application of Critical Thinking in a Complex and Uncertain Nursing-Care Environment

Contemporary nursing practice is dauntingly complex and uncertain. According to Schon[20]:

> The problems of real-world practice do not present themselves to practitioners as well-formed structures . . . they tend not to present themselves as problems at all but as messy, indeterminate situations. (p. 4)

However, stated Pless and Clayton[4]:

> Situations often occur as a hodgepodge of contextual factors rather than as a specific problem that can be solved in a linear fashion. (p. 427)

The design of the Suggested Exercises, in terms of critical thinking, is intended to foster what Miller and Malcom[10] referred to as:

> personalized solutions to unpredictable client circumstances (p. 71) [and to promote] an environment in which a student becomes "hooked" on the adventure of uncertainty. (p. 70)

As Waldrop[21] also noted, rather than simply assessing problems, one is "wading into them" (p. 21). In this approach, faculty serve as intellectual guides and as partners in the learning enterprise, rather than as the sources of answers.[14]

The chapter authors have employed a variety of strategies in designing the exercises to encourage critical thinking. The following list encompasses some of their techniques, as well as ones proposed by other authors. They are:

- Engaging in *argument* and *debate*[22,23]
- Exploring *cultural and recreational interests for analogies and metaphors* to expand frames of reference and to enhance clarity in communicating[17]
- Using *reflection, synthesis,* and *application*[10,24]
- Performing *case-study analysis* and writing *position papers*[10,23]
- Composing *professional-practice statements* (i.e., *position and job descriptions*)[23]
- Using *critical-thinking question cubes* and other *strategies for infusing games with academic concepts*[25]
- Determining the essential attributes of concepts by use of *structured concept analysis,*[26] and *concept clarification*[19]
- Performing *critique,* conducting *peer review,* and using *analogy*[27]
- Drawing *models* to depict relationships among concepts
- Engaging in *ethnographic techniques*[23]

Summary

This book is unique in several respects. First, because of recent revolutionary and ongoing changes in the American health-care delivery system and the associated potential for ever-greater utilization of all expanded professional-nursing-practice roles, it is timely to emphasize common concerns, with the expectation of enhancing the influence and opportunity of these advanced practice nursing roles. Ideally, introduction of such a collaborative model should begin during the formal educational preparation. Second, to our knowledge, this is the only book that addresses the *combined* advanced practice role concerns of NPs, CNSs, CNMWs, and CRNAs. Third, mastery or competency is directed toward the advanced level of synthesis and evaluation, with the intent of developing critical thinking as part of lifelong learning and clinical decision making. Fourth, the content, objectives, and exercises are not bounded or limited by peculiarities of individual states, but rather, they apply across the nation. This allows the many professional-role issues, which differ greatly by state (owing to the great diversity of practice acts), to be individualized across states. Finally, the book is a valuable supplement for others who seek to understand advanced practice nursing as it pertains to the interaction among the various roles and to organizational and regulatory contingencies. These include physicians and interdisciplinary colleagues and professionals in operations, such as chief executives, vice presidents, and clincal-service directors, and state boards of nursing.

We sincerely hope that this book furthers the progress of APNs at large, and welcome your comments.

CMS AND MM

REFERENCES

1. American Association of Colleges of Nursing: The Essentials of Master's Education for Advanced Practice Nursing: Report from the Task Force on the Essentials of Master's Education for Advanced Practice Nursing. American Association of Colleges of Nursing, Washington, DC, October 1995.
2. Bloom, BS, et al: Taxonomy of Educational Objectives: Handbook I. David McKay, New York, 1956.
3. Kintgen-Andrews, J: Critical thinking and nursing education: Perplexities and insights. J Nurs Educ 30:152, 1991.
4. Pless, BS, and Clayton, GM: Clarifying the concept of critical thinking in nursing. J Nurs Educ 32:425, 1993.
5. Tanner, CA: Thinking about critical thinking. J Nurs Educ 32:99, 1993.
6. Tanner, CA: More thinking about critical thinking and clinical decision making. J Nurs Educ 32:387, 1993.
7. Jones, SA, and Brown, LN: Critical thinking: Impact on nursing education. J Adv Nurs 6:529, 1991.
8. Watson, G, and Glaser, E: Watson-Glaser Critical Thinking Appraisal Manual. Harcourt, Brace World, New York, 1964.
9. Facione, P: Critical thinking: A statement of expert consensus for purposes of educational assessment and instruction: Research findings and recommendations. 1990. ERIC Document ED 315–423.
10. Miller, MA, and Malcolm, NS: Critical thinking in the nursing curriculum. Nursing & Health Care 11:67, 1990.
11. Sternberg, RJ: Teaching critical thinking: Eight easy ways to fail before you begin. Phi Delta Kappan 68:456, 1987.
12. Browne, MN, and Keeley, SM: Asking the Right Questions. Prentice Hall, Englewood Cliffs, NJ, 1981.
13. Dowd, SB: Teaching strategies to foster critical thinking. Radiol Technol 62:374, 1991.
14. Court, D: Teaching critical thinking: What do we know? The Social Studies 82(3):115, 1991.
15. Browne, MN, et al: Critical thinking in graduate economic programs: A study of faculty perceptions. Journal of Economic Education 26:177, 1995.
16. Brookfield, S: On impostership, cultural suicide, and other dangers: How nurses learn critical thinking. Journal of Continuing Education in Nursing 24:197, 1993.
17. Case, B: Walking around the elephant: A critical-thinking strategy for decision making. Journal of Continuing Education in Nursing 25:101, 1994.
18. Brooks, KL, and Shepherd, JM: Professionalism versus general critical thinking abilities of senior nursing students in four types of nursing curricula. J Prof Nurs 8:87, 1992.
19. Kramer, MK: Concept clarification and critical thinking: Integrated processes. J Nurs Educ: 32:406, 1993.
20. Schon, D: Educating the Reflective Practitioner: Toward a New Design for Teaching and Learning in the Professions. Jossey-Bass, San Francisco, 1987.
21. Waldrop, MM: Complexity: The Emerging Science at the Edge of Chaos. Simon & Schuster, New York, 1992.
22. Johnson, SD, and Weaver, RL: Groupthink and the classroom: Changing familiar patterns to encourage critical thought. Journal of Instructional Psychology 19:99, 1992.
23. White, NE, et al: Promoting critical thinking skills. Nurse Educator 15:16, 1990.
24. Watts, SM: Actions speak louder than words: Preparing our preservice and inservice teachers in the way we "expect" them to teach. 1993. ERIC document ED 386–710.
25. Williams, M: Playing is the thing: Three activities for school leaders. 1995. ERIC Document ED 387–911.
26. Walker, LO, and Avant, KC: Strategies for theory construction in nursing, ed 2. Appleton & Lange, Norwalk, Conn, 1988.
27. Toliver, JC: Inductive reasoning: Critical thinking skills for clinical competence. Clinical Nurse Specialist 2:174, 1988.

The Evolution of Advanced Practice in Nursing

PAULINE KOMNENICH, PhD, RN

Pauline Komnenich, PhD, RN, is currently a faculty member of the College of Nursing at Arizona State University. She received her baccalaureate from Stanford University in 1960 and her master's in nursing from the University of Washington in 1964. She also has a master's degree in anthropology and a doctorate in linguistics. Her doctorate was received through the Nurse Scientist Program at the University of Arizona in 1974.

During the past 35 years in nursing, Dr. Komnenich has made contributions to nursing as an educator, researcher in women's health and family caregiving for frail elders in the home, and clinical practitioner in elder care and nursing administration. Her major contributions have been to research and research development in nursing. More recently, she has become involved in care management of the elderly and parish nursing. She has a broad background of experience both nationally and internationally, having participated in nursing education and research in Eastern Europe and primary health care in Argentina.

Dr. Komnenich has conducted studies on the future of nursing, including perceptions of nurse practitioners and clinical nursing specialists. Her experience in nursing and in both quantitative and qualitative research provides a unique background for a unique chapter on the historical context of advanced practice nursing in four domains.

CHAPTER OUTLINE

CHAPTER OBJECTIVES

After completing this chapter, the reader will be able to:

1. Understand the evolution of advanced practice nursing within the historical context of each of the four practice domains of nurse midwives, nurse anesthetists, clinical nurse specialists, and nurse practitioners by reviewing the written historical accounts and reflections of "the lived experience" of six contemporary nursing leaders.

2. Identify and discuss the sociopolitical forces that stimulated the expanded role for nurses in each of these practice domains.

3. Evaluate critical trends in the educational preparation of nurses and the implications of those trends in preparing nurses for advanced practice roles.

4. Distinguish those characteristics that influence the scope of knowledge and skills within the practice domain.

5. Synthesize common or shared role parameters and concerns of advanced practice nurses from a historical perspective.

As Ford,[1] an influential leader in the nurse practitioner movement, has pointed out, myths and fallacies surround any movement. Therefore, the opportunity to directly interview those individuals who participated in the specific efforts to change the nursing profession provides a depth of understanding frequently not found in other historical narratives and helps to dispel some of the myths and fallacies. Built around the reflections of six contemporary nurses who have experienced firsthand the evolving role of the certified nurse midwife (CNM), certified registered nurse anesthetist (CRNA), clinical nurse specialist (CNS), and nurse practitioner (NP), this chapter not only provides a written and verbal account of events but also interjects the flavor and energy of the "lived experience" of these advanced practice nurses.

The contributors were selected based on their reputations in their respective practice domains as clinicians, educators, and leaders. Joyce Roberts, PhD, CNM, FAAN, FACNM, and Betty Bear, PhD, CNM, FAAN, FACNM, have worked skillfully through professional organizations to advance nurse midwifery education and professional development. John Garde, MS, CRNA, FAAN, has assumed a major role in the professional organization in nurse anesthesia and continues to work in that capacity today. Pamela Minarik, MS, RN, FAAN, has practiced as a psychiatric clinical nurse specialist liaison for nearly 20 years. She has contributed toward the professional development of the CNS movement through her practice and scholarly publications on the application of theory and research to practice as well as through her publications on political and policy implications for the CNS. Irene Riddle, PhD, MSN, RN, is a professor in nursing of children whose career as a pediatric nurse, master teacher, scholar, and researcher has included the mentoring of numerous CNS students and professional CNSs. Loretta C. Ford, EdD, MS, FAAN, professor and dean emerita, the University of Rochester, Rochester, New York, is a national leader in the NP movement and one whose contributions and vision of advanced practice for nurses have improved the quality of health care.

Developed through the use of semistructured telephone interviews and documented histories, the chapter describes the evolution of each domain from the perspective of history and sociopolitics, identifies key leaders and events, and discusses common role parameters. It concludes with a discussion of the common themes and distinguishing characteristics of each specific practice domain, as well as with some thoughts on the future, drawn from information obtained during the personal interviews.

Certified Nurse Midwives

According to Roberts,[2] as of 1996, there were 46 graduate nurse midwifery education programs in the United States. These programs included 34 master's-education programs, 9 certificate programs, and 3 certification programs. The development of these programs in the United States has a history dating back to the early 1900s. The period from 1900 to 1935 focused on the extension of education of midwives to the growth of nurse midwifery programs, which occurred from 1935 to the present. This development of nurse midwifery education programs has occurred with the placement of nurse midwifery education in post-nursing or post-baccalaureate programs within institutions of higher education.[3] The overall purposes of nurse midwifery education, as stated in the Carnegie Foundation for the

Advancement of Teaching report,[4] are the provision of better health care for mothers and babies and the promotion of midwifery as "a quality profession, requiring emphasis on caring, competence and public education" (p. 29).

HISTORICAL CONTEXT

While the established date for the inception of modern nursing is 1873, there are records of midwifery practice in the North American colonies dating back to 1630 and of attempts to educate midwives dating back to early 1762.[5,6] In these early times, the provision of obstetric care was outside the purview of medical practice and remained in the exclusive domain of midwives. According to Roberts,[3] efforts to establish formal midwifery schools, such as that of William Shippen, Jr., in Philadelphia in 1762, were unsuccessful, and throughout the 1800s, the native midwife was "self or apprenticeship-taught and was isolated from medicine, nursing or the hospital" (p. 123). Although interest in promoting education for midwifery practice renewed with the immigration of European midwives and physicians to the United States in the latter part of the nineteenth century, it was not sustained.

Many factors are considered by historians as contributing to the demise of midwifery's occupational identity. Of note is the fact that the medical specialty of obstetrics[7,8] arose against the backdrop of the lack of formal midwifery education[5] and the relatively inexact training requirements for midwives. Other social and economic events contributed to the decline of the native midwife.[9] Between 1900 and 1935, midwife deliveries dropped from 50 to 10 percent as the flow of immigration decreased and the emigrated midwife clients became integrated into the dominant society, as home deliveries were replaced with hospital deliveries, and as physicians became increasingly critical of the midwife.

An exception to this pattern of declining midwifery use in the United States existed among the Mormon pioneer midwives. During the late 1800s and early 1900s, the Mormons relied on midwives trained initially in their native lands and then further educated in the medical-obstetric arena available in the United States at that time.[3] In 1874, women who were able to travel to study at the Women's Medical College in Philadelphia returned to Utah and established midwifery courses. Licensure for practice was required in Utah from 1894 to 1932, during which time 208 midwives were licensed in Salt Lake City.

According to Roberts,[3] medical care in the early twentieth century was no better than midwifery care. A 1912 survey, carried out by J. Whitridge Williams, a professor of obstetrics at Johns Hopkins University in Baltimore, found that the lack of preparation of obstetricians rendered their practices as harmful as those of midwives, if not more so, and noted that more deaths occurred from improper operations than from infections at the hands of midwives. Carolyn van Blarcom's 1914 report to the New York Committee for the Prevention of Blindness acknowledged that women may have been better cared for by less-educated midwives than by the physicians, who were responsible for the eye infections and the puerperal septicemia that were occurring at that time.

Unfortunately, although major reform in medical education began to take place subsequent to the Flexner Report of 1910, no similar efforts to improve the education or preparation of the midwife took place. Roberts[2,3] perceived that the lack of education and opportunity for training further led to diminished opportunities for midwives. Furthermore, because midwives perceived childbirth as a "normal" phenomenon and within the female domain of competence, few of them sought formal education. Moreover, the predominantly male physicians' attitudes toward midwifery were that midwives were unsafe and that no "true" woman would want to learn the knowledge and skills needed for midwifery.[3]

Van Blarcom, instrumental in developing the Bellevue School for Midwives, became known as the first nurse in the United States to be licensed as a midwife.[10] She advocated the training, licensure, and control of midwives, while Williams, ironically, recommended the abolishment of midwives and better education of physicians. Even though this controversy led to a decline in midwifery deliveries, Roberts[3] noted that "the negative indicators surrounding childbirth actually rose with the decline of midwives" (p. 128). Lower maternal- and infant-mortality rates existed only where midwives were retained, notably Newark, New Jersey,[11] and New York.[12] If one considers that midwives were attending to poor, higher-risk women, these findings were even more impressive. Some of the poorer birth outcomes attributed to medicine were thought to be due to physicians' lack of training and experience with childbirth and to the techniques they used to hurry labor.

Fortunately, positive midwifery outcomes in Germany and England were noted by some American nurses who, according to Roberts,[2,3] believed that midwives should play a role in maternity care. This view led to the integration of the roles of the midwife and public health nurse into the preparation of the nurse midwife. American nursing leaders in the early 1900s did not consider midwifery to be a part of nursing preparation or practice. In 1901, Dock,[13] in a report on nursing education, pointed out:

> The nurse never takes up midwifery work and in private practice or district nursing goes only to obstetric cases where a doctor is in attendance. (p. 485)

Because so many births were being carried out in the community, nurses involved in the supervision of midwives predominantly worked in public-health and community nursing. During this time, nurses concerned with maternal-child health care who tended to be actively involved in social and health reforms included Lillian Wald, the founder of the New York Henry Street Settlement. One result of these reform efforts was the formation of a federal Children's Bureau. Established between 1909 and 1912, the Children's Bureau, according to Roberts,[3] was a "major force in health reforms and subsequent midwifery practice" (p. 130).

SOCIOPOLITICAL CONTEXT

During World War I, the limited fitness of men for military service resulted in legislative initiatives that were instrumental in leading to social and health-care reform and, eventually, to changes in maternity care.[14] The poor physical condition of potential recruits also captured the attention of physicians and public health officials, who noted that if one-half of these men were properly cared for during childhood, they would have qualified for military service. Interestingly, Tom[14] noted that the investment of state and federal funds into public-health programs was not stimulated by high maternal- and infant-mortality rates, but rather, by the concern for a fit fighting force to ensure the nation's security. According to Tom:

For the first time, children were recognized as future members of the military and thus deserving of federal funds. (pp. 4–13)

Childbearing women were considered to be producers of future fighting men; therefore, their health became a national resource.

The need for better maternity services in the context of opposition to midwives by physicians contributed to the controversy in nursing about the role of nurses in the practice of obstetrics. In 1909, the American Society of Superintendents of Training Schools for Nurses (ASSTSN) acknowledged that nurses' training in obstetrics should be included in the program, and in 1911, a resolution was passed to support that position (see Roberts[3] for more detail). However, the association directed that the training be limited to emergency preparation, observing symptoms, and reporting problems to a more general practice. In 1911, the ASSTSN passed another resolution to provide training for registration, licensure, and training in the practice of midwifery.

Around the same time, the Bellevue School for Midwives in New York City initiated a program to educate midwives. This occurred largely through the efforts of van Blarcom, who, as noted earlier, was a strong advocate for midwifery. Clara Noyes, Superintendent of Training Schools, Bellevue and Allied Hospitals, including the School for Midwives, also supported the education of nurses as midwives. The training program for midwives at Bellevue was supported by public monies from 1911 until 1935, when the diminishing need for midwives made it difficult to justify its existence.[3] Basically, the movement of maternity care into the hospitals excluded midwifery. The joint proposal of the Maternity Center Association (MCA) in New York and the Bellevue School of Midwifery to educate nurse midwives was opposed by medical and nursing leaders. Although the need for better maternal-child health services and midwifery practice continued, such opposition inhibited nurses from engaging in the practice of midwifery. Eventually, this continuing need led to the advanced preparation of public health nurses who could supervise midwifery practice and eventually prepare nurse midwives.

In 1921, the controversial Sheppard-Towner Act was enacted to provide money to states to train public health nurses in midwifery.[3] Although there was a major political effort to prohibit passage of the bill, according to Roberts,[3] the joint efforts of women represented "one of the most effective expressions of women's political influence" (p. 131). However, in 1929, major opposition by the American Medical Association (AMA) resulted in the lapse of the bill. Roberts[3] attributed the bill's demise to the desire of the AMA to "establish a 'single standard' of obstetrical care" (p. 131) and also to its concern that governmental regulation of midwifery would lead to regulation of medical practice.

According to Shoemaker,[15] despite this opposition to midwifery in nursing, the first school for nurse midwifery established in the United States was the Manhattan Midwifery School in 1928. Apparently the school, which was started by Mary Richardson, a public health nursing instructor who had taken a midwifery course in England, was short lived. Earlier, in 1925, Mary Breckenridge brought nurse midwives from England to help establish the Frontier Nursing Service. Two of the graduates from the school were identified as joining the Frontier Nursing Service in 1928.[3] The Frontier Nursing Service in Kentucky (service) in 1925 and the MCA (education) in New York City in 1932 were two public-health-oriented agencies that characterized the practice area for public health nurses prepared in nurse midwifery. According to Bear,[16] the Lobenstine Midwifery Clinic was established in 1931 to prepare public health nurses to be midwives. In contrast to the Manhattan School established by Richardson, this clinic was the first *recognized* nurse midwifery school.

After the opening of the Lobenstine Midwifery Clinic, the School of the Association for the Promotion and Standardization of Midwifery was established in 1932. Priority for attendance in the school was given to nurses from states that had high infant-mortality rates and many lay midwives. The intent was for the graduates to return to their home states to establish public-health-department programs for training and supervising "granny midwives."[3] In 1934, the school merged with the Lobenstine Clinic under the MCA and was known thereafter as The Clinic.

A key figure in the education of nurse midwives was Hattie Hemschemeyer, a public health nurse educator and graduate of the Clinic's first nurse midwifery class. She was later appointed as director of the Clinic, where the emphasis was on the provision of care to women during pregnancy and childbirth in neighborhood settings staffed by public health nurses and physicians. The MCA, a prototype of this type of service, developed about 30 centers in New York City in 1918.[3] Nurse midwives began to provide services in these centers around 1931, and hence, the role of the public health nurse as a nurse midwife emerged. At the same time, the role of the nurse in maternity care was evolving but appeared to be quite different from midwifery and medical practice.

In 1937, according to Roberts,[3] the National League of Nursing Education's (NLNE's) description of the role of the midwife in obstetrics was the "overall promotion of the health and comfort of the mother and baby" (p. 135), The obstetric nurse, in contrast, was described as a "bedside assistant" and "teacher of health."[17] Although preparation of the nurse in obstetrics was relatively poor in the early part of the twentieth century, development of programs in nurse midwifery during the 1940s demonstrated progress in the education for the role. According to Diers, as cited by Roberts,[3] nurse midwives have been described as

> the oldest of the specialized practice roles for nurses [and as providing] an unusually good example of the issues nurses face in addressing public policy considerations of manpower, economics, costs of care, quality and access to care, and interprofessional politics. (p. 136)

World War II had a significant impact on the development of nurse midwives. As a consequence of the war, there was a diminished supply of nurses; thus, an education program was initiated at the Frontier Nursing Service in Kentucky and was assisted by the MCA in New York. The positive publicity received by the Frontier Nursing Service brought nurse midwifery into public view. Interestingly, this recognition came largely from a Metropolitan Life report describing the first 10,000 Frontier Nursing Service deliveries from its initiation to the time of World War II. Dublin, as cited by Willeford in 1933,[18] reported that the Frontier Nursing Service protected the life of the mother and baby, saving 10,000 lives a year in the United States, preventing 30,000 stillbirths, and ensuring that there would be 30,000 more children alive at the end of the first month of life. According to Roberts[3]:

> There is an irony in the notion that an insurance company would serve to stimulate the expansion of nurse-midwifery services. (p. 141)

The formalization of nurse midwifery as an extension of public-health nursing continued after World War II. With increasing professionalization in nursing and health-care services, the progress of nurse midwifery education went hand in hand with the development of public-health education, which was considered to be essential for nurse midwifery practice. With the advocacy of clinical nursing specialization within universities, the nurse midwife or advanced maternity nurse became more qualified to work with physicians within a professional framework. Table 1–1 traces significant historical events that helped to shape the midwifery profession.

INFLUENCE OF GOVERNMENT AGENCIES AND PROFESSIONAL ASSOCIATIONS

In the 1970s and 1980s, efforts of both government and professional associations continued to advance the development of nurse midwifery. The Children's Bureau (later known as the Maternal Child Health Bureau), with leadership from Katherine (Kit) Kendall and Carmella Carvello, and the Division of Nursing, Bureau of Health Professions Education, was instrumental in facilitating the nurse midwifery movement by providing training grants.[2,16] According to Bear,[16] Senator Daniel K. Inouye of Hawaii assisted with lobbying efforts on Capitol Hill and with development of contacts between nursing and other key people. During the same time, Senator Daniel Patrick Moynihan of New York sponsored the Civilian Health and Medical Program for the Uniformed Services (CHAMPUS) in the Omnibus Reconciliation Act of the Defense Appropriations Bill.

Helen Varney Burst was the first president of the American College of Nurse-Midwives (ACNM) to serve two consecutive terms.[2] This event was particularly significant because her tenure occurred during a time when there were no provisions for nurse midwives in federal programs. Therefore, consistent leadership was needed to maintain intense lobbying efforts for key legislation that influenced programs such as Medicare, Medicaid, and CHAMPUS. These lobbying efforts opened the door for more autonomous nursing practice, the po-

TABLE 1–1
Significant Historical Events in Midwifery

Year	Event
1762	Unsuccessful attempt by William Shippen, Jr., was launched to establish formal midwifery schools in Philadelphia.
1874	Mormon midwives who were trained at Women's Medical College in Philadelphia returned to Utah to establish midwifery courses.
1892–1932	License to practice midwifery was required in Utah.
1911	American Society of Superintendents to Training Schools for Nurses passed a resolution to provide for registration, licensure, and training in midwifery.
1921	Sheppard-Towner Act was passed, providing money to states to train public health nurses in midwifery.
1928	Manhattan Midwifery School, the first school for nurse midwifery, was established.
1929	American Medical Association opposition allowed for the lapse of the Sheppard-Towner Act.

tential for third-party reimbursement, and greater recognition of the CNM as a health-care provider.

The medical-malpractice crisis was a key sociopolitical event that occurred in 1985 to slow the growth of nurse midwifery. Insurance carriers, fearing financial drains associated with litigation, dropped malpractice coverage for nurse midwives. This created a difficult challenge for the American Nurses' Association (ANA), the ACNM, and the Nurse Association of the American College of Obstetrics and Gynecology, all of which stepped in and worked to assist the ACNM in getting the Risk Retention Act passed. Passage of this law allowed independent carriers to provide malpractice insurance to individuals on a state-by-state basis.

Under Bear's presidency,[16] further movement toward professional development occurred during 1987 to 1989, when ACNM developed a Division of Research.[16] Joyce Thompson, who succeeded Bear and was the second person to serve two consecutive terms (1989 to 1993), oversaw a time of marked growth in the number and quality of educational programs. As the deputy director for the International Confederation of Nurse-Midwives (ICNM), Thompson also was involved in the international development of midwifery. During her term, a formal liaison developed between the ICNM and the Royal College of Midwives in London, England.

Among international organizations, the Agency for International Development and the World Health Organization (WHO) were probably most influential in promoting midwifery in developing countries. The ICNM,[19] founded in Europe in 1919, also worked to advance education in midwifery, with the aim of improving the standard of care provided to mothers, babies, and their families throughout the countries of the world. The confederation is the only international midwifery organization that has official relations with the United Nations and works closely with the WHO and the United Nations International Children's Emergency Fund (commonly known as UNICEF) to achieve common goals in maternal and child care.

Although its activities were interrupted during World War II, the first World Congress of Midwives began a new era and the start of a series of triennial meetings. These meetings brought together midwives from all over the world to share ideas and experiences and to improve knowledge in the field. The first triennial meeting, hosted by the United States, was held in 1972 in Washington, D.C.,[16] during the presidency of Lucille Woodville. Currently, there are nine other organizations that work with the confederation, including the International Council of Nurses and the International Federation of Gynecology and Obstetrics.[19]

INFLUENCE OF PRIVATE FOUNDATIONS, COLLEGES, AND UNIVERSITIES

The Carnegie Foundation served as a definite stimulus for the nurse midwifery movement. Ernest Boyer, president of the Carnegie Foundation until his recent death and whose wife was a nurse midwife, strongly supported nurse midwifery programs. However, at an exploratory meeting convened by the Carnegie Foundation in July of 1989, he posed a critical and continuing question regarding the issue of accreditation of a program designed for individuals who were not first educated as nurses. Basically, the ACNM responded by saying that accreditation of a program for nonnurse midwives would require identification of all the relevant knowledge, skills, and competencies that nurses bring to a nurse-midwifery education and would require that those essential competencies be acquired by completion of the midwifery education program.

A key principle underlying the ACNM, Division of Accreditation (DOA) program, was that[3]

> the ultimate competencies attained in an ACNM accredited midwifery program for non-nurses would be the same as those required of graduates of DOA-accredited nurse-midwifery programs. (p. 1)

According to Levy,[11] the ACNM further articulated this principle by stating that ACNM standards for nurse midwifery education and practice would "have to be maintained and upheld by every accredited program" (p. 1). However, until recently, the mechanism for taking the ACNM Certification Council (ACC) examinations has not been open to non-nurse midwives, the requirement being that those who took the ACC examination be registered nurses (RNs) licensed in the United States. Now, that avenue is open for both nurses and non-nurses. Although there is general concern regarding this issue, the ACNM points out that only those individuals graduating with a minimum of a baccalaureate degree from an ACNM-accredited midwifery program would be eligible to take the ACC examination. Thus far, no midwifery-education program for non-nurses has been accredited through the ACNM.

Nurse midwifery programs have received notable and growing support from a number of major colleges and universities throughout the United States. Support for doctoral education for nurse midwives who hold positions within university-based programs as well as for the preparation of leaders with the skills of scientific inquiry, knowledge of health-policy formulation, educational administration, and research also has become increasingly important.

FORCES INFLUENTIAL IN MARKETING AND EFFECTIVE UTILIZATION

According to Bear,[16] the professional association and legislative support have encouraged the use of nurse midwives by consumers. Although nurse midwives have been involved in health-maintenance organizations (HMOs) since 1980, consumer support was probably the most influential in the marketing and effective utilization of their services. Once the recipients of health care became aware of what nurse midwives could do, earlier misconceptions about midwifery were dispelled. The benefits of midwifery practice, especially among the underserved populations, were appreciated and disseminated.

KEY LEADERS

There has been a long debate on the content and structure of the curricular content that constitutes adequate education for nurse midwives and an effort by leaders to maintain the quality of education and care of mothers and children. Notable for their contributions to nurse midwifery practice and education were Mary Breckenridge, inducted into the Women's Hall of Fame in 1995,[3,16] and Hattie Hemschemeyer, the first president of the ACNM. These early leaders were dedicated to improving the quality of education for nurse midwives and to establishing institutions for monitoring midwifery care through the ACNM.[2,16] For example, the ACNM has been influential in formulating standards for education and practice that currently reflect the major differences between nurse midwives and traditonal midwives.

More contemporary leaders in the discipline include Ruth Lubic, formerly general director of the MCA in New York; Irene Sandvold in the Division of Nursing, Bureau of Health Professions (BHPr), Department of Health and Human Services (DHHS); Dorothea Lang, a former president of ACNM and director of maternal and infant projects in New York City; Joyce Cameron Foster of the University of Utah, who established a nurse midwifery graduate program and certified nurse midwife licensure; Katherine (Kit) Kendall, who was with the Maternal Child Health Bureau, DHHS; and Elizabeth Sharpe of Emory University and a graduate of Yale University. Joyce Roberts and Betty Bear are among those active leaders who continue to address nurse midwifery education and practice issues and the challenge to maintain the professional standards of midwifery practice that have been established through the ACNM.

Other prominent players featured in the long-standing movement toward the professional status of nurse midwives include Sister Mary Stella, past president of ACNM; Vera Keane, a professor from Yale University who coauthored the book on the perception of patients and their obstetric-care providers titled *Nurse Patient Relationships in a Hospital Maternity Service*; and Ernestine Weidenbach, author of *Family Centered Maternity Nursing*. Joyce Cameron Foster and Judith Fullerton also were instrumental in developing the National Certification Examination for nurse midwives.[16]

As with every profession, there are many unsung heroes and heroines in the nurse midwifery movement whose commitment, support, and leadership have contributed to its success and are a part of the unwritten history. Among others who worked steadfastly to establish a professional standard for nurse midwifery were Sister Nathalie Elder and Sister Jeanne Meurer, faculty members in the School of Nursing at St. Louis University, St. Louis, Missouri.

INTERFACE WITH NURSE ANESTHETISTS, CLINICAL NURSE SPECIALISTS, AND NURSE PRACTITIONERS

According to Roberts,[2] the focus of the nurse midwife is primarily on maternal-infant care within the context of the family and thus differs from the focus of the obstetric-gynecological (OB-GYN) practitioner, who is oriented more toward women's health. Nurse midwives probably identify more closely with nurse anesthetists, who have followed a similar path and positioned themselves within an area of practice that allows them to maintain a degree of autonomy within the medical community. As with nurse anesthesia, there is also differentiation between the specialist and educator, specifically with the initial requirement of certification for the practice of the specialty and the evolving requirement of a master's-level education.

Bear[16] has noted that a blending of the roles of advanced practice nurses in maternity care is beginning to occur. Many agree that roles probably overlap, because both the OB-GYN practitioner and the nurse midwife do primary care and care for the woman in labor. However, the primary focus of the midwife extends from pregnancy through the birth experience with responsibility for the conduct of the delivery. Nurse midwifery has developed into a professional discipline in the United States while retaining its identity as a specialty practice in nursing. In addition, it has retained its identity with midwifery internationally,[2] in comparison with the other specialties that constitute advanced practice nursing.

Nurse Anesthetists

Although midwifery as a vocation dates back to the 1600s, nurse anesthesia predates nurse midwifery as a specialty area of nursing in the United States. From the perspective of world history, the history of women attending other women in labor can be documented in pre-Christian times. Nurses attending patients in surgery to administer anesthesia is more recent in the historical context.

HISTORICAL CONTEXT

Anesthesia in the United States reportedly dates back to the mid-nineteenth century, with rival claimants to its discovery. Allegedly, William T. G. Morton successfully demonstrated anesthesia in surgery on October 16, 1846, at a centennial event held at Massachusetts General Hospital. This demonstration was followed by a number of reported studies, all of which failed to mention any involvement of nurse anesthetists. In response to this apparent oversight, Thatcher[20] emphasized the role of the nurse specialist in her book *History of Anesthesia*. In the preface to the book, she stated:

> If the place of the nurse as an anesthetist receives special emphasis in this history, it is because she has been derogated or ignored. (p. 15)

Bankert[21] also described the difficulty associated with identifying the first nurse anesthetist and the limited recognition of the prominence of nurses in anesthesia.

According to Thatcher,[20] church records of 1877 identify Sister Mary Bernard as being called on to function as an anesthetist within a year of enrolling in St. Vincent's Hospital, in Erie, Pennsylvania. As a result of this recording, Sister Bernard has been recognized as the first nurse anesthetist to practice in the United States. The further contribution of members of the religious orders to the development of the field of anesthesia was illustrated by many others, including Sister Aldonza Eltrich (1860 to 1920) and certain religious nursing orders.

According to Bankert,[21] the Hospital Sisters of the Third Order of St. Francis managed five hospitals that served employees of the Missouri Pacific Railroad between 1884 and 1888. During this period, nuns from the order served as anesthetists for the five settings. In 1912, Mother Superior Magdalene Wiedlocher, an anesthetist, developed a course in anesthesia for sisters who were graduate nurses. In 1924, this course was made available to secular nurses. Based on Thatcher's research, Bankert[21] has detailed the contributions of Catholic and Protestant nursing orders whose members served as nurse anesthetists since the 1850s, providing poignant narratives of these committed women. Included in this group are Alice Magaw, known as the "Mother of Anesthesia," and Sister Secundina Mindrup (1868 to 1951), both of whom were described as most "touching figures."

The emergence of nurse anesthesia in the United States cannot be considered outside the context of the development of nursing itself. In 1873, three nurses' training schools were established in New York, New Haven, and Boston. These American schools were referred to as "Nightingale Schools" and were credited with bringing the art of nursing into a more reputable view. At that time, there was some controversy over the philanthropic desire to make nurses' training attractive to the middle-class American woman. Some physicians supported the idea while many did not. According to Starr, as quoted by Bankert,[21] physicians were concerned that

> educated nurses would not do as they were told—a remarkable comment on the status anxieties of nineteenth-century physicians. (p. 20)

Fortunately, women reformers paid little attention to these remarks and, like Florence Nightingale, moved forward. The schools were established to attract respectable women and were modeled after the Saint Thomas Hospital Training School for Nurses founded in 1860 by Nightingale.

Eventually, physicians were forced to accept nurses who were trained to carry out the more complex work that hospitals were assuming. Shyrock, as quoted by Bankert,[21] described this change in attitude toward nurses rather vividly:

> All of this related to the public opinion of medical service in general, since the nurses came into more continuous contact with the patient than did any other figure in the whole range of medical personnel. Good nursing was invaluable from a technical point of view. It might make all the difference in the outcome of the individual case, and patients sometimes realized this. Better nursing was an essential feature in the gradual improvement of hospitals, and this in turn modified the earlier popular attitude toward these institutions. . . .The whole spirit of hospitals changed. (p. 21)

Baer, as quoted by Bankert,[21] made yet a stronger statement when she asserted that "nursing made medicine look good" (p. 21). She goes on to further illustrate this point:

> Medicine's ultimate success, technological advances, and subsequent impressive social power were achieved through hospitals, and nurses made those hospitals work. Nurses made them reasonable choices for sick-care, providing the environment in which patients felt safe enough to permit medical instrumentation to occur. The development of medical practice, education, therapeutics, etc. proceeded from that point. Happily, one prominent physician understood that and reminded his contemporaries in 1910: "Now one must have some understanding of the value of the profession of nursing in modern medicine. . . . It has changed the face of modern medicine: it is revolutionary in its influence upon the progress of modern medicine." (p. 21)

SOCIOPOLITICAL CONTEXT

The advent of anesthetics occurred simultaneously with the acceptance and promotion of asepsis and the emergence of nursing in hospital care[21]; thus, the elements "were in place for a removal of the remaining obstacle in the path of the advancement of surgery" (p. 22). Discussion concerning problems associated with anesthesia delivery began at the time of Morton's first successful induction and continued without resolution for some 40 years. Most anesthesia was given by novice interns who were more interested in the surgery than in the safe administration of anesthesia. In 1898, Saling, as quoted by Bankert,[21] illustrated the rather nonchalant attitude toward anesthesia characteristic of the times:

> Unfortunately, in most hospitals one of the younger interns is, as a rule, selected to administer the anaesthetic. The operator accustomed to having a novice give chloroform or ether for him is kept on the *qui vive* while performing the operation and watching the administration of the anaesthetic. Such a condition of affairs is not conducive to the best work of the surgeon. (p. 23)

One of the hospitals established by the Sisters of St. Francis played a particularly noteworthy role in the development of anesthesia care. Established in 1889 as St. Mary's Hospital, it later became known as the Mayo Clinic. During the early years at the Mayo Clinic, no interns were available to assist in surgery. Therefore, the clinic relied on nurse anesthetists, initially as a matter of necessity and, later, as a matter of choice.

The Mayo Clinic's first nurse anesthetists were Dinah and Edith Graham, sisters who had graduated from the school of nursing at the Women's Hospital in Chicago. To train the Graham sisters while continuing to support the work of the clinic, five staff nurses took over the patient-care nursing and housekeeping duties, while the Grahams administered anesthesia and did general office and secretarial work. According to Bankert,[21] Dinah's career as a nurse anesthetist at the clinic was brief, but her sister Edith continued there until she married William W. Mayo in 1893. Edith was succeeded by Magaw (1860 to 1928), reported to be brilliant not only as an anesthetist but as a scholar and researcher as well.

Bankert[21] noted that although Magaw "won more widespread notice than that of any other member of the Rochester group apart from the [Mayo] brothers" (p. 30), because she was a nurse, she was not given membership in the medical society. According to Garde,[22] Magaw administered anesthesia, kept data, and wrote articles. She was a meticulous data collector, and although her papers are not listed in the *Physicians of the Mayo Clinic Bibliography,* one of her studies was included in the *Collected Papers by the Staff of St. Mary's Hospital, Mayo Clinic, Rochester, Minnesota, 1905–1909.*[21] A 1941 catalogue by Clapesattle of Magaw's papers revealed that her first comprehensive paper, reporting more than 3000 cases, was titled "Observations in Anesthesia," and was published in *Northwestern Lancet* in 1899.[21] In 1900, the *St. Paul Medical Journal* published Magaw's update of the year's work, which included observations of 1092 cases reported. In 1906, Magaw published another review of more than 14,000 successful anesthesia cases. According to Bankert,[21] Magaw made numerous recommendations that shaped contemporary anesthesia practice. She stressed individual attention for all patients and identified the experience of the anesthetist as a critical element in quickly responding to the patient. Magaw's success also was attributed to her attention to the psychological dimension of the anesthetic experience. In her words, she believed that "suggestion" was a great help "in producing a comfortable narcosis" (p. 32).

The model of nurse anesthesia at the Mayo Clinic drew the attention of medical people from all over the United States and the world. The Mayo Clinic's reputation gave credibility to the movement, and Magaw's efforts provided a particular advantage to careful documentation and publication. As Garde[22] noted:

> We lose so many opportunities in clinical areas because people do not take the time to write articles that could be major contributions to the literature. [By her writing], . . . Alice Magaw really made a name for the nurse anesthetists.

In 1936, Crile,[23] hailed as one of America's greatest surgeons, praised the nurse anesthetist movement. In these nursing professionals, he found a special quality of "finesse" for administration of anesthesia not present in medical interns. His choice for the prototype nurse anesthetist was Agatha Cobourg Hodgins, a native of Canada. According to Bankert,[21] she "proved herself to be not only a brilliant anesthetist, but a woman of vision" (p. 39) in her dedication to the development of professional nursing and the establishment of a national nurse anesthesiology association.

A graduate of the Boston City Hospital Training School for Nurses at age 21, Hodgins went to Cleveland to work as a head nurse at Lakeside Hospital. There she was selected by Crile to administer anesthesia. She avidly read all she could about anesthesia, and "walked the wards" at night listening to sleeping patients' breathing to detect subtle differences. According to Crile, as quoted by Bankert[21]:

> Miss Hodgins made an outstanding anesthetist for she had to a marked degree, both the intelligence and the gift. (p. 41)

Crile and Hodgins inaugurated the Lakeside School of Anesthesia, which at once was recognized as an organized center for teaching anesthesiology, contributing to the education of nurse anesthetists, and furthering the work of the graduates.[21]

Not surprisingly, World Wars I and II, the Korean conflict, and the Vietnam War all had a significant impact on the development of anesthesia. Crile and Hodgins were part of the Lakeside Unit at the American Ambulance at Neuilly in 1914.[21] After 2 months, Crile returned to the United States to present a plan to the U.S. Surgeon General for the creation of hospital units composed of doctors, nurses, and anesthetists for service internationally. Hodgins stayed on in Neuilly to teach nurses, dentists, and physicians how to administer anesthesia. She later returned to Cleveland to resume her work at the Lakeside School of Anesthesia. The first graduating class consisted of six physicians, two dentists, and 11 nurses. After the formal declaration of war by the United States on April 6, 1917, the Lakeside Hospital Unit, Base Hospital No. 4, was mobilized. Hodgins did not accompany the unit at the time, instead remaining as director of the school and engaged in training nurse anesthetists for military service.

In addition to training at the Mayo Clinic, preparation of nurse anesthetists was also occurring in other parts of the country.[21] For example, Sophie Gran Winton (1887 to 1989), a graduate of Swedish Hospital in Minneapolis, had trained as an anesthetist. After garnering 5 years of anesthesia experience and having established a record of more than 10,000 cases without a fatality, she joined the Army Nurse Corp. Winton and other nurses from the Minneapolis Hospital Unit No. 26 were assigned to Mobile Hospital No. 1 in the Chateau-Thierry area of France. Working with the physician anesthetist James T. Gwathmey, the unit succeeded in pioneering anesthesia in mobile hospital units.

As suggested, a repeated theme in the nurse anesthetist movement has been that of an acknowledgment of the intelligence and dedication of women while pointing out, with some bias, that the gender differences made anesthesia a natural place for women to display their intelligence and feminine attributes. Bankert[21] described the following expectations as characteristic of persons administering anesthesia in 1896. She notes that these qualities were found in women who were recruited into a field shunned by physicians. According to Bankert, women of that period, as perceived by physicians such as Dr. Frederic Hewitt, should:

(a) have been satisfied with the subordinate role that the work required; (b) not have made anesthesia their one absorbing interest; (c) not have looked on the situation of anesthetist as one that put them in a position to watch and learn from the surgeon's technic; (d) have accepted comparatively low pay; and (e) have had the natural aptitude and intelligence to develop a high level of skill in providing the smooth anesthesia and relaxation that the surgeon demanded. (p. 50)

As Bankert[21] suggested, this "glorified handmaiden" image was part of the expectation of the surgeon and was one that came to be associated with nursing. The first battle between nurse anesthetists and medicine was waged in the 1920s. At that time, Francis Hoeffer McMechan, a third-generation Cincinnati physician, began to promote the organization of physician anesthesia. But before nurse anesthetists could assume McMechan's challenge to "cease and desist" practice, they first had to win a battle of acceptance within the profession of nursing. Again, it was Hodgins who led the movement to integrate nurse anesthetists into mainstream nursing through the ANA.

For years, the nurse anesthetist movement had met resistance from organized nursing. In 1909, nurse anesthetists were stunned when Florence Henderson, a successor of Magaw's, was invited to present a paper at the ANA with the unmet expectation of an invitation to join the association. In 1931, Hodgins initiated a formal effort for nurse anesthesia to become a section within the ANA (see Bankert,[21] p. 65, for a comprehensive account of this effort). According to notes in Bankert,[21] Hodgins mobilized the Lakeside alumnae as well as other nurse anesthetists around the country to "attend a meeting for the purpose of considering the organization of [a] nurse anesthetist group" (p. 67). She was committed to separate nurse anesthetists from hospital service but to retain nurse anesthesia within the ANA framework. The ANA eventually rejected this proposal, accepting nurse anesthetists only into the Medical-Surgical Nursing section. According to Bankert,[21] when the ANA rejected the affiliation of nurse anesthetists, Hodgins made a profound statement that led to an alliance with the American Hospital Association (AHA). The following words, excerpted from Bankert, are part of the speech Hodgins made to nurse anesthetists:

It seems to us that anesthesia, being in no sense nursing, could not be absorbed into a strictly nursing group such as the ANA, as we hope to include in our sustaining membership surgeons, hospital superintendents, and others interested in advancing the cause. (p. 73)

The nonacceptance by organized nursing stimulated nurse anesthetists to form the International Association of Nurse Anesthetists (later changed to the National Association of Nurse Anesthetists [NANA] in an effort to merge with the ANA). By 1938, the NANA had changed its name to the American Association of Nurse Anesthetists (AANA) and had moved to its new one-room office at the AHA's offices in Chicago. The affiliation with the AHA proved to provide a home that fostered the profession of nurse anesthesia.

The recognition by the AHA and the subsequent onset of World War II, with its need for an increased number of military nurses trained in anesthesia, stimulated further development of the nurse anesthetist movement and later prompted other efforts to standardize nurse anesthetist education and to establish a national certification examination.[21] According to Bankert,[21] Gertrude Fife addressed the first national convention of the NANA in 1933, calling for a committee to

> investigate nurse anesthesia schools for the purpose of accreditation and for a national board examination for nurse anesthetists. (p. 96)

Fife's stand on the direction for nurse anesthetist education was different from Hodgins and ultimately was opposed by Hodgins. Although Fife had the support of prominent physicians and the help of Dr. Howard Karsner, professor of pathology at Western Reserve University, in the development of national accreditation and procedures, opposition by Hodgins was based on the perception that under Fife's plan, the nurse anesthetist would not have a separate legal status.

Despite being ill and semiretired, Hodgins continued to influence the progress of the professional movement of the nurse anesthetists. However, it was Fife who carried the ball, later giving credit to John Mannix, assistant director of University Hospitals at Western Reserve. At the urging of Mannix, Helen Lamb and Walter Powell joined Fife to produce a nurse anesthesia program and move forward to achieve the following objectives[21]:

> (a) advance the science and art of anesthesiology; (b) develop educational standards and techniques in the administration of anesthetic drugs; (c) facilitate efficient cooperation between nurse anesthetists and the medical profession, hospitals, and other agencies interested in anesthesiology; and (e) promulgate an educational program to help the public understand the importance of the proper administration of anesthetics. (pp. 76–77)

Although Hodgins died before the first qualifying examination for membership in the AANA was held on June 4, 1945, and before the first Institute for Instructors of Anesthesiology was convened in Chicago later that same year, her efforts, along with those of other leaders, came to fruition in peacetime after World War II. Education became the primary goal of the association, and an increased effort was made to form standards and to develop a standardized curriculum to teach nurses to be nurse anesthetists.

The move toward accreditation of schools of anesthesia was approved in September 1950 with the encouragement of the AHA's Council on Professional Practice and under Lamb's leadership as chair of the Advisory Committee of the AANA.[21] The AANA accreditation program for schools of nurse anesthesia became effective on January 19, 1952. Although the program allowed for an interim period during which schools in existence could meet the accreditation criteria, new schools were required to meet accreditation requirements from the outset.

Unfortunately, the rift between organized nursing and nurse anesthesia continued as deans of nursing schools and colleges resisted the inclusion of nurse anesthetist academic programs into their curricula. According to Garde,[22] this dilemma of nonacceptance led to the development of many anesthetist programs in colleges of allied health and education. Although allied health was most receptive to nurse anesthesia, the profession wanted and needed more than a certificate program.

The 1970s witnessed pivotal and profound changes in society: the nation's economic recession, the energy crisis, inflation, involvement in Vietnam, and President Nixon's articulation of a "health-care crisis," to name but a few. The general direction of nursing-education preparation was changing as well. As the educational requirement in nursing moved from diploma to a baccalaureate degree, the requirement for nurse anesthesia moved from certification to a baccalaureate and master's framework. A major breakthrough in nurse anesthesia preparation occurred when Rush University decided to offer a master's of science in nursing for anesthesia. Another major move to higher education for nurse anesthetists was the establishment of the first master's program in nurse anesthesia through the Department of Nursing at California State University, an effort promoted through the leadership of Joyce Kelly, a nurse anesthetist affiliated with Kaiser Permanente.

In the 1970s, the AANA experienced a change in leadership and a continued controversy with organized medicine. Although Florence A. McQuillen ("Mac") had single-handedly held the organization together since 1948, the time had come for a new approach, marking the end of an era for the Association. The conflict between American Society of Anesthesiologists and the AANA centering on issues of control and autonomy has not yet been fully resolved.

INFLUENCE OF GOVERNMENT AGENCIES

The various state boards of nursing, who worked closely on licensing issues with the National Council of State Boards of Nursing and the U.S. Department of Health, were most influential in supporting nurse anesthesia. Controversy over the authority and licensing of nurse anesthetists continues to the present day. The consensus is that the state boards of nursing should regulate nursing, including advanced practice nursing. According to Garde,[22] the Association of Nurse Anesthetists is monitoring the recommendations of the Pew Commission very closely as they pertain to advanced practice. The association views the report as a way of collapsing barriers and opening doors to allow nurse anesthetists to practice unencumbered.

KEY LEADERS

The succession of key national leaders began with Alice Magaw, who was recognized for her techniques in the administration of anesthesia as well as for her brilliant documentation of anesthesia. Her papers, though not identified as research, probably merit being identified, along with Nightingale's, as an early effort to systematically document patient outcomes and report those outcomes in scholarly publications.

Agatha Hodgins, the second most prominent nurse anesthetist, was noted for contributions stemming from her work with and support from Crile and for their combined efforts to improve the education and professional status of nurse anesthetists. She was the impetus behind the movement for professional development of nurse anesthetists and was elected the first president of the AANA

(1931 to 1933). Other leaders who appeared repeatedly in the literature included not only Fife (Hodgins' successor) but also the following past presidents of the Association of Nurse Anesthetists: Hilda Solomon, Helen Lamb, Hazel Blanchard, Lucy Richards, and Verna Rice.

In addition, the following were recipients of the association's Award of Appreciation for their contributions to the profession: Barnes Hospital, part of Washington University in St. Louis, Missouri, a site where much of the educational progress for nurse anesthetists took place (1948); and individuals such as George W. Crile, MD (posthumously 1948); Gertrude L. Fife (1956); Mae B. Cameron (1951); Agnes McGee (1953); Hospital Sisters of the Third Order of St. Francis, Springfield, Illinois (1954); Helen Lamb and Lucy Richards (1956); Hilda Solomon (1958); and Verna Rice (1959). Honorary memberships (nonanesthetist) were extended to Cameron W. Meredith and Betty A. Colitti for their contributions, and a special recognition award was given to John R. Mannix for his assistance in establishing licensing examinations.[21]

INTERFACE WITH CERTIFIED NURSE MIDWIVES, CLINICAL NURSE SPECIALISTS, AND NURSE PRACTITIONERS

Although the role of nurse anesthetists has been more akin to that of nurse midwives, who struggled to maintain an identity with nursing while preserving their own practice in an autonomous role outside medicine, there are shared goals with other advanced practice nurses. Garde[22] envisions commonly shared roles, with advanced practice nurses practicing to their fullest potential without artificial barriers, with direct and fair reimbursement, and with services marketed to managed-care organizations. As health care is becoming more business oriented, nursing in general and advanced nurse practice in particular will be facing major challenges to identify the breadth and depth of advanced practice nursing. According to Garde,[22] there must be a united effort to keep medicine and hospital administration on the same path with advanced practice in nursing to have a positive impact on health.

Clinical Nurse Specialists

According to Hamric and Spross,[24] the concept of nurse specialties is not new in the profession of nursing. Minarik[25] referred to DeWitt's article in the American Journal of Nursing (see Bibliography), in which DeWitt attributed the development of nursing specialties to present civilization and modern science (p. 14).

According to Sparacino, Cooper, and Minarik,[26] DeWitt's view of specialty nursing follows the medical model, basically responding within a limited domain to nursing patients with certain types of conditions or "working for a specialty physician" (p. 4).

HISTORICAL CONTEXT

During the first half of the twentieth century, the term "specialist" implied[24]

> a nurse with extensive experience in a particular area of nursing, a nurse who completed a hospital-based "postgraduate" course, or a nurse who performed with technical expertise. (p. 3)

Although, at that time, such nurses were recognized for their expert knowledge regarding nursing practice in a specific area, most postgraduate-nursing courses before World War II were limited to functional courses that prepared a nurse administrator and/or nurse educator. Although there is some controversy about when the title "clinical nurse specialist" was first used, there is clear agreement that, in 1943, Frances Reiter promoted the idea of the nurse clinician.[24,25,27] According to Hameric and Spross,[24] her perception of the nurse clinician was one of

> a nurse with advanced knowledge and clinical competence committed to providing the highest quality of nursing care. (p. 3)

She did not believe that a master's degree was the distinctive qualification to be a nurse clinician, but she did recognize that graduate education was the most efficient means of preparing such practitioners.

Norris[28] dated the inception of the CNS to 1944 and the NLNE's Committee to Study Postgraduate Clinical Nursing Courses. Smoyak[29] credited a national conference of directors of graduate programs, sponsored by the University of Minnesota in 1949, for the genesis of the clinical-nurse specialty. Even though the NLNE had recommended a plan to develop nurse specialists, urging qualified universities to undertake the experiment, one major difficulty with advancing the concept of the CNS was that the predominant level of education for nurses at the time was the diploma. Another was that many nurses in baccalaureate- and master's-level courses shared the same classroom in the 1950s. Eventually, psychiatric nursing was credited with being the first specialty to develop graduate-level clinical experiences.

SOCIOPOLITICAL CONTEXT

Several factors inhibited the growth of specialization in nursing. After World War II, there was both an increased demand for nurse generalists and an increased demand for the advanced education of such nurses because of the numbers of veteran nurses who were eligible for educational benefits under the GI Bill. Factors such as these, as well as the focus of preparation of the early graduate leaders in nursing at Teachers' College, Columbia University, and the post–World War II increase in hospital care, resulted in nursing shifting from a private-duty model to a supervisory model within a hospital bureaucracy. In response, the National Mental Health Act was passed, which provided research and training funds for advanced study in core mental-health disciplines. Because psychiatric nursing was identified as a core discipline, both undergraduate and graduate education in this specialty were eligible for funding. Peplau,[30] a psychiatric nurse leader, educator, and clinician, developed the first master's program focused on advanced practice in psychiatric nursing.

Oncologic nursing was another area that early on developed graduate education for specialization. These efforts were spearheaded by the American Cancer Society and the National Cancer Institute. According to Hamric and Spross,[24] the American Cancer Society has continued its interest in the development of CNSs in oncology into the 1990s. The Oncology Nursing Society is credited with establishing cancer nursing as a specialty and with contributing to the development of the oncology CNS role and refining of the advanced practice role in oncology.

The Professional Nurse Traineeship Program of 1963 was a major force that stimulated the inclusion of education in the development of the CNS movement. This expansion, along with the increasing numbers of baccalaureate-prepared nurses and with the profession's interest in graduate education, led to the establishment of education for clinical specialization within graduate programs.[24] The shortage of physicians in the 1960s helped to create a milieu for expanding clinical specialization in nursing, and, in addition, opportunities were opening up within the health-care environment for more competent professionals prepared for advanced practice. By the 1970s, there were master's-level programs to prepare CNSs for a variety of practice settings and specialty areas. However, without a clear mandate for entry-level preparation, confusion remained over the use of multiple-role titles such as nurse clinician, nursing specialist, expert clinician, clinical nurse scientist, and CNS. Also during this time, questions were raised regarding the purpose, preparation, function, responsibility, and practice setting for the CNS.

According to Minarik,[25] the role confusion began to resolve somewhat with the publication of the ANA social policy statement, which defined specialization in nursing. Clarification of the various issues provided a public declaration of criteria for the title of CNS. Other groups embraced the definition and supported the characteristics, but without a doubt, the strongest support came from the ANA in 1980.[31] Specialty organizations and state nurses' associations then reinforced this definition by formally describing the requisites and competencies of nurses assuming the CNS role (e.g., American Association of Critical Care Nurses' [AACN] position statements [1987],[32] ANA [1986],[33] and California Nurses' Association [1984][34]). According to Sparacino, Cooper, and Minarik,[26] further validation of acceptance of the CNS role within the ANA became a reality with the publication of a study undertaken by the Council of Clinical Nurse Specialists reporting that 19,000 RNs functioned as CNSs. A clear definition of the CNS role appeared in the ANA publication *The Role of the Clinical Nurse Specialist*, published when Sparacino was chair of the CNS Council.[36]

Funding for advanced-nursing education occurred through federal government agencies, such as the National Institute of Mental Health and the BPHr, Division of Nursing. Private foundations, such as The Robert Wood Johnson Foundation, also provided funding.

Minarik's[25] perception of the evolution of the CNS role was that it grew out of needs recognized by nurse educators and clinicians, in contrast to the NP role, which grew out of recognition of a need to provide services for well children in primary care. Before the development of the CNS role, there were no rewards or opportunities for advanced study and practice in clinical nursing; a graduate student had two role selections: educator or administrator.

The social forces noted by Minarik[25] that had a significant impact on the CNS movement included growing specialization, growing use of technology, growing acuity of care, and in a phrase coined by Cooper,[35] a growing need for "attendance" in nursing. The CNS was similar to the attending nurse who, by virtue of confidence and skills gained through years of direct clinical contact with patients, was a refined expert in providing care and guidance to others. Unlike the generalist nurse, the CNS had to be more than just a safe practitioner. As the ANA Social Policy Statement[31] emphasized, the CNS was expected to have master competence in a clinical specialty over time. In addition, the role reflected the additional components of educator, consultant, and researcher.

In conversations with Minarik[25] and Riddle,[27] one gains a view of the CNS as a special kind of nurse who is able to view the patient from a well-developed knowledge base in a specialized area of nursing. According to Riddle,[27] who is not a CNS but a master teacher and clinician in nursing of children, the CNS could be viewed as a pioneer. These clinicians learned how to present themselves in a professional manner and to work with nursing service in innovative and creative ways. The CNS programs helped nursing students learn to upgrade the quality of the care that they delivered. The CNS has a broader set of responsibilities than the non-CNS in the service setting and, thus, needs a broader educational experience.

According to Minarik's personal experience,[25] inherent and invaluable in the CNS educational experiences are collegial relationships that can be sustained over time. Minarik described her experience as follows:

> The beautiful thing that happened to me was being at the University of California at San Francisco because of the colleague relationship. . . . There were strong clinicians, strong thinkers. This resulted in my colleagues being editors for each other's work. We struggled through the thinking involved, it was a wonderful exciting process of co-mentorship, editing and learning together.

These comments by Minarik reflect the collegiality, collaboration, and creativity that developed as these clinicians worked together to provide expert patient care in teams of nurses and physicians. Emerging from these collegial, creative, and collaborative relationships was a need to communicate through writing what occurred with patients. The shared experience resulted in innovative nursing care in which the individuals learned from one another and shared that knowledge with others.

INFLUENCE OF GOVERNMENT AGENCIES, A PRIVATE FOUNDATION, AND PROFESSIONAL ASSOCIATIONS

The Robert Wood Johnson Foundation was a major funding agency, as was the Division of Nursing of the BHPr. A particular influence in the marketing of the role has been the students themselves.[25,27] CNSs have generated a vast number of publications in which they have described patient care within their specialties and have attempted to clarify areas of responsibility, specialization, and the multiplicity of the roles. However, according to Minarik,[25] because they did not write about their roles as CNSs, they remained invisible as CNSs. The ANA remained a strong marketing force, working hard to increase the visibility of the CNS. The Oncology Nursing Society and the AACN also focused on clinical practice problems and efforts.

KEY LEADERS

A list of the key leaders in the CNS movement begins with Frances Reiter,[24,25,27] who introduced the title "nurse clinician." Hildegarde Peplau is known for opening the door to clinical specialization in psychiatric nursing. Riddle[28] also would include on this list the many students who should be credited for opening doors by marketing their skills and collaborating with other health-care providers. The students were risk takers and innovators.

Minarik,[25] after 20 years of experiencing the role, has identified other influential contributors to the CNS movement. For example, Pauline Beacraft was recognized for the creation of the CNS journal and for providing a forum for discussion of CNS issues. Beverly Malone implemented the role and a consultation service of CNSs at the University of Cincinnati. Linda Cronowett was a key player in introducing the use of research in practice. Pat Sparacino provided leadership through her practice and publications as well as through her activities as chair of the ANA Council of Clinical Nurse Specialists. Helen Ripple, director of nursing at the University of California Hospitals in San Francisco and former president of the American Organization of Nurse Executives, strongly supported the CNS role and, as an administrator, implemented mechanisms within the service setting to fully use the expertise of CNSs. She also actively supported 14 years of annual CNS conferences, sponsored by the University of California at San Francisco, that brought together leaders in the field to grapple with key issues and promote the CNS role.

Other notable contributors to the role include Joyce Clifford at Beth Israel Medical Center in Boston and, more recently, Brenda Lyon and her group. Barbara Siefert has focused on the professional question and Dorothy Brooten has focused on research outcomes.

INTERFACE WITH NURSE MIDWIVES, NURSE ANESTHETISTS, AND NURSE PRACTITIONERS

Minarik[25] believes that the four roles of nurse midwife, nurse anesthetist, CNS, and NP have more similarities than differences. The CNS's expertise is in the identification and intervention of clinical problems and in the management of those problems within the larger health-care system. The challenge of the future will be the ability of the advanced practice nurse to be prepared to serve in a variety of roles. Leadership, flexibility, responsiveness to change, and depth and breadth in theoretical knowledge, all combined with fully developed expertise and advanced clinical judgment, are critical in all four areas of practice. According to Minarik,[25] defining the expertise and how we educate students will be the greatest challenge. She feels strongly that it cannot be done without graduate preparation and that it is important to understand that preparation of the expert is not only in learning facts and content but in developing critical thinking and judgment.

Nurse Practitioners

The NP movement—the most modern of the four advanced practice roles—arose against the backdrop of the 1960s and in response to needed changes in the health-care environment and in the education of graduate nurses.

HISTORICAL AND SOCIOPOLITICAL CONTEXT

The time of transition from the post–World War II generation to the baby boomers' developmental years was one of social activism and scientific advancement. The assassination of President John F. Kennedy created a sense of deep national commitment to public service among young people, and according to Ford,[37] there was a true concern for both the "haves and have nots." While the war in Vietnam was accelerating, President Lyndon Johnson declared the war on poverty. As the increase in technology was driving the need for knowledge, information systems began to emerge, and the pace of life began to accelerate.

During this time, society exhibited a sincere concern about the maldistribution of health resources, especially physicians. The increasing concerns relating to health care and the emerging emphasis on health promotion made it a good time for change in the profession of nursing. Ford[37] described the time as one in which nurses were able to try new things. Although there was some uncertainty and resistance to change, the window of opportunity was clearly open.

In a candid interview reported in the *Journal of the New York State Nurses Association*, Ford[1] described the NP movement as an

> outgrowth (a) of the Western Interstate Commission on Higher Education for Nursing (WICHEN) Clinical Content study on Master's preparation in Community Health Nursing in which I was involved from 1963 to 1967 and (b) an experience that pediatrician Henry K. Silver had at a Child Health Nursing Conference which was organized in the mid-1960s by the public health nurses and the Colorado State Health Department. (p. 12)

The WICHEN project provided the stimulus for the change needed in the health-care environment and the education of graduate nurses, and Dr. Silver's involvement provided the mechanism for that change.

Ford[1] has identified seven myths that have hampered the NP movement and that continue to the present day. The first myth is that the development of the NP role was solely in response to a proclaimed physician shortage existing at the time. The reality is that the rationale for the development of the NP role came from nursing leaders who were committed to preparation of graduate nurses for clinical specialization. Four groups of faculty, representing 13 western states, had worked together to identify the clinical content for a master's degree in nursing. Stimulated by both social and professional developments and aided by the maldistribution of medical personnel, an "opportunistic" environment for changes in well-child care in ambulatory settings was created.[1,37] The aim of the clinical-content model was not only to prepare graduate students for clinical specialization but also, according to Levy,[11] to "reclaim a role that public health nurses had historically held" (p. 12).

To reclaim that role, nurses needed to be able to work in an autonomous and collegial way with physicians. The experience with Silver provided an opportunity for Ford and Silver to promote an experiment that would allow nurses to reclaim the role. Dr. Silver, who had been introduced to Ford by Henry Kemp, a pediatrician known for his identification of the battered-child syndrome, had not been enthusiastic about the idea of NPs. However, he returned from his attendance at the Child Health Nursing Conference with a new and enthusiastic view of nurses. Thus, the liaison began.[1,37]

This association between Ford and Silver led to a collegial relationship in which the role of nursing in well-child care was tested to determine if nurses could competently care for well children in community-based settings. The NP model was far from the "medical model" that is frequently attributed to the practitioner program; it was fashioned after the nursing profession's criteria for clinical practice, as set forth by the ANA. The emphasis was on professional, direct client care, health and wellness, collegiality with physicians, and prevention-oriented care, including consumer education.

The initial NP program at the University of Colorado began as part of a demonstration project in which a post-master's student worked in an expanded role for nursing. Ford[37] dated the inception of the practitioner program to the admission of the first student to the University of Colorado's program in the fall of 1965. The demonstration project tested the scope of practice by building on what had existed as part of community-health nursing and doing it more thoroughly. A survey of health needs identified major problems commonly encountered by nurses in the community.

More than just collecting data, the survey also focused on data interpretation and management of the well child. Results of the demonstration project helped to extend the focus of practice toward[38]

> testing a nursing role in well-child care to determine whether nurses could competently deliver care to well children in community-based settings.

Included in the project were efforts to increase the sensory input of nurses and to increase the nurse's ability to share that input with parents, thus assisting the parents in making decisions for themselves that were based on an informed consideration of both options and consequences.[38] As a result, the observations of the nurse and her decision-making abilities were sharpened.

The intent of the project was not only to teach nurses how to provide care competently and confidently but also to establish an advanced nursing practice grounded in, and held to, a postbaccalaureate academic standard. The program was successful and led to the establishment of nine accredited programs, with the standard for entry being a baccalaureate in nursing. The program attracted nurses with international experience, including mission work and broader community experience.

Although the myths about the program may have been negative, the outcomes were very positive. It was not, as suggested by the second myth identified by Ford, a medical model with nurses performing as junior physicians. According to Ford,[1,37] the model was anything but medical: it was based on well-child care, health promotion, and disease prevention, and it afforded the nurse an opportunity to assess autonomously, innovate, and work collaboratively with physicians and families in providing care. Ford also considered the National League of Nursing's statement[39] that the early programs

> have been considered a means of controlling costs by introducing lower-paid health care providers . . . as an answer to distribution problems in geographic areas short of physicians. (p. 2)

Ford[1] believed that the distribution problems provided an opportunity to test the expanded role of nurses.

The third myth focuses on the educational pattern followed to prepare NPs, suggesting that[1]

> short-term continuing education courses were the educational pattern used to prepare nurse practitioners from any nursing background. (p. 12)

Ford clarified that the first pediatric NP program at the University of Colorado, which had been funded through the Medical Research Fund at the University of Colorado and began admitting students in 1965, required a baccalaureate in nursing and qualifications to meet graduate-school admission requirements. Findings from this experimental program were to be incorporated into collegiate nursing programs at the appropriate degree level.[42]

The fourth myth, according to Ford,[1] is that the "innovations in expanded roles came from professionals other than nurses" (p. 12). The fifth myth addresses the issue of laws governing practice. Ford emphasized that the model was within the practice of nurses and did not necessitate changing nurse-practice acts. The sixth myth, according to Ford,[1] is that "physician supervision was necessary for nurse practitioners" (p. 12). Ford pointed out that the University of Colorado program was collegial; it was only when academic standards were compromised that the NP role became confused with the physician assistant role and control by the medical profession became an issue.

The seventh myth surrounds the acceptance or lack of acceptance of the NP by physicians and patients. Again, according to Ford,[37] once collegiality was experienced, problems between or among groups apparently diminished, resulting in the mutual acceptance of roles.

INFLUENCE OF GOVERNMENT AGENCIES

Federal support came a little late to the movement, mainly for political reasons. Without the strong support of the professional organizations, it was difficult to promote the developing programs. The first attempt to gain federal support for the demonstration project at the University of Colorado was through the Children's Bureau. However, this approach was unsuccessful because the perception was that the project did not fit the mold or mission of the Children's Bureau. According to Ford,[37] the bureau's rejection turned out to be fortunate because it motivated a search for other funding sources that proved to be very productive. The other source of federal funding was through the Division of Nursing of the BPHr.

INFLUENCE OF PRIVATE FOUNDATIONS, COLLEGES, AND UNIVERSITIES

Despite the lack of support and the resistance of the professional associations, the practitioner movement made continued progress through the support of private foundations and specialty organizations. The Robert Wood Johnson Foundation and The Commonwealth Fund were very supportive of the NP role. Through their efforts, including both moral and financial support, the program, according to Ford, was "put on the map."[37] Unfortunately, university nursing faculty were slow to do more than challenge the ideas; it appeared that faculty were more interested in preparing the CNS. In addition, the few faculty who were in practice feared medical control.

Curriculum was the most important aspect of this movement, according to Ford[37]; however, in many schools, that preparation did not include physiology, had a behavioral focus, and did not include research. Ford[37] thought that the practitioner movement was doing what it should be doing: testing the "boundaries of knowledge." The ANA stated that clinical studies should be undertaken, but it was using the model of the CNS, including the nursing process with a focus on clinical judgment and nursing management.

Given that the ANA and the schools did not support the early NP effort, the NP went to the American Academy of Pediatrics for sponsorship and certification. From 1970 and into the 1980s, NPs persisted in their attempts to be recognized by nursing organizations and academies, making repeated demands of the traditional organizations. Now in the 1990s, according to Ford[1]:

> The goals of the first nurse practitioner educational programs—to be integrated and institutionalized in collegiate nursing programs are coming to fruition. (p. 13)

The NP is clinically competent, well accepted by patients and health-care professionals, cost effective, and professionally credentialed.[37,42] The NP has continued to expand into new settings and new specialty areas as needs, demands, and opportunities have increased. The NP has also been influential in academic settings, introducing the concept of faculty practice and influencing graduate and undergraduate curricula.[42]

FORCES INFLUENTIAL IN MARKETING AND EFFECTIVE UTILIZATION

From Ford's perspective,[37] the use of pilot projects, spurred by the academic credentials and success of Ford and Silver, helped to keep programs afloat. The Colorado Health Department and private pediatricians helped to study the process and to identify outcomes by following students into the practice areas. Ford served on the State Board of Nursing in Colorado and, as president, helped to keep the health community informed. She made visits to the medical and nursing boards and described what NPs were doing, reassuring the boards that the nurses were not changing the nature of practice but remaining within its scope.

The students themselves were probably most influential in marketing and communicating the effective use of NPs.[37] Articles, published books, personal testimonies, and invitations to visitors for direct observation at practice sites contributed to highlighting the progress and distributing the message of the NP. As health-care issues assumed a larger part of the public agenda, newspapers begin to pick up on the trend.

An obstacle to the marketing and effective use of NPs has been the lack of uniform credentialing. Apparently, 43 states have special NP legislation, and 34 states have laws providing prescriptive privileges. Ford[1] prefers that the ANA confer NP certification and that the states' nurse-practice acts not be altered. Ford[1] believes that every professional nurse should be required to read Safriet's scholarly analysis (see Bibliography) of the legal "mishmash created by nurse practitioner legislation" (p. 13).

KEY LEADERS

The movement toward expanding the NP role included leadership from nurses and physicians alike. In addition to Ford and Silver, the following is a brief list of some of the prominent figures who were engaged in the expanding scope of practice through collaboration with physician colleagues: Priscilla Andrews, RN, John Connelly, MD, and others in Massachusetts[40]; Barbara Resnick, RN, and Charles Lewis, MD, in Missouri[43]; Harriet Kitzman, RN, and Evan Charney, MD, in Rochester, New York.[44] According to Ford[1]:

> These maverick nurses were pioneering innovators; but most of all, they were nurses." (p. 12)

Ingeborg Mauksch, PhD, FAAN,[45] who became an NP in 1972, published a paper with a physician colleague on joint practice and later became an ANA representative to the National Joint Practice Commission, where she served for 4 years. She also served as director of the Robert Wood Johnson Faculty Fellowships in Primary Care program, helping to prepare 100 fellows in primary-care leadership, teaching, and practice. In addition, many nursing leaders in key positions throughout the country supported the movement. These leaders include Margaret Arnstein; Fay Abdellah; Mary Kelley Mullane; Florence Blake; and Esther Lucille Brown, whose favorite quote regarding NPs was "I have seen nursing in its finest."[37] The Center for Human and Child Development also strongly supported the development and positioning of the NP movement.

Leaders such as these served to explode the last four myths about the NP, which implied that practice laws would need to be expanded, that increased supervision of NPs would be necessary, that patients and physicians would have a difficult time accepting the NP, and that NPs would become extinct once the physician shortage was over. Again, according to Ford,[1,37] due in part to the leadership of such nurses, none of these notions was true. In addition to the positive pilot projects, publicity, and the rapidly changing health environment that were a continuous stimulus to the movement's development, these nurses committed the NP to a high quality of education during a time when government and professional support was lacking. For a more comprehensive list of exceptional NPs and "Who's Who" among NPs, refer to the special anniversary issue of *Nurse Practitioner*, September 1990.[46]

INTERFACE WITH THE NURSE MIDWIVES, NURSE ANESTHETISTS, AND CLINICAL NURSE SPECIALISTS

According to Ford,[37] the nature of nursing is "timeless and enduring." The role of the NP is similar to that of the other three advanced practice roles in its emphasis on practice autonomy, interdisciplinary collaboration, and its continuing efforts toward a barrier-free practice. At the same time, there are distinguishing characteristics among the three role components. In general, the NP is focused on health and wellness in a community-based primary-care setting, autonomy in clinical decision making, systematic and orderly collection of data through history taking and the provision of feedback to the client, and advocacy on the client's behalf. The collaborative element of the NP role affords not only an opportunity for consumer choice but also for effective resource allocation and follow-up.

Joining Forces: Role Parameters and Concerns

Within the historical and sociopolitical contexts of the evolution of the four advanced domains of CNM, CRNA, CNS, and NP, certain similarities and differences are evident. From the educational perspective, the most common theme is the fact that all four domains were influenced by the early development of nursing, which, through the Nightingale Schools, stimulated better education and professional development for nurses. As each practice area has evolved, education has been a significant force in enabling greater autonomy in practice.

Trends in educational preparation gradually have moved toward postbaccalaureate preparation, with the CNS and NP requiring master's-level preparation and a strong move in the other two domains toward a similar level of preparation. Nonetheless, the controversy surrounding entry-level education for nursing continues to persist. Moreover, because there were no clear paradigms for advanced practice, each role has evolved within its own framework. For instance, faculty in the western United States have not yet agreed on a definition of advanced nursing and its scope of practice.

As has been illustrated, progress in advanced practice nursing has been hampered by the profession's history, medicine's concern for competition, the lack of acceptance of nursing both externally and internally as a discipline with its own body of knowledge, and by the tendency toward a lack of mutual support as each movement has moved forward. As Minarik[25] pointed out, nurses tend to be territorial, holding on to their areas of practice. Even nursing faculty have been separated by their own agendas in these advanced practice areas, with each having a strong orientation or bias.

Table 1–2 compares historical information and the views of the nursing leaders interviewed for this chapter. The historical developments of nurse midwifery and nurse anesthesia are clearly more alike in their association with the medical community and their competition with medicine. The CNS movement and the NP movement are more recent and have been focused on comprehensive health care in acute- and primary-care settings.

In each of the four practice areas, interviewees noted the recognition of the move toward autonomy in decision making and professionalism by the medical community as consistently important in operationalizing each role. For nurse midwives, nurse anesthetists, and NPs, acceptance of the autonomous nature of their roles by the medical community helped connect responsibility and accountability to authority in independent decision making in areas of assessment and care normally requiring medical management under the purview of the physician. The CNS, in contrast, needed similar autonomy but was not so closely aligned to medical management as were the other three. Responsibilities of the CNS were broader within the specialty and focused more on nursing management of illness in acute care, consultation, education, and research.

In all four domains, support from medicine, from state and federal legislatures, and, most important, from the consumer, was of significant consequence. The nurse midwives' primary source of consumer support came from the underserved populations who benefited from their attendance at home deliveries. Nurse anesthetists gained recognition through physicians and patients, especially because of their impeccable records with survival rates through surgery. Similarly, but in different practice arenas, CNSs and NPs have been their own best advocates. Consumer satisfaction and physician advocacy have proved to be powerful stimuli for both of these movements. Unlike the NP and CRNA movement, the CNS movement had the benefit of unyielding support from the ANA. All four groups were actively involved in scholarly and lay publications as their specialties developed, keeping both professionals and the public informed.

With the exception of the NP role, a state of war acted as a catalyst to the expanded use, and consequential favorable opinion, of the advanced practice nursing role. Other significant outside influences included both public and private initiatives. The Children's Bureau was significant in the nurse midwifery movement. The National Council of State Boards was important for maintaining standards for the CRNA, and Robert Wood Johnson, Pew, and the Division of Nursing, the BPHr, helped to support educational programs that moved the CNS and NP movements forward. While the ANA focused its support on the CNS movement, The Commonwealth Fund was a particularly helpful source of support for the NP movement. In addition, advancing technology and growing acuity in care gave further impetus to the need for clinical specialization, thus assisting the CNS movement. In contrast, the current emphasis on primary care and community-based illness prevention and health promotion have created greater opportunities for the NP.

Each of the domains has experienced its own struggle in establishing credibility and acceptance by the profession and public. Educational preparation, certification, licensure, and credentialing are overriding concerns for all four domains. Increasing competition in the health-care market in the 1970s and 1980s has been a concern to those practicing in each of the areas, but especially to the emerging NP, who is particularly susceptible to the issues of equitable economic reimbursement for services, hospital privileges, and prescriptive authority. Collaboration, interdisciplinary emphasis, and mutual support are emerging as key common elements in a changing health-care environment. Garde[22] pointed out that it will be necessary for artificial barriers to communication within the profession to be removed and for each practice area to join forces in identifying the best ways to provide services in a managed-care environment in a way that recognizes each other's area of practice.

The distinguishing characteristics of the four domains are presented from a multitude of perspectives in the literature. Roberts[3] does an excellent job of summarizing the various events influencing CNMs and their move to professionalism. Bankert[21] and Thatcher[20] are two authors who have done an outstanding job in capturing the history of the CRNA from its inception. Sparacino, Cooper, and Minarik,[26] Hamric and Spross,[24] and Menard[47] have provided historical and clinical descriptions of the role of the CNS. Ford[1] has contributed to dispelling myths that have been perpetuated in the literature regarding the NP, as well as clearly articulating the NP's role.

The distinctive feature of the nurse midwifery practitioner is the focus on the health and comfort of mothers and babies during the birthing experience, both in the home and in the hospital. Like the nurse midwives, CRNAs may require medical support, but in the acute-care hospital-based environment. Both CRNAs and nurse midwives have engaged in systematic data collection through key leaders to demonstrate competency. Direct care is probably the most distinctive feature of the CNS, followed by coordination, evaluation, and planning for the individual within the broader context of acute and to some extent, community-based health care. According to Sparacino, Cooper, and Minarik,[26] the CNS role incorporates theory, clinical-practice content, and research in a particular specialty area, thus promoting the "integration of education, consultation, and

TABLE 1–2
Comparison of Four Specialty Domains

Characteristics	Certified Nurse Midwife	Certified Nurse Anesthetist	Clinical Nurse Specialist	Nurse Practitioner
Mechanisms that helped operational- ize the role	Autonomy Professional de- velopment War Medical support Access to con- sultation Legislative sup- port	Autonomy Professional de- velopment War Medical support Access to con- sultation	Autonomy Professional de- velopment War Medical support Access to con- sultation Legislative sup- port (primarily ANA lobby)	Autonomy Professional de- velopment Medical support Access to con- sultation Legislative sup- port
	Consumer sup- port (dealing with under- served popu- lations)			Consumer sup- port
	Publications	Publications	Publications Managing ill- ness in acute care Growing spe- cialization	Publications Academic sup- port of Ford and Silver Communication with state board (Col- orado)
			Increased use of technology in acute care created need for an attend- ing nurse	Pilot projects
Forces that in- fluenced marketing and effec- tive utiliza- tion	Wars Focus on im- proving edu- cation Federal initia- tives (Frontier Nurs- ing Service)	Wars Focus on im- proving edu- cation Certification Department of Health National Coun- cil of State Boards	Federal initia- tives	Federal initia- tives (not ini- tially but later)
	Development of the American College of Nurse- Midwives Malpractice cri- sis 1985	Private Founda- tions Pew HCFA	Private founda- tions (The Robert Wood John- son)	Private founda- tions (The Common- wealth Fund and The Robert Wood Johnson Foun- dation)
	Consumer sup- port		Students Consumer sup- port	Students Consumer sup- port

HCFA = Health Care Financing Administration

TABLE 1–2
Comparison of Four Specialty Domains (Continued)

Characteristics	Certified Nurse Midwife	Certified Nurse Anesthetist	Clinical Nurse Specialist	Nurse Practitioner
Distinguishing characteristics	Health and comfort of mothers and babies	Medical focus nature of	Support of nursing service administration	
			Direct care broad within the specialty	Good public relations
	Distinctive medical support	Distinctive medical support	Filled the gap for the need for attending nurse to coordinate care within the specialty in the acute-care setting	Health and wellness focus within a community-based primary-care context
	Development of core competencies in 1978	Systematic and orderly data collection		
	Well grounded in childbirth after normal delivery			Systematic and orderly data collection with feedback
	Community based and hospital based	Hospital based	Depth and breadth of clinical knowledge in one specialty	Consumer advocacy within the independent role
			Fully developed specialty	
Interaction with other specialties	National Organization for Specialty Nurses	National Organization for Specialty Nurses	National Organization for Specialty Nurses	National Organization for Specialty Nurses
	Frontier Nursing Service			
Common shared roles	Autonomy in practice	Autonomy in practice	Autonomy in practice	Autonomy in practice
	Interdisciplinary emphasis and sharing of each other's skills	Interdisciplinary emphasis and sharing of each other's skills	Interdisciplinary emphasis and sharing of each other's skills	Interdisciplinary emphasis and sharing of each other's skills
	Joint effort to practice without artificial barriers	Joint effort to practice without artificial barriers	Joint effort to practice without artificial barriers	Joint effort to practice without artificial barriers
	Recognition of each other's areas of expertise	Recognition of each other's areas of expertise	Recognition of each other's areas of practice	Recognition of each other's areas of practice
	Practice in acute-care and community-based settings	Shared role in selling services in managed care	Movement to community-based care, potential for merging of role with NP	Movement to acute care, potential for merging of roles with CNS
	Movement to graduate preparation	Movement to graduate preparation	Graduate preparation	Movement to graduate preparation

leadership with the clinical practice component" (p. 7). The hallmarks of the NP role are an emphasis on primary care and health promotion that may occur in an independent or collegial setting and the fact that the NP role appears to offer the best opportunity for independence and innovation in practice.

Trends indicate that the future of advanced practice nursing will be community-based primary care in a managed-care environment. For the NP and the nurse midwife, this trend will probably increase the scope of practice and the potential for new growth. The nurse anesthetist has been, and will continue to be, affected by the health-care changes, with more emphasis on one-day outpatient surgery. The implications of this type of surgical experience in a changing environment will create a need for continuity and better communication between providers. The future of the CNS is less clear.

Recently, 25 NPs were interviewed about the movement's evolution and the future challenges for the role. The question of the future curriculum for NPs for the next decade resulted in mixed opinions. While the need for "advanced practice" preparation was recognized, the question of integration of the CNS and NP roles resulted in differing opinions. Mauksch[45] envisions a retitling of the NP to CNS in primary care for consistency with ANA nomenclature for the appropriate master's-level preparation in the specific field. Ford,[48] along with others,[36] sees the need to merge these two roles, with a general effort made to increase the assessment skills of all nurses and to provide for clinical learning that may not be appropriate for graduate credit. Ford[48] also promotes postmaster's level continuing education for CNSs and a "retooling and retraining [of] faculty" (p. 28).

Minarik[25] and Riddle[27] hold a different view of the future of the NP and CNS roles. Although many NPs foresee the CNS role eventually being absorbed into the NP role, both authors question who "will provide direct care in the acute care setting" and express concern that the "broad responsibility and creative nursing care of the CNS" may be lost in the transition. Whether there will be a true blending of CNS and NP roles or an emergence of a coordinator of health care based on the scholarly, sensitive, patient-centered approach that has been so much a part of the CNS role is yet to be determined.

The current state of uncertainty surrounding the American health-care delivery system may present the greatest window of opportunity for advanced nurses to unite and be heard as a vital force in care during health and illness. A response to the rapid changes in medical technologies worthy of nursing's history, the concerns over health-care resources, and the ethical considerations inherent in the pressure to deliver high-quality, cost-effective health care will require collective strength that demands a joining of forces of these four autonomous domains of practice.[44] Although, in the past, disputes over nursing's "identity" created internal conflicts and diverse opinions on what is best for nursing, these histories reflect a collective commitment by the profession to remain true to its essence while continuing to develop. With our predecessors as prototypes, the secure and successful future of nursing in the emerging model of health care can best be accomplished by collaboration and cooperation and by drawing on the intellect, integrity, and vigor that has marked the best of nursing's past.

Suggested Exercises

1. Briefly trace the historical development of the four domains of advanced practice nursing discussed in this chapter. From a historical perspective, identify the forces that have influenced progress in each of these areas of practice. From your perspective, which of these forces do you view as having the most significant impact and why?

2. Identify three key players in each of the domains and discuss their major contributions to the advanced practice movement.

3. Describe the role of the federal government and private foundations in the advanced practice movement. Compare and contrast the similarities and differences of these organizations in moving advanced practice forward in each of the four domains.

4. After reading this chapter and thinking about the four domains of practice and your personal experience, where do you perceive the need for joining forces and what mechanisms would you identify as critical in enabling these four areas of practice to move forward in a unified way?

5. Create a scenario in which representatives from each of these domains have been called forward to testify at a congressional hearing to convince members of Congress to continue to support advanced practice nursing. What points would you identify that each representative could make unique to each domain and collective to all four domains that would support continued funding?

6. Consider yourself a consumer advocate for each of the four domains. Describe what you consider the strengths of each of these specialties and how they contribute to improving health care of the U.S. population.

7. How would you respond to a layperson who asked you why one might select an advanced practice nurse as a primary-care provider?

8. On the basis of this chapter, what roles do you see merging and which do you view as remaining separate? In your thinking, take into account the historical context in which these roles emerged.

9. This chapter incorporated interviews from the "lived experience" of key players in each of the four domains of practice. What role does the lived experience play in historical documentation of nursing movements and what did you learn that you might not have learned if the chapter included only written documentation versus personal communication?

10. In what ways can our lived experiences be preserved to document the historical progress of nursing?

REFERENCES

1. Ford, LC: Nurse practitioners: myths and misconceptions. Journal of the New York State Nurses Association 26:12, 1995.
2. Roberts, J: Personal communication, March, 1996.
3. Roberts, J: The role of graduate education in midwifery in the USA. In Murphy-Black, T (ed): Issues in Midwifery: 119. Churchill Livingstone, Tokyo, 1995.
4. American College of Nurse-Midwives: Background on the AENM/MAWA uterorganization workgroup on midwifery education (IWG). Quickening 24:29, 1993.
5. Hiestad, WC: The development of nurse-midwifery education in the United States. In Fitzpatrick, ML (ed): Historical Studies in Nursing. Teachers' College Press, Columbia University, New York, 1978.
6. Chaney, JA: Birthing in early America. J Nurse Midwifery 25:5, 1980.
7. Litoff, JB: American Midwives: 1860 to the Present. Greenwood Press, Westport, Conn, 1978.
8. Litoff, JB: The midwife throughout history. J Nurse Midwifery 27:3, 1982.
9. Stern, CA: Midwives, male-midwives, and nurse-midwives. Obstet Gynecol 39:308, 1972.
10. Hawkins, JW: Annual Report of the ANA Council on Maternal-Child Nursing. American Nurses Association, Kansas City, June 1987.
11. Levy, J: The maternal and infant mortality in midwifery practice in Newark, NJ. Am J Obstet Gynecol 77:42, 1968.
12. Baker, J: The function of the midwife. Woman's Medical Journal 23:196, 1913.
13. Dock, LL: In Robb, IA, Dock, LL, and Banfield M (eds): The Transactions of the Third International Congress of Nurses with the Reports of the International Council of Nurses. JB Savage, Cleveland, Ohio, 1901.
14. Tom, SA: The evolution of nurse-midwifery 1900–1960. J Nurse Midwifery 27:4, 1982.
15. Shoemaker, MT: History of Nurse-Midwifery in the United States. The Catholic University of America Press, Washington, DC, 1947. Dissertation.
16. Bear, B: Personal communication, February, 1996.
17. Hall, CM: Training the obstetrical nurse. Am J Nursing 27:373, 1927.
18. Willeford, MB: The frontier nursing service. Public Health Nurs 25:9, 1933.
19. International Confederation of Midwives. Fact sheet. nd.
20. Thatcher, VS: History of Anesthesia, with Emphasis on the Nurse Specialist. Lippincott, Philadelphia, 1953.
21. Bankert, M: Watchful Care: A History of America's Nurse Anesthetists. Continuum, New York, 1989.
22. Garde, J: Personal communication, February, 1996.
23. Crile, GW (ed): George Crile: An Autobiography. Lippincott, Philadelphia, 1947.
24. Hamric, AB, and Spross, JA: The Clinical Nurse Specialist in Theory and Practice, ed 2. WB Saunders, Philadelphia, 1989.
25. Minarik, PA: Personal communication, March, 1996.
26. Sparacino, PA, Cooper, DM, and Minarik, PA: The Clinical Specialist: Implementation and Impact. Appleton & Lange, Stamford, Conn, 1990.
27. Riddle, I: Personal communication, February, 1996.
28. Norris, CM: One perspective on the nurse practitioner movement. In Jacox, A, and Norris, C (eds): Organizing for Independent Nursing Practice. New York, Appleton-Century-Crofts, 1977.
29. Smoyak, SA: Specialization in nursing: From then to now. Nurs Outlook 24:676, 1976.
30. Peplau, HE: Specialization in professional nursing. Nursing Science 3:268, 1965.
31. American Nurses' Association. Nursing: A Social Policy Statement. American Nurses' Association, Kansas City, 1980.
32. American Association of Critical Care Nurses: AACN Position Statement: The Critical Care Clinical Nurse Specialist: Role Definition. American Association of Critical Care Nurses, Newport Beach, Calif, 1986.
33. American Nurses' Association. Clinical Nurse Specialists: Distribution and Utilization. American Nurses' Association, Kansas City, 1986.
34. California Nurses' Association. Position Statement on Specialization in Nursing Practice. California Nurses' Association, San Francisco, 1984.
35. Cooper, DM: A refined expert: The clinical nurse specialist after five years. Momentum 1:1, 1983.
36. Sparacino, P: The clinical nurse specialist. Nursing Practice 1:215, 1986.
37. Ford, LC: Personal communication, February, 1996.
38. Ford, LC, Cobb, M, and Taylor, M: Defining Clinical Contact Graduate Nursing Programs: Community Health Nursing. Western Interstate Commission for Higher Education, Boulder, Colo, 1967.
39. National League of Nursing: Position Statement on the Education of Nurse Practitioners. National League of Nursing, New York, 1979, publication 11–1808.
40. Ford, LC, and Silver, HK: The expanded role of the nurse in child care. Nurs Outlook 15:43, 1967.
41. Shoultz, J, Hatcher, PA, and Hurrell, M: Growing edges of a new paradigm: The future of nursing in the health of the nation. Nurs Outlook 40:58, 1992.
42. Ford, LC: The contribution of nurse practitioners to American health care. In Aiken,

LH (ed): Nursing in the 1980's: Crises, Opportunities, Challenges. Lippincott, Philadelphia, 1982.

43. Lewis, CE, and Resnik, BA: Nurse clinics and progressive ambulatory patient care. N Engl J Med 277:1236, 1967.

44. Charney, E, and Kitzman, H: Child-health nurse (pediatric nurse practitioner) in private practice: A controlled trial. N Engl J Med 285:1353, 1971.

45. Mauksch, I: Special anniversary issue: 25 years later 25 exceptional NPs look at the movement's evolution and consider future challenges for the role. Nurse Pract 15:28, 1990.

46. Special anniversary issue: 25 years later 25 exceptional NPs look at the movement's evolution and consider future challenges for the role. Nurse Pract 15:28, 1990.

47. Menard, SW: The Clinical Nurse Specialist: Perspectives on Practice. John Wiley & Sons, 1987.

48. Ford, LC: Special anniversary issue: 25 years later 25 exceptional NPs look at the movement's evolution and consider future challenges for the role. Nurse Pract 15:28, 1990.

BIBLIOGRAPHY

Aiken, LH: Health Policy and Nursing Practice. McGraw-Hill Book Co, 1981.

American College of Nurse-Midwives: Background on the AENM/MAWA uterorganization workgroup on midwifery education (IWG). Quickening 24:29, 1993.

Baker, J: The function of the midwife. Woman's Medical Journal 23:196, 1913.

Bankert, M: Watchful Care: A History of America's Nurse Anesthetists. Continuum, New York, 1989.

Barry, PD: Psychosocial Nursing Care of Physically Ill Patients and Their Families, ed 3. Lippincott, Philadelphia, 1996.

Bear, B: Personal communication, February 1996.

Breckenridge, M: Wide Neighborhoods. Ross Laboratories, Columbus, Ohio, 1967, p 117.

Burnside, I: A scarce professional: The geropsychiatric clinical nurse specialist. Clinical Nurse Specialist 4:122, 1990.

California Alliance of Advanced Practice Nurses: October 1, 1995.

California Nurses' Association: Position Statement on Specialization in Nursing Practice. California Nurses' Association, San Francisco, 1984.

Campbell, ML, et al: An advanced practice model: Inpatient collaborative practices. Clinical Nurse Specialist 9:175, 1995.

Chaney, JA: Birthing in early America. J Nurse Midwifery 25:5, 1980.

Charney, E, and Kitzman, H: Child-health nurse (pediatric nurse practitioner) in private practice: A controlled trial. N Engl J Med 285:1353, 1971.

Clapesattle, H: The Doctors Mayo. University of Minnesota Press, Minneapolis, 1941, p 427.

Clinical Nurse Specialist Survey. State of California, Board of Registered Nursing, Sacramento, December, 1994.

Cooper, DM: A refined expert: The clinical nurse specialist after five years. Momentum 1:1, 1983.

Corbin, H: A nurse looks ahead. Am J Obstet Gynecol 59:899, 1946.

Crile, GW (ed): George Crile, An Autobiography. Lippincott, Philadelphia, 1947, p 168.

DeWitt, K: Specialties in nursing. Am J Nurs 1: 14, 1900.

Diers, D: Future of nurse-midwives in American healthcare. In Aiken, L (ed): Nursing in the 1980s: Crises, Opportunities, Challenges. JB Lippincott, Philadelphia, 1982.

Dock, LL: In Robb, IA, Dock, LL, and Banfield, M (eds): The Transactions of the Third International Congress of Nurses with the Reports of the International Council of Nurses. JB Savage, Cleveland, Ohio, 1901, p 485.

Education and Practice Collaboration: Mandate for Quality Education: Practice, and Research for Health Care Reform. American Association of Colleges of Nursing, Washington, DC, October 25, 1993.

The Essentials of Master's Education for Advanced Practice Nursing. American Association of Colleges of Nursing, 1995.

Faut-Callahan, M, and Kremer, M: Nurse anesthesia: An established advanced practice nursing specialty. Unpublished manuscript, 1996.

Fenton, MV, and Brykczynski, KA: Qualitative distinctions and similarities in the practice of clinical nurse specialists and nurse practitioners. Professional Nurse 9:313, 1993.

The first nurse anesthetist. BNANA 7:63, 1939.

Fitzpatrick, ML (ed): Historical Studies in Nursing. Columbia University, New York, 1978, p 68.

Forbes, KE, et al: Clinical nurse specialist and nurse practitioner core curricula survey results. Nurse Pract 15:43, 1990.

Ford, LC: The contribution of nurse practitioners to American health care. In Aiken, LH (ed): Nursing in the 1980's: Crises, Opportunitites, Challenges. JB Lippincott, Philadelphia, 1982, p. 231.

Ford, LC: Nurse practitioners: Myths and misconceptions. Journal of the New York State Nurses Association 26:12, 1995.

Ford, LC: Personal communication, February, 1996.

Ford, LC: Special anniversary issue: 25 years later 25 exceptional NPs look at the movement's evolution and consider future challenges for the role. Nurse Pract 15:28, 1990.

Ford, LC, Cobb, M, and Taylor, M: Defining Clinical Contact Graduate Nursing Programs: Community Health Nursing. Western Interstate Commission for Higher Education, Boulder, Colo, 1967.

Ford, LC, and Silver, HK: The expanded role of the nurse in child care. Nurs Outlook 15:43, 1967.

Freeland, T: Letters to the Editor. Clinical Nurse Specialist 8:289, 1994.

Galloway, DH: The anesthetizer as a specialist. The Philadelphia Medical Journal, p 1175, May 27, 1899.

Garde, J: Personal communication, February, 1996.

Gleeson, RM, et al: Advanced practice nursing: A model of collaborative care. MCN 15:9, 1990.

Guidelines and Standards for Nurse Anesthesia Practice. American Association of Nurse Anesthetists, Park Ridge, Ill, 1992.

Guyette, MI: Letter to the Editor. Clinical Nurse Specialist 9:424, 1995.

Hall, CM: Training the obstetrical nurse. Am J Nursing 27:373, 1927.

Hamric, AB, and Spross, JA: The Clinical Nurse Specialist in Theory and Practice, ed 2. WB Saunders, Philadelphia, 1989.

Hawkins, JW: Annual Report of the ANA Council on Maternal-Child Nursing. American Nurses Association, Kansas City, June 1987.

Hemschemeyer, H: A training school for nurse-midwives established. Am J Nurs 32:374, 1939.

Hiestad, WC: The development of nurse-midwifery education in the United States. In Fitzpatrick, ML (ed): Historical Studies in Nursing. Teachers' College Press, Columbia University, New York, 1978, p 86.

Hoyer, A: Sexual harassment: Four women describe their experiences: Background and implications for the clinical nurse specialist. Arch Psychiatr Nurs 8:177, 1994.

Is primary care the answer? Nurses respond. The American Nurse, 1994.

Jackson, PL: Advanced practice nursing: II. Opportunities and challenges for PNPs. Pediatr Nurs 21:43, 1995.

Keane, A, and Richmond, T: Tertiary nurse practitioners. Image J Nurs Sch 25:281, 1993.

Kobrin, FE: The American midwife controversy: A crisis of professionalization. Bull Hist Med 40:350, 1966.

Kupina, PS: Community health CNSs and health care in the year 2000. Clinical Nurse Specialist 9:188, 1995.

Lerner, G: The Majority Finds Its Past: Placing Women in History. Oxford University Press, New York, 1979.

Levy, J: The maternal and infant mortality in midwifery practice in Newark, NJ. Am J Obstet Gynecol 77:42, 1918.

Lewis, CE, and Resnik, BA: Nurse clinics and progressive ambulatory patient care. N Engl J Med 277:1236, 1967.

Litoff, JB: American Midwives: 1860 to the Present. Greenwood Press, Westport, Conn, 1986.

Litoff, JB: The midwife throughout history. J Nurse Midwifery 27:3, 1982.

Long, KA: Master's degree nursing education and health care reform: Preparing for the future. Prof Nurs 10:71, 1994.

Magaw, A: A review of over fourteen thousand surgical anesthesias. BNANA 7:63, 1939.

Magaw, A: Observations in anesthesia. Northwestern Lancet 19:207.

Mauksch, I: Special anniversary issue: 25 years later 25 exceptional NPs look at the movement's evolution and consider future challenges for the role. Nurse Pract 15:28, 1990.

Mason, G, and Jinks, A: Examining the role of the practitioner-teacher in nursing. British Journal of Nursing 3:1063, 1994.

Medicaid Waiver Programs: Lessons for the Future or Time-limited Experiments. State Initiatives in Health Care Reforms, May/ June, 1994.

Menard, SW: The Clinical Nurse Specialist: Perspectives on Practice. John Wiley & Sons, New York, 1987.

Minarik, PA: Alternatives to physical restraints in acute care. Clinical Nurse Specialist 8:136, 162 1994.

Minarik, PA: Cognitive assessment of the cardiovascular patient in the acute care setting. Cardiovasc Nurs 9:36, 1995.

Minarik, PA: Collaboration between service and education: Perils or pleasures for the clinical nurse specialist? Clinical Nurse Specialist 4:109, 1990.

Minarik, PA: Editor's response. Clinical Nurse Specialist 8:289, 1994.

Minarik, PA: Federal action on prescriptive authority. Clinical Nurse Specialist 7:46, 1993.

Minarik, PA: Graduate education and health care. Clinical Nurse Specialist 246, 1996.

Minarik, PA: Health Care Financing Administration (HCFA) instructions clarify Medicare reimbursement eligibility. Clinical Nurse Specialist 8:16 46, 1994.

Minarik, PA: Incorporating imagery in clinical practice. Clinical Nurse Specialist 7:234, 1993.

Minarik, PA: Legislative and regulatory update: DEA registration for midlevel practitioners. Clinical Nurse Specialist 7:319, 1993.

Minarik, PA: Legislative and regulatory update: Federal reimbursement revisited. Clinical Nurse Specialist 7:102, 1993.

Minarik, PA: Legislative and regulatory update: Health care reform and managed competition: Implications for CNSs. Clinical Nurse Specialist 7:105, 1993.

Minarik, PA: Legislative and regulatory update: Priorities for clinical nurse specialists. Clinical Nurse Specialist 6:168, 1992.

Minarik, PA: Legislative and regulatory update: Reimbursement and health care reform legislation introduced. Clinical Nurse Specialist 7:245, 1993.

Minarik, PA: Legislative and regulatory update: Second license for advanced practice? Clinical Nurse Specialist 6:1, 1992.

Minarik, PA: Medwatch: Medical products reporting program. Clinical Nurse Specialist 8:74, 1994.

Minarik, PA: Mind-body connection: Enhancing healing through imagery. Clinical Nurse Specialist 7:169, 1993.

Minarik, PA: Personal communication, March, 1996.

Minarik, P, and Learith, M: The angry demanding hostile response. In Riggel, B, and Ehrenreich, D (eds): Psychological Aspects of Critical Care Nursing. Aspen Publishers, Rockville, Md, 1989.

Montemurd, MA: The evolution of the clinical nurse specialist: Response to the challenge of professional nursing practice. Clinical Nurse Specialist 1:106, 1987.

National League for Nursing: Position statement on the education of nurse practitioners. National League for Nursing, New York, 1979, publication 11–1808.

New York Adopts Pure Community Rating: Other States Take Incremental Approach. State Initiatives in Health Care Reform, July/August, 1994.

Norris, CM: One perspective on the nurse practitioner movement. In Jacox, A, and Norris, C (eds): Organizing for Independent Nursing Practice. New York, Appleton-Century-Crofts, 1977, p 21.

Nursing Education's Agenda for the 21st Century. American Association of Colleges of Nursing, Washington, DC, March 22, 1993.

Nursing's Agenda for Health Care Reform: Final Draft.Lf:021. American Nurses Association, Kansas City, Mo, April 24, 1991.

Owen, H, and Wangensteen, SD: The Rise of Surgery. University of Minnesota Press, Minneapolis, 1978, p 353.

Peplau, HE: Specialization in professional nursing. Nursing Science 3:268, 1965.

Pew Health Professions Commission: Health Professions Education for the Future: Pew Professions Committee, UCSF Center for the Health Professions, San Francisco, Calif, February, 1993.

Pew Health Professions Commission: Policy Papers. University of California, Center for Health Professions, San Francisco, April 1994.

The professional anesthetizer (editorial). Medical Record, p 522, April 10, 1897.

Public Education Crucial to Health Care Reform: Citizens Bombarded with Special Interest Messages. State Initiatives in Health Care Reform, September/October 1994.

Qualifications and Capabilities of the Certified Registered Nurse Anesthetist. American Association of Nurse Anesthetists, Park Ridge, Ill, 1992.

Reid, ML, and Morris, JB: Perinatal care and cost effectiveness: Changes in health expenditure and birth outcome following the establishment of a nurse midwife program. Med Care 17:491, 1979.

Riddle, I: Personal communication, February, 1996.

Robb, IAH: Nursing: Its Principles and Practice for Hospital and Private Use. W.B. Saunders, Philadelphia, 1893.

Roberts, J: The role of graduate education in midwifery in the USA. In Murphy-Black, T (ed): Issues in Midwifery: 119. Churchill Livingstone, Tokyo, 1995.

Roberts, J: Personal communication, March, 1996.

The Role of the Clinical Nurse Specialist. American Nurses' Association, Kansas City, 1968.

Roush, RE: The development of midwifery: Male and female, yesterday and today. J Nurse Midwifery 24:27, 1979.

Safriet, BJ: Healthcare dollars and regulatory sense: The role of advanced practice nursing. Yale Journal on Regulation 9:417, 1992.

Shoemaker, MT: History of nurse-midwifery in the United States. The Catholic University of America Press, Washington, DC, 1947. Dissertation.

Shoultz, J, Hatcher, PA, and Hurrell, M: Growing edges of a new paradigm: The future of nursing in the health of the nation. Nurs Outlook 40:58, 1992.

Shyrock, R: The Development of Modern Medicine. Kropt, New York, 1947, pp 346–347.

Sloan, PE: Commitment to equality: A view of early black nursing schools. In Fitzpatrick, ML (ed): Historical Studies in Nursing. Columbia University, New York, 1978.

Smoyak, SA: Specialization in nursing: From then to now. Nurs Outlook 24:676, 1976.

Sparacino, P: The clinical nurse specialist. Nurs Practice 1:215, 1986.

Sparacino, PA, Cooper, DM, and Minarik, PA: The Clinical Specialists: Implementation and Impact. Appleton & Lange, Stamford, Conn, 1990.

The Specialist Role of the ICN. Nursing Times 90:63, 1994.

Spenceley, SM: The CNS in multidisciplinary pulmonary rehabilitation: A nursing science perspective. Clinical Nurse Specialist 9:192, 1995.

Starr, P: The Social Transformation of American Medicine. Basic Books, New York, 1982, p 155.

Stern, CA: Midwives, male-midwives, and nurse-midwives. Obstet Gynecol 39:308, 1972.

Strunk, BL: The clinical nurse specialists as change agent. Clinical Nurse Specialist 9:128, 1995.

Thatcher, VS: History of Anesthesia with Emphasis on the Nurse Specialist. Lippincott, Philadelphia, 1953, pp 27–28.

Tierney, MJ, Minarik, PA, and Tierney, LM: Ethics in Japanese health care: A perspective for clinical nurse specialists. Clinical Nurse Specialist 8:235, 1994.

Tom, SA: The evolution of nurse-midwifery 1900–1960. J Nurse Midwifery, 27:4, 1982.

Van Blarcom, CC: Midwives in America. Am J Public Health, 4–6:197, 1914.

Webster's New Collegiate Dictionary. G and C Merriam, Springfield, Mass, 1979.

Willeford, MB: The frontier nursing service. Public Health Nurs 25:9, 1933.

Williams, JW: Medical education and the midwife problem in the United States. J Am Med Assoc 58:1, 1912.

CHAPTER 2

Advanced Practice Nursing in the Current Sociopolitical Environment

Advanced Practice Nursing in the Current Sociopolitical Environment

LUCILLE A. JOEL, EdD, RN, FAAN

Lucille Joel, EdD, RN, FAAN, is a professor at Rutgers—The State University of New Jersey, College of Nursing, and director of the Rutgers Teaching Nursing Home Program. Dr. Joel is editor-at-large of the *American Journal of Nursing*. She is past president of the American Nurses' Association and the North American representative to the Board of Directors of the International Council of Nurses, with headquarters in Geneva, Switzerland. Dr. Joel is a certified clinical specialist in psychiatric–mental health nursing and maintains a private practice. She has been involved in the education of advanced practice nurses since 1976.

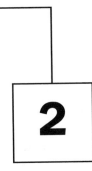

2

CHAPTER OUTLINE

THE AMERICAN PEOPLE AND THEIR HEALTH
Our aging and changing society
Our economic issues and problems
Our ethnic makeup
Our future selves
Our health and lifestyle
THE HEALTH-CARE DELIVERY SYSTEM: ORIGINS OF CHANGE
DOMINANT TRENDS IN AMERICAN HEALTH CARE
THE ADVANCED PRACTICE NURSE AND THE EMERGENT DELIVERY SYSTEM

Advanced practice nursing: Beyond primary care
BARRIERS TO ADVANCED NURSING PRACTICE
Internal disputes
External obstacles
Reimbursement
Prescriptive authority
Professional staff privileges
Assuring competency
Professional liability insurance
SUMMARY
SUGGESTED EXERCISES

CHAPTER OBJECTIVES

After completing this chapter, the reader will be able to:

1. Estimate those qualities of the advanced practice nurse (APN) most valued by the public.
2. Articulate current barriers to advanced practice that may become more formidable obstacles as the health-care delivery system evolves.
3. Formulate a strategy for facilitating the practice of APNs.
4. Critique the sociopolitical tactics used by organized nursing to promote the advanced practice nursing agenda.

What advanced practice nursing is and what it will become are largely dependent on the choices that the American people make about their health care. Ideally, public opinion is a major force in determining governmental policy, and consequently, the form and function of the health-care delivery system. However, with the dramatic shift in public opinion from the urgent call for government-initiated health-care reform in 1993 to the clarion call for balancing the budget through 1997, it is clear that the public vision for its new health-care system remains in a formative stage.

With the election of President Clinton in 1992, dramatic and immediate reforms in the American health-care system were predicated. Commissions were formed, congressional committees were convened, and the electronic and paper media reported constantly on the public's demand for health-care reform. Then ____, the American people handed over control of the Congress to the Republic ____ directly, endorsed that party's "Contract with America." Waste in ____ ned, balancing the budget became a priority, and so- ____ ere scrutinized with an objective (or mean-spirited) eye (depend____ ____litics) toward cost containment. Health care ceased to be a concern, except ____ he extent that public entitlement programs represented a large target for budget cuts.

The sequence of events by which the sociopolitical environment forges public policies is familiar. These policies or their absence will shape the health-care industry, including the role of APNs as participants in the industry. That being the case, we must move cautiously to assure a future for advanced nursing practice. An understanding of the preferences of American consumers, their attitudes toward health services, and an appreciation of the economic and political forces that continue to influence the form and function of our emerging health-care delivery system can enable the nursing profession to decide how and if it fits into the emerging delivery system. The focus of this chapter is advanced practice, but the implications go well beyond this one segment of nursing.

The American People and Their Health

A health-care system is the product of political, sociological, economic, cultural, and demographic trends of the time. Change in every aspect of our lives is the norm, but never has change been as quick and penetrating as in recent years. Given this reality, it is amazing that the health-care industry has not undergone an even more radical transformation. It is impossible to identify all of the factors that have conspired to maintain the status quo and equally challenging to define all of the reasons for those that have compelled the recent changes. Political, sociological, and economic perspectives provide the backdrop for this chapter.

Demographics are presented here, albeit briefly, to illustrate current population trends, because any discussion of health-care services must begin with an appreciation of the people they serve.

OUR AGING AND CHANGING SOCIETY

The U.S. population is aging rapidly, with a 40 percent increase in the number of those 84 years of age and older anticipated by the year 2000. Americans have become more urbanized over time, but there is some indication that this trend has slowed. More generous public assistance and agricultural subsidies, the decline of industry and manufacturing, and the negative image of many cities are said to have caused a disenchantment with migration to the cities.[1]

OUR ECONOMIC ISSUES AND PROBLEMS

The deterioration of the family, poverty, and hopelessness continue to be major social problems with implications for health care. As of 1993, 47 percent of households with children had two parents who were employed, but only 26 percent of households with children under 18 included a married couple.[2] The decline in the size of the American household has slowed, as younger members of the baby boom generation start families, and women in their 30s and 40s eagerly plan for parenthood. Half of women with infants hold jobs, highlighting the need for child care arrangements and flexibility in working hours. One in every seven Americans lives below the poverty level, with one in every four children younger than 3 years being poor. One of every two African-American children and two of every five Hispanic children are poor. The fact that those who are already poor, undernourished, undereducated, and underemployed tend to have the most children increases social consequences. Almost 2 million Americans are homeless at any one time, with the fastest growing group being single mothers and children.[3] Where middle class Americans once had a great deal of sympathy for these needy people, sympathy has turned into backlash, with financial pressures, crime, unemployment, and international hostilities all testing their patience.

OUR ETHNIC MAKEUP

The United States is also experiencing a dramatic shift in ethnic and racial diversity. Immigration is at an all time high, rivaling the numbers of people who entered this country around the turn of the century. One notable difference is that, unlike the great European migrations of earlier times, the new immigrants are primarily of Hispanic and Asian origins (Table 2–1). The Asian population grew by 70 percent in the 1980s, and the Hispanic population is increasing five times

TABLE 2–1
Highest Ranking Countries of Birth of
U.S. Foreign-Born Population, 1994

Country	Number (in thousands)
Mexico	6264
Philippines	4003
Cuba	805
El Salvador	718
Canada	679
Germany	625
China	565
Dominican Republic	556
Korea	533
Vietnam	496
India	494

Source: The World Almanac and Book of Facts 1996. Funk & Wagnalls, Mahwah, NJ, 1995, p 393.

as fast as the general population. Hispanic-Americans tend to be relatively young, with one-third being younger than 18 years and one-half being younger than 26 years. For the first time in history, most immigrants speak one language—Spanish.[4] Many of the newest immigrant groups tend to live in ethnic enclaves or neighborhoods, where they sometimes are immune to assimilation. These observations provide insights essential for the design and location of health-care systems and for the education of providers.

OUR FUTURE SELVES

To anticipate the future of our health-care delivery system from socioeconomic and sociopolitical perspectives, it is important to remember that each generation is a product of its times. Today's "twenty-something" adults are the subject of much commentary. Many were raised by surrogates while their baby boomer parents were caught up in the perceived need for dual incomes and the all-too-common eventuality of divorce and the "supermom" phenomenon. At least half of these Generation X'ers, so called because they have yet to establish their unique group identity, are college educated and have expressed resentment at having to pay the price for the uncontrolled spending and environmental indiscretions of their parents. Also labeled "13ers" because they are the 13th generation in American history, the group may well suffer a loss in living standard compared with that of their parents, a situation contrary to the American tradition. Most analysts predict that the 13ers will fight to regain what they claim they have lost. They will strengthen the family, look suspiciously on public assistance, support conservative public policy, and favor the needs of the young over the old, who, ironically, will be their boomer parents. They will support volunteerism, long-term commitment as opposed to "adhocracy," and will have a no-nonsense attitude about social welfare programs.[5]

OUR HEALTH AND LIFESTYLE

In the midst of all this turbulence, some things remain constant. Heart disease, cancer, stroke, personal injury, and chronic obstructive pulmonary disease continue to claim the most lives. Minority distinctions in morbidity and mortality continue to be notable in all areas, and become an issue of conscience. The life expectancy for the African-American male population is 67.8 years, in contrast to almost 73 years for the white male population. Similar ethnicity-based differences are evident in maternal-child health statistics, such as the high incidence of low-birth-weight babies and in mortality and morbidity from acquired immuno-deficiency syndrome (AIDS) among nonwhite populations.[1]

Factors contributing most significantly to death and disability in this country are associated with lifestyle: smoking, diet, lack of exercise and activity, substance abuse, stress, firearms, risky sexual behavior, vehicular accidents, and environmental pollution. Appreciating the wisdom of investing in health, in 1991, the U.S. Department of Health and Human Services initiated the Healthy People 2000 project.[6] The aim of the project was to increase the years of health and to decrease the disparities in health among the American people.

The Healthy People 2000 project involves periodic monitoring of quality-of-life indicators. By the middle of the decade, decreases were noted in cigarette smoking and alcohol-related vehicular accidents and deaths. Americans were noted to be consuming less fat and salt and were using more supplementary vitamins and minerals. At the same time, industrial accidents, homicides, and teenage pregnancies had increased, and Americans were more overweight than ever before. Deaths were slightly down from heart disease, cancer, and stroke, but deaths from chronic obstructive pulmonary disease and AIDS, which had become the leading cause of death for women between ages 25 and 45 years had increased.[1] By 1993, almost 11 percent of the population was disabled by chronic disease,[7] a direct result of the sophisticated medicine we practice and the lives we lead.

Our unique American health-care system, with its blend of private- and public-sector resources, its taste for specialization, and its state-of-the-art technology, is envied both here and abroad. At the same time, consumers' expectations of freedom of choice in health care and our allegiance to states' rights have created serious problems with regard to access, cost, and quality. Approximately 40 million residents of this country have no guarantee of health care, and an equal number have inadequate assurances of such care. These observations have not escaped the notice of the public. Americans are highly critical of this country's health-care system, and that criticism is creating an awakening of conscience.

The American public's attitude about health care and the health-care industry is well documented. There is agreement that the health-care system is flawed and needs to be fixed. Many consumers believe that the major problems are greed and waste. There is general suspicion about all of our traditional leaders, including doctors, lawyers, clergy, and politicians. More Americans feel powerless once they enter the health-care delivery system. Because of the prevalence of employer-based health insurance, many Americans feel trapped in their jobs, often afraid to seek more challenging and satisfying work because of preexisting conditions that jeopardize insurance coverage and because of fear that an illness will threaten their financial security. The Medicare "final directives" requirement and the Congress's request that the Agency for Health Care Policy and Research develop clinical guidelines are no coincidence. The result of both is pressure on the federal government to return to consumers some control over decisions influencing life and death in the health-care delivery system.

Despite apparent discontent with the system, most Americans seem to prefer inaction. For the most part, the voting public has access to health care, even if it is limited and of questionable value. President Clinton's Health Security Act of 1993 provided the vehicle for broad, sweeping change. After much debate, this legislation failed in September of 1994. There are lessons to be learned from the experience. To begin, Americans are not willing to jeopardize one-sixth of the domestic economy. According to Joel[8]:

> Incremental reform—proceeding with caution, building on successes, allowing one change to be assimilated before requiring that another be accommodated—may be the only option, however distasteful to some. (p. 7)

Furthermore, Americans also tend to guard tenaciously their freedom of choice in health care, even though most do not realize that their health-care choices have already been limited. States Joel[8]:

> They want options, but they also want the safe haven associated with relinquishing some of those options. (p. 7)

Managed care plans have responded to this sensibility by offering the opportunity to "buy out at the point of service"—the assured access to health-care services with the right to choose providers outside the plan's network for an additional out-of-pocket cost. The American passion for freedom of choice in health care is closely associated with a distaste for the heavy hand of government. The Clinton plan seemed to guarantee a bloated bureaucracy and federal mandates that would have preempted states' rights. The plan seemed to call for a mushrooming social-welfare state, funded by heavier taxation on the middle-class majority. The government's response was to propose reduced funding for entitlement programs, notably Medicare and Medicaid. An intuitive public recognized that the private sector would ultimately be required to subsidize the funding deficit created in these programs.

The 105th Congress, though responding to public sentiment, gives cause for concern. Deep financial cuts into both Medicare and Medicaid have been urged by both Democrats and Republicans. Cost containment will most likely be accomplished through increased copayments and deductibles for the aged, limitations on routine increases in funding linked to the cost-of-living index, and fewer matching dollars to states to subsidize the poor. Administration of the Medicaid program could be decentralized totally by awarding block grants to the states with few, if any, federal pass-through requirements. The result could be a license to institute significant inequities on a state-by-state basis, while the federal government takes credit for reducing bureaucracy.

The Health-Care Delivery System: Origins of Change

Enactment of Titles 18 and 19 of the Social Security Act created Medicare and Medicaid more than 25 years ago. After a very few years of experience operating the programs, the federal government began to anticipate a serious financial crisis. Hoping to find some solution that would contain the rapidly accelerating cost of health care, the government supported a variety of demonstration projects. By 1982, this period of experimentation had produced the Medicare prospective payment system incorporating diagnoses-related groups (DRGs) as the "case-mix" model for payment to hospitals. Targeted at hospitals, the most costly offenders in the system, this model's use began an era of technical gameplaying to reduce cost, while the issue of quality care became secondary.

Although the financial pressure on hospitals was first applied by Medicare, other public and private sector insurers quickly adopted the same or similar reimbursement strategies. The health-care industry responded with a rapid migration to community-based services. The variety of clinical situations managed in physicians' offices and the supportive technology in those settings grew rapidly and probably was the first stage in restructuring. Many office-based practices began to resemble mini-hospitals, although largely unregulated. Concentrating their practices in these settings allowed physicians to circumvent the utilization constraints and oversight of hospitals.

The all-inclusive DRG rate for one hospitalization made internal monitoring of the prescriptive practices of physicians a necessity. Physicians who remained insensitive to the length-of-stay limitations and who ordered expensive diagnostic tests and therapeutic regimens, when less expensive options were available and appropriate, were considered a liability and pressured to rethink their practice patterns. Yet physicians continued to be essential to hospital survival, given their virtually exclusive ability to admit patients.

Observing the escalating cost of Part B of Medicare, the Health Care Financing Administration began the search for algorithms (similar to DRGs) that would place reimbursement limits on the out-of-hospital activities of providers. Common procedural technology codes and the resource-based relative value scale were developed for this purpose. So far, these algorithms have been unsuccessful; they do not appear to control volume but only seem to fuel discontent in the medical community.

Still lagging in its ability to control cost, government looked to private-sector models, notably managed care. While fee-for-service (payment for each activity or service) and episode-of-illness (DRG) models continued, further economies were deemed unachievable. The longstanding success of managed care in the private sector piqued the interest of government and politicians. Although managed care comes in many structural forms and financial arrangements, the goal is to encourage (more often require) the least costly (and sometimes the least aggressive) diagnostic and treatment approaches. A transition to managed care was a major ingredient in President Clinton's Health Security Act.

Dominant Trends in American Health Care

The nature of health-care delivery continues to change in response to both economic and social forces at work in the community. The prescriptive practices of providers are being reshaped to ration limited resources. This comes as a harsh blow to an American public that reveres specialization and technology and that has come to expect aggressive clinical management. Attempts to introduce reason into clinical decision making have been branded as rationing. Unwilling to accept any scrutiny of their practice, many physicians with a robust following, in turn, have rejected managed care arrangements. In contrast, physicians with fewer patients often see managed care as an opportunity, resulting in a stereotype of managed care as a second-class option.

Ignoring an initial (and often persistent) negativism, managed care plans continue to flourish as the only option that promises a more cost-efficient future. Medicare and Medicaid have contributed to a growing managed care market by offering incentives to relinquish most of traditional fee-for-service insurance in favor of managed care. Although not all managed care plans are capitated, this form appears to promise the best value. Whether quality will be sacrificed remains an unanswered question. By the end of 1995, 49 percent of Americans with private-sector health plans were using managed care.[9]

Primary care is the backbone of most managed care programs regardless of their form. The literature contrasts older models of primary care with a hybrid that incorporates a broader view of health, patient, and community. Contemporary practice will include the intense use of information systems, active patient participation, appreciation of limited resources vis-à-vis the concept of value (the relationship of quality to cost), and an interdependence among a variety of providers. Providers will be as concerned with populations as with individuals, promising a renewed commitment to public health.[10]

The primary care provider (PCP) is the linchpin in the system, filling the subroles of direct care provider, first contact at point of entry into the system, and coordinator of continuing care. Referral to a specialist is the exception rather than the rule. The PCP is expected to shape the health behavior of patients. Often gaining access to patients through the management of minor acute illness and chronic conditions, the PCP seizes the opportunity to prevent disease and develops consumers' attitudes and skills for healthy living. Although this philosophy may be inconsistent with the medical model, it is totally consistent with the orientation of nursing.

In the managed care environment, multiple levels of care come together in a vertically integrated system. Primary and specialty, acute, subacute, long-term, ambulatory, and home care, and rehabilitation services are combined into a seamless continuum of services. Patients may enter at any point and move with fluidity in and out of any component in the system. This essential characteristic creates the need for alliances and has prompted an industry merger-and-acquisition frenzy to build a full range of services.

The Advanced Practice Nurse and the Emergent Delivery System

The form of tomorrow's health-care system is certain, but not firmly set. All the actors have not yet been cast, and statements of philosophy and beliefs are often contradictory. The system is still maturing, and part of that process requires public education about, and socialization into, managed care. The value of health promotion, disease prevention, and self-sufficiency is gaining momentum. Consumers are demanding more control over their health-care decisions, even if the freedom of choice in providers is limited to those with the financial ability to seek and purchase care outside of a provider's plan.

Routinely, each person's access to the system will be through the PCP, who will continue to coordinate services and manage those problems that can be resolved at the PCP's level of competence. In the ideal situation, the PCP is not only a skilled clinical generalist but also a developer of people. Counseling and teaching must be the forte, and consumer satisfaction is a requisite outcome. Managed care plans strive to guarantee the consumer a sound relationship with a PCP, but these relationships can often be strained by the emphasis on appropriate, but not unlimited, care. Adequate enrollment in the plan is always a concern: A testy encounter with a PCP could result in the loss of a plan subscriber. The inability to retain subscribers and develop self-reliance ultimately increases costs. APNs are well suited to the PCP role given their clinical competence, their philosophy of health promotion, and their comittment to the goal of increasing the independence of their clients.

Although a window of opportunity still exists for APNs in managed care arrangements, it may soon close. Physicians historically have been more interested in specialization and subspecialization than in generalist practice and health. This is not a criticism, but a simple observation based on the past. APNs, more specifically nurse practitioners (NPs), clinical nurse specialists (CNSs), and certified nurse midwives (CNMs), are the natural competitors with physicians for the PCP role. While only a handful of physicians select primary-care practice, the government has been offering incentives for them to select this option. These incentives and the current physician surplus must be considered in any strategy to increase the presence and prominence of APNs in managed care. The policies of these plans should also be carefully monitored. For example it is becoming common to allow female subscribers to have a relationship with two PCPs, one for women's health and a second for general health concerns. This trend has strategic implications and should cause the APN to reflect on the CNM role and the nature of our specialty preparations. Women's health becomes an attractive clinical choice and CNMs are logical as PCPs.

The future of APNs is closely associated with the concept of value: the value of caring in its own right, the economic value of APNs as physician substitutes, and the inherent value of primary care and APNs' exceptional suitability for the PCP role. Given the urgency implicit in today's health-care debate, APNs must be open to a broad range of interpretations of value. The efficacy of nurses in advanced practice has been proved many times over. APNs are safe and therapeutically effective.[11] Although nursing should continue to support research that verifies APNs' credibility and value, efforts should not end there. The research focus should shift to the value of caring in its own right and, more specifically, the value of nursing's performance in the PCP role.

ADVANCED PRACTICE NURSING: BEYOND PRIMARY CARE

The acceptance of primary care as a valued component of an evolving health-care system is significant but should not cause nursing to ignore traditional markets for nursing services. The increased complexity of patients at every level of care creates the need for APNs in a variety of direct care roles, including case management, patient advocacy, triage, and development of the practice of staff nurses. Satisfaction and success in these roles require certain requisite skills. A "mental set" that integrates clinical and financial information is necessary. Information systems that justify the APN's salary must be established. If patient outcomes cannot be attributed directly to APNs, they must become a master of inference. Much of the frustration facing those who practice in the CNS role derives from the fact that it is a highly mediated role. Positive patient outcomes are frequently accomplished by other nurses but only because the CNS has developed the nurses' capacity for more sophisticated practice.

The advanced practice role often removes the "critical-mass" advantage that staff nurses have found so useful in their campaign for a higher quality workplace. The educational and experiential background of the APN should result in peer status in a multidisciplinary environment. This background also assumes that the practitioner is above parochialism and ready to join in interdisciplinary practice. Seeing some role activities as equally fit for a number of providers is a relatively novel attitude for many nurses. Case management is a good example of a situation in which the physician, nurse, or social worker (among others) may be equally suited to the role.

Barriers to Advanced Nursing Practice

INTERNAL DISPUTES

Advanced practice nurses include the CRNA, CNM, CNS, and NP. Today's APN requires the knowledge, skills, and supervised practice that comes only through graduate study in nursing (the master's or doctorate). In the past, these educational requirements were often satisfied through certificate programs with no specific entry requirements other than licensure. Nurses from these certificate programs continue to practice today and should be commended for their leadership contributions to the advanced practice movement. All CNS and most NP educational programs award the master's degree. For the NP, preferential federal funding and certification requirements have hastened the movement toward graduate education. Although the trend is toward the master's degree, postlicensure programs that do not require a baccalaureate degree still exist for the study of nurse midwifery. Of the 94 accredited nurse anesthesia programs in the United States, 85 percent offer the master's degree, and all are required to do so by 1998.

The CNS and NP roles are in a state of transition. These roles evolved almost simultaneously. The CNS established the credibility of clinical-nursing practice at the graduate level, and the NP legitimized the concept of practice autonomy in those border areas of practice shared with medicine.[12] NPs were most commonly found in primary care, and CNSs in secondary and tertiary settings. Over time, these roles have started to overlap in response to consumer need.

An apparent merger of these roles was responsible for the consolidation of the American Nurses' Association's (ANA) Councils of NPs and CNSs into the Council of Nurses in Advanced Practice. This merger was significantly influenced by a 1990 curriculum study that found the education for these roles to be more alike than different.[13] Many APNs also saw the roles as interchangeable and claimed that maintaining the distinction was an impediment to career mobility. Whether those who clamored for change were a representative sample of APNs is subject to challenge. Further, the rigor with which the survey's validity and conclusions were scrutinized is subject to debate. I am not implying that nursing has taken the wrong route, but I merely am suggesting that milestone events often go unrecognized.

The merger of the CNS and NP roles originated with the legislative and regulatory strategy of the ANA. In the 1980s, the ANA began to link the NP and CNS in public policy language. Legislators already understood the NP role and its benefit to the public. This appreciation was based largely on the NP's ability to substitute for the physician, offering the same services at a lower cost. Linking the less commonly understood CNS with the NP in public policy hastened progress toward recognition of both groups. In the early 1990s, the term *advanced practice nurse* was chosen to additionally include the CRNA and CNM. The purpose of this language was political and directed largely toward the reimbursement agenda.

While there is agreement that both the CNS and NP are advanced practitioners, there is less support for the use of the single title of APN. Debate continues over the body of knowledge and skills common to both. Many of the most prestigious university schools of nursing have ignored these internal debates and have begun to blur the distinctions between these two roles. Meanwhile, APNs in one category or another continue to question whether role crossover is possible without additional education. The disparity in the views of educators and practicing APNs surfaces, one basing action on logic (as they see it) and the other on experience (as they live it). Meanwhile, the good job market for NPs has created a demand for post-master's and second master's degree programs for the CNS preparing for NP practice. Some of these changes can be traced to state laws that require graduate education to specify NP preparation. In this case, role crossover is no longer left to the discretion of the profession or the professional.

These observations tend to highlight the critical need for advisory relationships between education and practice, and a combined effort to control the sometimes illogical behavior of government agencies.

Such internal disputes are a part of the politics of nursing. NPs question the ability of CNSs to diagnose and treat the common illnesses that are a major part of generalist practice. CNSs suspect that NPs are socialized into the medical model and therefore are less able to negotiate and manipulate systems of care on behalf of their patients or to develop the clinical sophistication of the nursing staff. No such disputes have arisen around CRNA or CNM practice; each of these groups seems to be in control of its clinical area.

Such differences of opinion have seriously hampered the ability of APNs to move into the vanguard of health care. Foresight is often rare. While nursing debates the details, it ignores the fact that the merger of NP and CNS roles is becoming more useful as society is confronting growing numbers of the chronically ill who need primary care. The best PCP for these situations may be the CNS because the patient also needs the sophistication of a specialist. NPs are valuable in acute, critical, long-term, ambulatory, and home care for their abilities in health assessment and clinical management. The market for NPs in acute care will increase as graduate medical-education funding decreases or disappears. Rather than responding with arrogance or infighting regarding the assumption of some medical responsibilities, nursing should seize the opportunity to bring advanced practice nursing to new populations and to further establish autonomy in border areas of practice.

EXTERNAL OBSTACLES

Most external obstacles to advanced practice have, in one way or another, been associated with public policy. Although doors open slowly, nurses have made good legislative and regulatory progress. The goal has been for the APN to secure direct access to the public. In our fragmented, litigious, and medicalized system, this requires direct reimbursement, prescriptive authority, clinical privileges, adequate professional liability insurance, and nursing practice acts and credentialing systems that attest to our competency. Anticipating the future, providers who bring these indicators of autonomy with them will assume roles of clinical prominence in managed care.

REIMBURSEMENT

Achieving reimbursement for advanced practice nursing services has been a tortuous and costly agenda. Progress has been slow but steady. By the early 1990s, some categories of advanced practice nursing services were reimbursable in every federal entitlement program. Medicaid includes mandatory reimbursement of family and pediatric NPs and CNMs but defers to state discretion for CRNAs and CNSs. Medicare has been the most resistant. CRNA and CNM medical reimbursement has been recognized, but NP and CNS reimbursement has been limited to rural and medically underserved areas and to nursing homes for certain services provided by gerontological nurse practitioners. Extensive reimbursement privileges are allowed in the Federal Employees' Health Benefits Program and the Civilian Health and Medical Program for the Uniformed Services (CHAMPUS), which is the health program for nonuniformed employees, dependents, and retirees of the military. However, CHAMPUS restricts CNS reimbursement to the psychiatric-mental health CNS.

A noteworthy gain has been the federal Department of Transportation's recognition that NPs and CNSs may perform and be reimbursed for the physical examination needed to qualify for a commercial driver's license. The latest incident with federal reimbursement occurred in 1996, as legislation for broad advanced practice reimbursement under Medicare was released from committee. The victory was bittersweet, however: The categorical designation of APN had been dropped, with only the recognition of NPs being retained (CRNAs and CNMS were included previously). Of course, this incident should not be treated lightly, but it can be best understood if analyzed in its sociopolitical context. Primary care is assured prominence in the emergent delivery system, and NPs have established themselves in that area. CNSs have had less visibility and are seen by many as an add-on cost as opposed to a more cost-efficient option. The laws or statutes of 40 states currently include CNSs within the APN category, but seven of those only recognize the CNS in psychiatric-mental health nursing.[14]

Indemnity and commercial insurance is governed by state laws, and these laws recognize advanced practice nursing to varying degrees. The picture is confusing, however, and changes from day to day. APNs report reimbursement in 34 states,[15] and many APNs report reimbursement "incident to" the practice of a physician by both federal and state programs, as well as private-sector plans. In this situation, the nurse is paid a fee equal to what a physician would have received for the same services. If the APN bills independently, the fee is anywhere from 65 to 85 percent of the physician's reimbursement amount.

Reimbursement is honeycombed with social bias and self-serving behavior. A particularly blatant example can be seen in the work of the Physician's Payment Review Commission (PPRC). Charged with proposing a rate structure for Part B of Medicare, the PPRC based its fee-setting techniques on the service to the patient, as opposed to the identity of the provider. The commission justified this move by alleging the need to increase the attractiveness of primary care for physicians by reducing the financial differential between generalists and specialists. However, when it came time to apply the same standard to nonphysician providers, the PPRC recanted and proposed that the extent of the provider's education should be built into the reimbursement formula for this group.[4]

There has been a recent surge in the NP job market associated with growth in community-based services and primary care. The fact that NPs are very comfortable in the employee role and excel in their ability to work within systems has not been lost on employers. Furthermore, NPs are seen as lower-cost physician substitutes. In contrast, the CNS is often undervalued, even by nurses themselves, and considered expendable when money gets tight in health-care institutions. The fact that CNSs are not a luxury but a necessity is theirs to prove. It is painful, but true, that the activities sanctioned by nursing licenses traditionally have not been reimbursable, but priorities are changing as the medical model becomes less dominant. Managed care could be the catalyst for this metamorphosis. Disease prevention, health promotion, and self-care promise more value than earlier paradigms. Reimbursement may soon become a nonissue with the rapid domination by managed care. APNs must be included within managed care networks and as members of approved provider panels. State prohibitions that limit the ownership of medical offices to physicians and other select providers must be challenged.

PRESCRIPTIVE AUTHORITY

Almost every American entering the health-care system receives a prescription for drug therapy. Historically, the right to prescribe medications has been the exclusive domain of the physician. Even as NPs become more established, many continue to manage illness, including the prescription of medication, in a joint practice or a collaborative relationship (a euphemism for supervision) with a physician. The reasoning is warped. NPs are proposed as a physician substitute because they represent a better value at lower cost, but with equal or better outcomes. This rationale loses its credibility when medical management cannot proceed without physicians' approval. Physicians who accept the responsibility for an APN's practice are confronted with an increase in their liability-insurance premiums. Naturally, the cost is passed on to the consumer. If APNs are to be PCPs, they must have full prescriptive authority and the right to prescribe medications (including controlled substances) on their own signature.

The authority to prescribe independent of any physician involvement exists for one or more categories of APNs in 14 states; 37 others (the District of Columbia is treated as a state for this analysis) maintain the caveat of physician oversight of some type. Only one state, Illinois, totally rejects prescriptive authority.[14] Prescriptive authority for nurses may be controlled in a variety of ways. The range of drugs permitted to be prescribed by nurses is sometimes limited to a formulary developed jointly by state boards of nursing, medicine, and/or pharmacy. Prescriptive authority may be limited to drugs common to a specialty area. The variety of constraints is creative and often obviously self-serving. It appears that the medical community is bound and determined to maintain its control over access to drug therapy for nurses.

The ANA documents 300,000 nurses who are likely candidates to move into the PCP role and, consequently, pursue prescriptive authority. While physicians direct their energy and money toward foiling the attempts of APNs to expand their practice into the once exclusive domain of medicine, other nonnursing professional groups are making inroads, which could ultimately establish precedent. Psychologists and pharmacists argue that they are qualified to prescribe. Eleven states now allow pharmacists to initiate or modify drug therapy.[16] Physicians' assistants have the authority to write prescriptions without a cosignature in approximately 40 states.[4] As each occupational group evolves, it will expand its scope of practice and seek more rights and responsibilities.

With characteristic patience and tenacity, nursing has made progress related to prescriptive authority by accepting physician oversight. Strategically this can be a first step toward autonomy. In 1990, New Hampshire nurses were successful in "carving out" the requirement for physician supervision from their prescriptive authority statute. This scenario, which could be repeated often in the future, is contingent on electing legislative representatives sympathetic to nursing, thus creating a public demand for nurses to offer these services. The best source of detail on state-to-state variations in prescriptive authority can be found each year in the January issue of *Nurse Practitioner*.

In the interim, prescriptive authority contingent on oversight can be workable. Joint practice arrangements between nurses and physicians could be the expected norm in primary care centers. The inherent value of this arrangement may be appealing particularly where these centers are owned, operated by, or contracted with managed care plans. Community nursing centers usually employ a medical director who could be relied on to fill the oversight requirement until the time when such oversight is unnecessary.

PROFESSIONAL STAFF PRIVILEGES

Criteria for the approval and accreditation of health-care programs and facilities have been fairly consistent in adopting an expanded definition of the term *professional staff*. This expanded definition awards professional staff privileges to a variety of providers. However, health-care systems often impose more specific restrictions for the expressed purpose of denying privileges to emerging or non-traditional providers, such as APNs, podiatrists, chiropractors, and dentists. According to Kelly and Joel[4]:

> It remains to be tested whether the withholding of privileges is an act of discrimination or restraint of trade. (p. 326)

Because the survival of any health-care organization will depend on its ability to negotiate managed care contracts, nursing must now be willing and able to educate managed care plan administrators to the value of APNs as full-fledged professionals.

Professional staff privileges often recognize the right to admit, treat, or consult on the clinical management of patients. In effect, withholding privileges denies patient access to excluded providers once they are admitted to a particular system. The nursing staff organization has been proposed by some as the counterpart of the medical staff organization (more currently renamed the professional staff organization). However, such arrangements could be confused with the organized nursing staff who come together for purposes of negotiating conditions of employment (with or without a formal collective bargaining agreement). This is an unacceptable solution for many reasons. One reason is parity and a need for appropriate recognition within a multidisciplinary environment. A second concerns a technicality of labor law. An organized effort such as this could be misconstrued and later create a challenge to the right of nurses to choose a collective bargaining agent and/or unionize.

Several beginning prototypes can provide the APN some guidance. Currently 19 states report nurses with hospital privileges of some variety.[14]Access to these privileges does not include all APNs, but usually is limited to a specific category (NP, CNS, CRNA, or CNM). Eleven percent of NPs and CNSs report having privileges of some variety.[18] In some situations, privileges are associated with joint or collaborative practice with a physician. Specialty-dependent limitations remain (e.g., psychiatric-mental health CNS, gerontological nurse practitioner, and so forth). Other dynamics and dilemmas will be contingent on whether the APN with privileges is an employee or an independent contractor. Physicians are empowered by their ability to admit patients to a system, thereby contributing to its financial stability. To the extent that an APN is viewed by an institution as a "mere employee," the power of the admitting privileges could be minimized. This issue is more important as APNs become prominent in rural and medically underserved areas.

CMNs are a contrasting story of success. Just 20 years ago, few states permitted nurse midwives to practice.[4] Between 1975 and 1991, the number of hospital births attended by CNMs increased by sevenfold. CNMs' mandatory access to Medicaid recipients ensures practice viability in every state and territory. The preferred practice setting for CNMs has become the hospital, perhaps due to the legal requirement to maintain a collaborative arrangement with an obstetrician.

CRNAs have the legal authority to practice anesthesia in all 50 states without anesthesiologist supervision. Although there is a growing market for anesthesia in ambulatory practice, the hospital remains a major practice site for CRNAs. These observations seem to support the prevalence of practice privileges among these groups.

ASSURING COMPETENCY

The issue of assuring competency has surfaced with a vengeance as APNs and, more specifically, NPs and CNSs have become more aggressive in the pursuit of reimbursement and prescriptive authority. Leaders in both medicine and nursing caution that specialty practice should be regulated internally by the profession as opposed to externally by the government. This opinion is based on the clinical complexity of specialization and the fact that the science advances through research conducted in specialty areas. For the discipline to advance, the specialty edge must remain unencumbered by public policy and the inevitable bureaucracy that it attracts.

For nursing, it is already too late to hold firm to this standard of autonomy for the practice. Forty-nine states currently address advanced practice in public policy. For the most part, state boards of nursing hold the authority and require a nationally recognized certification in the specialty and sometimes additional education in pharmacology where the prescription of medications is a sanctioned activity. By this arrangement, state boards of nursing have deferred to the profession's right to recognize its specialists through certification and to develop and promulgate the standards of practice on which certification is based. This position is being actively questioned. Critics see the standards as vague and call for precise competency statements on which to build certification. At its annual meeting in the summer of 1995, the National Council of State Boards of Nursing (NCSBN), an association of state and territorial boards of nursing, postponed action on a motion to move forward on a certification program for NPs and CNSs under the aegis of the state boards themselves. This remains an ongoing issue.

The regulatory process for CNMs and CRNAs seems to have attracted less scrutiny. This could be in part due to the fact that the CNM is commonly recognized in the law through amendment to the Medical Practice Act, which legally requires CNMs and CRNAs to practice collaboratively with a physician. The CRNA has a long history of credibility but is currently defending against medicine's attempts to require anesthesiologist supervision of their practice. Some attempts at regulatory change have proposed a one-on-one supervisory relationship between the CRNA and the anesthesiologist. Rather than inserting this oversight requirement in the CRNA licensing law, an alternate tactic has been to insert language in the regulations for facility licensing. Obviously, this degree of dependency would make the use of CRNAs inefficient and, at the very least, would result in increased cost to the consumer and, more ominously, loss of anesthesia practice to nurses.

Motivated primarily by a sense of public stewardship and to some degree by the aggressive position of NCSBN, both the American Association of Colleges of Nursing (AACN)[19] and the National Organization of Nurse Practitioner Faculty (NONPF)[20] have developed program standards for NP and advanced nursing practice education that give direction for competency statements (these standards are not relevant to anesthesia practice or nurse midwifery). Although these documents were developed separately, each group proceeded with an awareness of the other's work as seen in the cross-referencing.

The result has been the inference that there is a core curriculum for both graduate study in nursing and advanced practice, with some unique requirements for competency as an NP in primary care settings. This was the first occasion for the AACN to speak on advanced practice education. The NONPF expanded and validated statements first issued in 1990. The next logical step would be for the National League of Nursing (NLN) to incorporate competencies in its accreditation process and/or for the certification boards to design their examinations on these competencies. This is not merely an option, but a necessary step for the profession to maintain any control over advanced practice. Application of the same standard by both the accrediting and the certifying agency would provide the best assurances for the consumer. The fact that these competency statements originated with practitioners would show a united front.

Because the U.S. Department of Education has deferred action on the NLN's petition for continued recognition as nursing's accrediting body, NLN participation would seem difficult at this time. The NLN was only one among many accrediting groups caught in new and more stringent requirements for educational surveillance included in 1992 federal legislation but not strictly enforced until many years later.[21] Given the significant resources required for the NLN to address these governmental standards, competency assurance may be better linked with certification. Although the public good provided through this system of checks and balances is incontestable, the dynamics demonstrate the "tug of war" between professional and public policy.

Medicine has assured the credibility of its specialists (advanced practitioners) by the creation of an oversight board, the American Board of Medical Specialties (ABMS). The ABMS recognizes specialty boards that conform to specific standards defined by their specialties, the process and testing instruments used to assure the competency of their diplomates, and the quality of their residencies among other program aspects. In 1992, nursing established the American Board of Nursing Specialties (ABNS) for the purpose of assuming a similar leadership role in certification. However, the ABNS has not become prominent. Given the threat of increased government oversight, the ABNS could be a vital link between internal and external regulation of the specialties.

PROFESSIONAL LIABILITY INSURANCE

A liability insurance crisis occurred in 1985, when CNMs sustained an increase in their premiums so great that it could not be absorbed by their incomes. CNMs were assumed to represent a liability risk equal to obstetricians, who have the highest claims experience in the medical field. Nurse midwives, with their long-standing mandatory relationship with physicians to assure back up in the event of intrapartum complications, have been tainted by physicians' malpractice experience. The ANA, negotiating on behalf of CNMs, secured temporary and affordable coverage through the ANA carrier until a more permanent solution was possible. That solution was a self-insured arrangement involving the American College of Nurse-Midwives and a consortium of insurance companies. CRNAs, NPs, and CNSs have not had similar experiences. Their claims experience is low and coverage is available at reasonable rates, though higher than the rates for staff nurses.

Many skeptics choose to ignore the safe, effective, and satisfying service provided by APNs. Instead of interpreting their low claims experience as an indication of quality, critics prefer to agree that a litigant will target providers with assets (deep pockets) in hope of greater financial recovery. Regardless of the past, we are entering an era of tort reform in which financial recovery may be based on a new standard. The personal danger that litigation holds for the provider will also be different in a managed care environment where many providers are employees.

Summary

To date, NPs have achieved the greatest autonomy working with underserved populations. CRNAs are the sole anesthesia providers in the majority of rural hospitals but have been less dominant in areas where physicians' presence is high. CNSs are the unsung heroes, best known for their work with the seriously ill. Today, it is the middle-class majority (many, from urban areas, are relatively healthy and financially secure) whose acceptance and demand for APNs could establish their credibility. The difficulty is that these potential clients do not know about APNs and advanced nursing practice. The exception may be the CNM whose popularity has grown with Americans of moderate and substantial means. Because midwifery services are not always reimbursable, those who can pay out of pocket represent the largest share of midwifery clients. In resisting challenges to midwifery practice and the operation of birthing centers, CNMs have succeeded in mobilizing the support of the influential middle and upper classes on their behalf.

Many APNs who wish to serve the middle-class market have joined physicians in their practices as employees. These opportunities are not always readily available and must be initiated and developed. Often, positions appear to be cast in the medical model, and therefore, many APNs may be reluctant to secure them. The decision for the APN remains whether to walk away from a challenge or to work for change from within.

In presenting themselves to the middle class, the clinical competency of APNs must be beyond question. Resentment over the need to be better, brighter, and more giving holds little weight. There is no one so condemning as the advocate for advanced practice nursing who provides APNs with access to patients and then receives reports of inept clinical management. The most painful incidents occur when APNs are displaced in favor of physicians, unfortunately a frequent occurrence with today's physician surplus. APNs often do not document the value they represent, nor do they routinely mobilize patients or the community in communicating their value.

Nurse-managed centers are an ideal setting in which to prove and promote APN excellence. More than 250 primary care nursing centers exist in the United States. These centers are managed and staffed by nurses. Nurse-managed centers may be free-standing, entrepreneurial enterprises or affiliated with a college of nursing or a health-care institution. They are strong candidates for partnerships with managed-care networks. A fuller discussion of nurse-managed centers can be found in *Dimensions of Professional Nursing*.

Educated risk-taking, commitment to excellence, and courage of convictions must become watchwords as APNs shape a future that is good for nursing and good for the American public.

Suggested Exercises

1. Propose a strategic plan to assure the competency of APNs to the public. Include the roles of both the profession and the government.

2. Develop a career plan for an NP intent on the role of a PCP in a geographic area that has never experienced an advanced nursing practice.

3. Identify the reimbursement and prescriptive authority rights of APNs in your state. What should the next stage in policy development be to increase APNs' access to the public?

4. Anticipate the opportunities for advanced practice nursing in the emerging health-care delivery system and the areas of resistance that APNs will encounter.

5. Propose a plan to create an American middle-class following for APNs.

REFERENCES

1. Kelly, LY, and Joel, LA: The Nursing Experience, ed 3. McGraw-Hill, New York, 1996.
2. The World Almanac and Book of Facts 1994. Funk & Wagnalls, Mahwah, NJ, 1993.
3. Foster, C, et al: The Homeless in America. Information Plus, Wylie, Texas, 1993.
4. Kelly, LY, and Joel, LA: Dimensions of Professional Nursing, ed 7. McGraw-Hill, New York, 1995.
5. Quinn, JB: The Luck of the Xers. Newsweek, p. 66, June 1994.
6. Institute of Medicine, National Academy of Science: Healthy People 2000: Citizens Chart the Course. National Academy Press, Washington, DC, 1990.
7. McGinnis, JM, and Lee, PR: Healthy People 2000 at mid-decade. JAMA 273:1123, 1995.
8. Joel, LA: Health care reform: Getting it right this time. Am J Nurs 95:7, 1995.
9. American Hospital Association, Information Services: Personal communication, February, 1996.
10. Geoppinger J: Renaissance of primary care: An opportunity for nursing. In Hickey, JV, et al (eds): Advanced Practice Nursing. Lippincott, Philadelphia, 1996, p 70.
11. Brown, S, and Grimes, D: Meta-Analysis of Process of Care: Clinical Outcomes and Cost-Effectiveness of Nurses in Primary Care Roles: Nurse Practitioners and Nurse Mid-

wives. American Nurses Association, Kansas City, 1992.
12. Stafford, M, and Appleyard, J: Clinical nurse specialists and nurse practitioners. In McCloskey, JC, and Grace, HK (eds): Current Issues in Nursing, ed 4. Mosby, St. Louis, 1994.
13. Forbes, KE, et al: Clinical nurse specialist and nurse practitioner core curricula survey results. Nurse Pract 15:43, 1990.
14. Pearson, LJ: Annual update of how each state stands on legislative issues affecting advanced nursing practice. Nurs Pract 21:11, 1996.
15. Pearson, LJ: Annual update of how each state stands on legislative issues affecting advanced nursing practice. Nurs Pract 20:11, 1995.
16. AACP committee examines state practice acts. The American College of Clinical Pharmacy (ACCP) Report. American College of Clinical Pharmacy, Kansas City, October 1995.
17. American Nurses' Association: States with Some Form of Nurse Privileging. American Nurses' Association, Washington, DC, 1993.
18. Washington Consulting Group: Survey of Certified Nurse Practitioners and Clinical Nurse Specialists: December 1992 Final Report. USPHS, Division of Nursing, Rockville, Md, February 1994.

19. American Association of Colleges of Nursing: The Essentials of Master's Education for Advanced Practice Nursing. American Association of Colleges of Nursing, Washington, DC, October 1995.
20. National Organization of Nurse Practitioner Faculty: Advanced Nursing Practice: Curriculum Guidelines and Program Standards for Nurse Practitioner Education. National Organization of Nurse Practitioner Faculty, Washington, DC, 1995.
21. Brider, P: New accrediting regs pose issues for nursing schools: NLN. Am J Nurs 96:63, 1996.

ANNOTATED BIBLIOGRAPHY

American Nurses' Association: Nursing's Agenda for Health Care Reform. American Nurses' Association, Washington, DC, 1991.
An overview of ANA's public-policy agenda for health-care reform. This agenda is endorsed by over 80 nursing and allied-health associations.

Bullough, B, and Bullough, V: Nursing Issues. Springer, New York, 1994
Strong and creative thinking on a selected group of controversial issues.

Harrington, C, and Estes, CL (eds): Health Policy and Nursing. Jones and Bartlett, Boston, 1994.
Good chapters on finance, the delivery system, outcomes of care, the nurse labor market, and implications for nursing in every issue area.

Howe, N, and Strauss, B: The 13th Generation: Abort, Retry, Ignore, Fail? Vintage Books, New York, 1993.
Presentation of the unique characteristics, history, and predicted future of today's twenty-something young adults.

Kovner, A (ed): Health Care Delivery in the United States, ed 5. Springer, New York, 1995.
An overview of the U.S. delivery system, its providers and settings for care, funding, historical development, and emergent trends.

Lee, P, and Estes, CL (eds): The Nation's Health, ed 4. Jones and Bartlett, Boston, 1994.
Recent statistics and chapters that allow basic understanding of the delivery system and its issues.

Mason, DJ, et al (eds): Policy and Politics for Nurses, ed 2. Saunders, Philadelphia, 1993.
Chapters on policy and politics in a broad range of situations, including the politics of nongovernmental organizations and workplace policies.

McCloskey, JC, and Grace, HK (eds): Current Issues in Nursing, ed 4. Mosby, St Louis, 1994.
A variety of papers on current issues organized in sections that are introduced by a debate relevant to the particular topical area.

Corporate Health and Managed Competition: Implications for Advanced Practice Nursing in the New American Health-Care System

MARIANNE McCARTHY, PhD, RN, CS
JUDITH A. BERMAN, JD, RN

Marianne McCarthy, PhD, RN, CS, is an assistant professor of nursing at Arizona State University. Dr. McCarthy is prepared as both a geriatric nurse practitioner and as a gerontological clinical nurse specialist and has completed a multidisciplinary Geriatric Fellowship Program at the San Francisco Institute of Aging. Dr. McCarthy has practiced extensively in a variety of settings as an advanced practice nurse for almost 20 years. Currently, she is involved in clinical practice in long-term care and coordinates and teaches theory and practicum courses in the Adult Advanced Practice Nursing Program at Arizona State University.

Judith A. Berman, JD, RN, is a 1975 graduate of The Mount Carmel School of Nursing, Columbus, Ohio. After a nursing career in adult oncology and hematology, she obtained her law degree from Ohio State University in 1988. She is associated with the law firm of Doyle, Winthrop, & West, PC, Phoenix, Arizona, and practices in the areas of health-care and professional liability litigation.

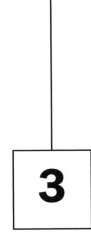

3

CHAPTER OBJECTIVES

After completing this chapter, the reader will be able to:
1. Analyze the influence of economics on the restructuring of the health-care delivery
   system in the United States.
2. Compare and contrast various challenges facing both publicly and privately financed health care.
3. Synthesize information regarding cost-containment efforts as they affect advanced
   practice nursing.
4. Compare and contrast various models proposed for the delivery and financing of
   health care.
5. Debate the advantages and disadvantages of different reimbursement strategies
   as they might apply to the advanced practice nurse (APN) in a managed-care environment.
6. Delineate strategies that can be used by APNs to gain entry into competitively
   managed markets.

n Dr. Pauline Komnenich's ethnographic retrospective of the evolution of advanced practice nursing (see Chapter 1), several themes echo from the past with a message to today's APNs[1]:

- Times of change create opportunities for APNs to define and shape themselves.

- Forces outside the profession of nursing—often economic—have been the stimulus for this development.

- At the same time, the professional establishment—both within nursing and within medicine—have at times erected barriers to independent advanced nursing practice.

A similar time of change exists for APNs in today's "managed-care revolution." To position themselves as leaders in the reform movement, APNs must become sensitive to the various forces that have stimulated the movement toward health-care restructuring. Health-care reform is not only about who is going to pay for coverage—businesses, individuals, and families as taxpayers—but also about who is going to manage the plan—private companies, the government, and/or consumers themselves. To compete, APNs must better understand factors as they relate to payment and reimbursement mechanisms and the aggregate resources necessary for this new order.

This chapter provides a brief history of the evolution of this "time of change" in health-care financing and describes the current state of what has come to be known as "corporate health care." It also sets forth the theoretical basis of "managed competition" so that the reader can appreciate the difference between what has come to be and what could be.

The American Health-Care Revolution

It is likely that the 1990s will be remembered as the decade in which the nation acknowledged, although grudgingly, that the demand for medical services is apparently unlimited—but that the capacity of the society to pay for such services is not.
JOURNAL OF PSYCHOSOCIAL NURSING[2]

The 1990s will also be remembered as the decade during which Americans set out on a path of health-care reform from which there appears to be no return, yet no agreement on exactly what that reform will become. Although Congress failed to adopt President Clinton's proposal for national health-care reform, it served as a catalyst that sparked a revolution within the health-care industry. Publicity surrounding the proposal served to drop the health-care crisis squarely into the laps of the American people by focusing attention on the major culprits of the crisis: greed and waste.

Americans began to realize that our nation was spending more per capita on health care than any other nation in the world.[3] Although health-care costs were soaring, the number of American people without health-care coverage had climbed to an all-time high. Americans were introduced to the notion that they could have universal insurance coverage without incurring added expense. However, to do this, we need to begin to spend money more wisely and efficiently.

Driven by newly heightened public sentiment (even in the absence of national reform), the private and public sectors began to make sweeping changes, altering the ways in which health care is delivered and financed in the United States. These changes are reshaping traditional medical care into what Dr. Lucille Joel describes as something "uniquely American." As we stand on the threshold of the twentieth century, Americans are witnessing a transition from industrial medicine to the emergence of a new system of health care with managed competition and corporate health as its cornerstones.[4] How we got to this point is instructive.

Financing Health Care

The problem of soaring health-care costs is not a new one. From 1970 to 1990, health expenditures in the United States increased at a yearly rate of 12 percent.[5] Americans spent $42 billion on health care in 1965, representing 6 percent of the gross national product (GNP) for that year. In 1981, that figure rose to $287 billion, or 9.8 percent of the GNP. During that time, local, state, and federal government expenditures were responsible for an increased share of total health-care financing—from 26 percent in 1965 to almost 43 percent ($123 billion) in 1981. In 1991, $753 billion, or just more than 13 percent of the GNP, was spent for health-care purposes. The Commerce Department estimated that health-care spending totaled $838.5 billion for 1992, or more than 14 percent of the GNP for that year.[6]

These expenditures, representing over $2868 per year per person, far exceeded the overall inflation rates prevalent in the American economy at the time. According to current projections, annual national health expenditures may reach almost $1.7 trillion by the year 2000.[7]

The system for financing health-care services is a key factor that has shaped the delivery of health care in the United States. Unlike many European systems, which are largely publicly financed, the American system, as it has evolved during the past 30 years, involves a complex blend of private and public responsibilities.

WHAT THE HEALTH-CARE DOLLAR BUYS

To better understand health-care financing, one first must appreciate what is being achieved by the ever-increasing health-care expenditure levels. As measured by the federal Health Care Financing Administration (HCFA), national health expenditures are grouped into two categories[8]:

1. Research and medical facilities construction
2. Payments for health services and supplies

Five types of personal expenditures accounted for more than 75 percent of the 1991 total health-care spending[9] (Fig. 3–1).

Not included in the HCFA figures were medical-education costs, except insofar as they are inseparable from hospital expenditures, and biomedical research. These personal health-care expenditures (PHCEs) constituted the bulk of the national health care "bill"—more than $900 billion in 1993.[10] According to the

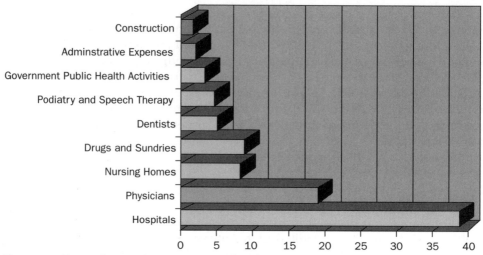

Figure 3–1   Types of personal expenditures for health care.

Department of Commerce, the figure for PHCEs is expected to grow by 12 to 15 percent annually during the next 5 years unless significant changes occur in the health-care delivery system.[11]

WHERE THE HEALTH-CARE DOLLAR COMES FROM

In the early part of this century, people paid for medical care "out of their own pockets," much like they would purchase any other service. Costs and utilization were kept at a minimum because, frankly, there was little in the way of medical care that physicians could offer and that money could buy. In the 1930s, with the introduction of ether as an anesthetic, and with the advent of other advances in surgical technology, physicians finally had more to sell. Consequently, resource utilization increased and the price of medical care climbed. In response to this increased demand and escalated cost for medical services, the first health insurance plan, Blue Cross, was jointly developed and offered by a group of hospitals and surgeons. Although the plan limited coverage to inpatient care, with physician services and medications remaining available only to those who could afford to pay for them, the third-party reimbursement system, with its attendant insensitivity to economics, was established.[12]

Although it is said that health-care monies come from different sources, what is really meant is that dollars take different routes on their way from consumers to providers. Ultimately, the American people pay all health-care costs, regardless of whether payment occurs via government, private insurance companies, or independent plans.

Moreover, these third-party costs are paid in addition to the out-of-pocket payments. For example,[13] in 1991, out-of-pocket costs represented nearly 22 percent of the PHCEs ($144.3 billion). At the same time, the government's share of personal health-care expenses was nearly 43 percent (about $283.3 billion), with federal government spending representing nearly three-fourths of that amount. Finally, almost 32 percent of such costs were paid by and through private insurance companies ($209.3 billion).[14]

Public Outlays

As suggested by the these figures, the increase in PHCEs, especially since 1965, is largely a result of greater federal expenditures. Proportionately, state and local government outlays have remained fairly constant over time. The significant rise in federal spending is accounted for by the Medicare and Medicaid programs, Titles XVIII and XIX, respectively, of the Social Security Act.[10]

MEDICARE The Medicare program, which provides a basic package of health insurance for most Americans aged 65 years and older, accounts for 45 percent of the national health-care outlay, making it the largest single source of payment for health care in the United States.[15] It is a federally funded health-insurance program created by Title XVIII of the Social Security Act of 1965 and originally was designed to protect people 65 years of age and older from the high cost of health care. The program was expanded in 1972 and again in 1973 to include permanently disabled workers eligible for old-age-, survivors-, and disability-insurance benefits and their dependents, as well as people with end-stage renal disease. A more recent attempt to expand the scope of Medicare was contained in the Medicare Catastrophic Insurance Act of 1988. In that legislation, Congress attempted to "improve" coverage by setting limits on the maximum out-of-pocket costs for which beneficiaries were responsible in the case of hospital care, physicians' services, and pharmaceuticals. The act was greeted unenthusiastically by many elderly who, under the terms of the bill, were to assume the costs of the program in the form of higher premiums and income-related surcharges on their federal income tax. The act was repealed in the fall of 1989,[16] but its effects, though diminishing, still linger.

As currently structured, Medicare comprises two programs, each of which has its own trust fund[17]:

1. Part A, the hospital insurance program, is financed by payroll taxes collected under the social security system. It provides coverage for inpatient hospital services, posthospitalization skilled nursing services, home health-care services, and hospice care.

2. Part B, a voluntary supplemental medical-insurance (SMI) program, pays certain costs for physicians' services, outpatient hospital services and therapy, and other health expenses. The SMI program is financed by monthly premiums collected from elderly enrollees and by general tax revenues. The general revenue share of SMI grew from about 50 percent in the early 1970s to approximately 70 percent in the 1980s. By 1990, the general revenue share accounted for 72 percent of the SMI program income.

MEDICAID Medicaid was established by the federal government in 1965 to provide health care to the poor.[18] Unlike Medicare, which is solely a federal program, the Medicaid program is jointly funded and administered by federal and state governments. The name "Medicaid" is more or less a blanket label for 50 different state programs designed specifically to serve welfare recipients. Different states give their individual Medicaid programs different names. For example, in California, Medicaid is known as MediCal, whereas in Arizona, the program is called Access.

Begun in January 1967, Medicaid provided federal funds to states on a cost-sharing basis according to each state's per capita income. This program was designed to ensure that health-care services would be fully afforded to the aged poor, the blind, the disabled, and families with dependent children if one parent was absent, unemployed, or unable to work.

The Medicaid program represents a high degree of decentralization in that the federal government requirements are only minimally restrictive. States exercise significant control over Medicaid eligibility and benefit packages within federal guidelines. For the most part, Medicaid is available only to very-low-income persons. Given that fact, Medicaid covers only 40 percent of the poor.[19] The program also has categorical restrictions; that is, only families with children, pregnant women, and those who are aged, blind, or disabled can qualify.

The basic set of services mandated by the federal government for Medicaid programs includes[20]:

- Inpatient and outpatient hospital care
- Other laboratory and x-ray services
- Physicians' services
- Nursing-facility care for persons older than 21 years
- Home health for those entitled to nursing-facility services
- Screening, diagnostic, and treatment services for persons younger than 21 years
- Family planning

Although states must provide the basic set of services, they can set their own rates based on how much they are willing to spend on their percentage of the cost. Generally, the federal government will reimburse states between 50 and 83 percent of what they spend. Because each state can determine how much it will pay for services under the Medicaid program, much variability exists. For instance, in Massachusetts, a physician might be reimbursed about $1500 for delivering a baby, while in New Mexico, a physicians might only receive about $900 for the identical service.

OTHER PUBLIC EXPENDITURES Medicare and Medicaid account for more than 76 percent of public outlays for personal health-care services. State and local government outlays represent the next largest expenditure category, but only account for about 10 percent of the total amount. The remaining four major personal health-care categories for which government monies are spent include:

1. Federal outlays for hospital and medical services for veterans
2. Department of Defense provision of care for the armed forces and military dependents
3. Workers' compensation medical benefits
4. Other federal, state, and local expenditures for personal health care

Finally, public spending for research and facilities construction totaled approximately $14 billion in 1991. Of this amount, public outlays for research totaled $11.7 billion, with the federal government representing the primary source for most of the money spent.[21]

The Current Challenge to Publicly Financed Health Care

Notwithstanding the ever-increasing infusion of monies into Medicare, neither part A nor part B offers comprehensive coverage. Deductibles and coinsurance are built into each program. Limitations on the amount of coverage exist as well. For example, hospital benefits cease after 90 days if the patient has exhausted the lifetime reserve pool of 60 additional hospital days, and extended-care facility benefits terminate after 100 days. Medicare payments represent approximately 65 percent of the total annual national expenditure of hospital services and 27 percent of physicians' services. Because Medicare clarified its conditions for nursing-home payment in 1988 with the Catastrophic Coverage Act, it seems likely that Medicare will maintain its current share of total spending for nursing-home care at 4 to 5 percent.[22]

As of 1990, approximately 25.3 million people received some type of Medicaid benefit, with approximately $71.3 billion of combined federal and state funds being spent for personal health care. As a result of this accelerated growth, Medicaid's share of the nation's PHCEs has increased significantly. Medicaid's expenditures are largely institutional, with more than 40 percent spent on hospital care and approximately 35 percent spent on nursing-home care annually. Medicaid continues to be the largest third-party payer of long-term care expenditures, financing almost 50 percent of nursing-home care annually.[23]

Confronted with increasing numbers of recipients and recent legislative expansions to the Medicaid program in the face of limited revenues available to finance the program, states have been pressured to control their individual Medicaid costs. Strategies used or proposed by states include:

- Overall spending cuts
- Reallocation of available funds from high-cost services to lower-cost services
- Rationing high-technology services to selected recipients to provide lower-cost services to a broader group of recipients
- Provider-specific taxes
- "Voluntary donations" from physicians and hospitals

Private Outlays

Although the amount of public funding for health care is staggering, the predominant source of funding for the American health-care system comes from private sources. The bulk is derived from individuals receiving treatment and from third-party insurers making payments on the behalf of individuals.

In 1929, private payment of PHCEs represented 88.4 percent of the total amount spent on PHCEs. In 1935, that figure dropped to 82.4 percent. In 1965, before the advent of Medicare and Medicaid, such private payments accounted for nearly 77 percent of the total. In 1991, private payment of PHCEs totaled $377 billion, or just over 57 percent of all PHCEs.[24]

The decline in the private share of PHCEs is primarily due to the sharp drop in out-of-pocket payments associated with federal spending. In 1965, 53 percent of the personal health-care expenditures was paid for by the patient, and in 1991, 22 percent. Yet because of inflation and other factors, the per capita dollar amount paid directly by a patient in 1983 was four times that in 1965.[25]

PRIVATE THIRD-PARTY REIMBURSEMENT Most Americans receive their health insurance as a tax-free benefit through their employers.[26] This employer-based financing of health care was started during World War II and has grown steadily ever since. The system relies predominantly on private, employment-based, insurance-type financing schemes that, at least until recently, divorced financing from the delivery of services.

Private health-insurance companies constitute one of the largest sectors of the health industry. The United States has more than 1000 for-profit, commercial health insurers and 85 not-for-profit Blue Cross and Blue Shield plans. These private insurance organizations, along with health-maintenance organizations (HMOs), preferred-provider organizations (PPOs), and other third-party payers, paid for 32 percent of the total health-care expenditures in 1988.[27]

While the data on the number of Americans covered by private insurance do not completely agree, according to the Health Insurance Industry of America,[28] more than 190 million Americans were covered by private health insurance in 1992. Of that number, 71 million were in self-funded employee plans run by major employers, 96 million were insured under for-profit group policies, and 10 million had individual or family insurance policies. Seventy-three million were insured by Blue Cross and Blue Shield. Almost 98 percent of Americans older than 65 years were covered by Medicare. Twenty-five million of those citizens had Medigap insurance to cover uninsured services.

Blue Cross and Blue Shield and the Rise of Indemnity Insurance

The term "insurance" originally meant, and often still refers to the contribution by individuals to a fund to provide protection against financial loss following relatively unlikely but damaging events. Thus, there is insurance against fire, theft, and death at an early age. All of those events occur within a group of people within a predictable rate, but are rare occurrences for any one individual in a group.

JONAS'S HEALTH CARE DELIVERY IN THE UNITED STATES,[9] p 272

Medical insurance was introduced in the mid-1800s to defray costs associated with unexpected disabilities. Essentially, it consisted of cash payments by some carriers to individuals to offset income losses attributed to accident-related disabilities. Medical insurance continued in this tradition until the 1930s when, coincident with the rise in available medical services, a number of prepayment plans that offered care at various hospitals were organized in several cities. These hospital insurance plans soon became known as Blue Cross.[29] Shortly thereafter, Blue Shield was developed independently as an insurer for physicians' services. With the organization of Blue Cross and Blue Shield, a new policy for reimbursing general health-care costs started.

The "Blues" were established as nonprofit membership plans that served state and regional areas and offered both individual and group membership. For many years, the Blues were committed to **community rating**.[30] In exchange for offering coverage to anyone in the community, the Blues were able to secure significant discounts in costs by way of negotiations and through regulations known as the "most-favored-nation status," which ensured that they would have the lowest rates given to any payer.

In recent years, this community-rating approach has placed the Blues at a disadvantage when competing with commercial insurers that have entered the health-insurance field adhering to a policy of **experience rating**. Experience rating has allowed commercial insurers to charge different individuals and groups different premiums, based on individual risk and on the use of services. Low-risk groups could secure benefits at lower premiums because of the "healthy-worker effect," whereas high-risk groups were only able to receive commercial insurance coverage at prohibitively high premium rates. Consequently, the Blues have been left as the insurers of last resort for those individuals who might have chronic illnesses and/or are unable to obtain employer-based group insurance coverage.

Commercial Insurance

Like the Blues, commercial insurance plans offer comprehensive coverage for hospital and physicians' services; however, they differ in that they also sell medical and cash-payment policies. The commercial portion of the industry has grown rapidly in this country, primarily because experience rating has allowed them to respond to consumer demand for reduced out-of-pocket costs for medical care and because of the "employer-based" model for financing health care that developed during World War II.

Initially, commercial insurance companies were slow to enter a market dominated by the Blues. However, during and after World War II, tax laws changed to permit employers to offer tax-free health coverage as part of employee benefit packages, allowing commercial companies that previously had offered limited coverage to individuals to offer hospital insurance to groups. Since that time, commercial insurance companies have acquired more than half of the health-insurance market from Blue Cross and Blue Shield. Currently, there are more than 1000 private insurance companies providing individual and group health coverage in the United States.[31]

Self-Insurance

To avoid high tax premiums, administrative overhead, and marketing expenses, a majority of large corporations have become self-insured. Commercial insurance companies have found themselves to be little more than transaction processors for these corporations, providing claims-payment services to the self-insured on a cost-plus basis. Consequently, these insurance companies are experiencing operating losses due to the shrinking fully insured market. To compete and survive, group insurance carriers are transforming themselves into managed-care companies, thereby improving internal operating and marketing efficiencies. However, it is estimated that only 25 of the nearly 500 group health-insurance carriers have the capability, financial support, management, and customer volume to accomplish this task.[32]

Health-Maintenance Organizations and the Rise of Nonindemnity Insurance

As health-care costs escalated in the 1970s, Congress passed legislation that encouraged the formation of **health-maintenance organizations (HMOs),** or systems that would integrate the delivery and financing of health care. These operate differently from traditional indemnity insurance plans that reimbursed on a fee-for-service basis. HMOs provide comprehensive health- "maintenance" care (and restorative care when necessary) for its enrollees at a flat prepaid fee. Although this "capitated" form of health insurance has been available for the past

20 years, it has only recently begun to reshape the way many Americans relate to the health-care arena.

Although several different types of prepaid plans are available, the basic notion of each is that an annual fixed payment is made by or for beneficiaries in exchange for the delivery of all necessary health care by a group of providers within the scope of their contracts. Distinctions among HMOs pertain to the ways in which fiscal agents or the financing organizations relate to groups of care providers.[33] Most prepaid plans contract with providers for scheduled reimbursement, capitated payments, discounted charges, or per episode payments. Currently, there are four distinct HMO models in operation in the United States (Table 3–1).

Regardless of the type of plan, a capitated annual insurance premium is paid in exchange for all necessary care, including preventive and routine services not generally covered under indemnity plans. Presumably, HMOs reduce health-care costs (owing, for the most part, to lower rates of hospitalization) while providing coverage that has fewer copayment features and uncovered services. These plans have grown popular with employers who are looking for ways to reduce health-care benefits spending.

In 1992, 41.1 million Americans received care through HMOs, nearly 7 times those in 1976, and the number of HMOs has grown from 174 in 1976 to 546 in 1992. In 1993, for the first time, the number of people covered by traditional indemnity medical insurance represented less than one-half (49.9 percent) of all people who had health coverage through employer-sponsored plans.[34]

Preferred-Provider Organizations

The success of the independent practice association (IPA) model of HMOs increased experimentation with varying levels of consumer and physician choice, eventually leading to the introduction of PPOs. **PPOs,** like HMOs, offer the consumer a choice of full coverage for ambulatory and inpatient services provided by a selected panel of providers, combined with a limited range of coverage for out-of-plan use.[35] Frequently, PPOs are established by groups of physicians who

TABLE 3–1

Health-Maintainence Organization Models in the United States

Model	Description
Staff model	In this traditional HMO system, the fiscal agent engages individual physicians who are paid a salary to deliver services to the HMO's enrollees.
Group model	This model is similar to the staff model; however, it varies in that a single group of physicians contracts with the fiscal agent to deliver services.
Network model	Fiscal agents contract with multiple groups of physicians to deliver services to enrollees. Physicians in this model do not have exclusive contracts with fiscal agents and generally provide services to non-HMO enrollees.
Independent practice association (IPA) model	Fiscal agents contract with a range of independent practice physicians or multispecialty group practices to deliver care to its enrollees. As in the network model, physicians in the IPA model provide services to HMO enrollees as well as to patients with other forms of insurance. Usually, HMO enrollees represent a small percentage of IPA physicians' practices.

are interested in maintaining patients and revenues in the face of competition from HMOs.

Preferred-provider organizations provide health care at a lower cost to those beneficiaries who use participating providers, who are paid on the basis of negotiated or discounted rates. Beneficiaries are usually given some type of incentive, such as lower insurance premiums or waivers of cost-sharing requirements, for selecting a preferred provider. PPOs are gaining popularity, especially in markets where there is significant competition among physicians and other health-care providers.[36]

In such competitive areas, providers can be persuaded more easily to offer discounted services in exchange for a larger share of the patient volume. In 1988, there were approximately 620 PPOs, with about 36 million members.[37] In 1992, PPOs accounted for 13 percent of the private insurance market. The enhancement in consumer choice afforded by PPOs mimics the freedom of choice found in traditional fee-for-service medicine. Overcoming barriers of restricted choice to consumer and physician acceptance has helped alternative delivery systems expand rapidly and, consequently, has resulted in reduced market share for indemnity carriers and Blue Cross and Blue Shield plans.[38]

The Current Challenge to Privately Financed Health Care

Although private health insurance coverage for Americans is extensive, it is far from complete. The Health Care Association reports that Americans aged 16 to 24 years had the lowest rate of coverage at 79 percent. The highest rate of coverage was reported for those individuals between ages 35 and 64 years. Within this group, Hispanics had the lowest rate of coverage (53.7 percent). African-Americans were covered slightly more often (58.4 percent). More than 80 percent of whites were reported to have private health insurance.[39] These data support the notion that the proportion of the population that has insurance is directly related to income and ethnic membership. At the same time, employers are applying pressure on insurers to pare down premiums. This trend was most evident in a recent push by a consortium of 11 large employers in San Francisco that joined together to negotiate premium reductions from 17 Bay Area HMOs.[40]

HOW THE MONEY IS PAID OUT

Until about 25 years ago, the predominant manner of payment to hospitals and providers was the retrospective fee-for-service method. However, with the spiraling costs associated with Medicare and Medicaid, the federal government began to exercise its prerogative in scrutinizing the value received for the health-care dollars it reimbursed hospitals and physicians. Commercial health-insurance companies were quick to follow the government's lead by adopting similar payment policies.

With the proliferation of HMOs and PPOs and with increased fee regulation by public programs, physicians and hospitals are now less able to freely set prices for their services. At this time, there are three basic approaches that insurers may use to pay physicians for their services:

1. Fee for service

2. The preferred-provider approach

3. Capitation and salary

Although there are many permutations within these hospital reimbursement categories, the two dominant approaches are retrospective and prospective payment. What follows is a description of those reimbursement methods and their development.

Federal Cost Control and Its Effect on Hospital Reimbursement

As early as 1972, the related issues of the cost and the quality of the care delivered under federal entitlement programs were addressed by the passage of legislative amendments. Professional standards review organizations (PSROs) were established in an effort to monitor the quality and quantity of institutional services delivered to Medicare and Medicaid recipients. Later amendments attempted to limit the continuing growth in health-care expenditures in a dramatically different way, that is, by changing the manner in which the amount to be reimbursed hospitals and physicians was calculated.

In 1982, Congress passed the Tax Equity and Fiscal Responsibility Act (TEFRA). Designed to provide incentives for institutional cost containment, it replaced the PSROs with a "utilization and quality-control peer review organization" (PRO). The TEFRA legislation introduced the cost-per-case reimbursement system known as diagnoses related groups (DRGs) and, simultaneously, placed limits on the rates of increase in hospital revenues. Additional legislation mandated that hospitals covered under Medicare's new case-based reimbursement system contract with a PRO by 1984.[41]

The 1983 amendments to the Social Security Act further refined the case payment system by establishing a prospective payment system. These amendments created a revolutionary method of reimbursing hospitals for inpatient care to Medicare patients based on DRGs. Under the **prospective payment system,** hospitals are paid a pre-fixed amount per case treated. Research exploring the impact of DRGs suggest that the utilization patterns of hospitals are changing as a result of the reimbursement system. Most notably, hospital admissions and length of hospital stays have significantly decreased, and a sharp increase in posthospital care, including the use of home health services and nursing homes, has sharply increased.[42]

While prospective payment represents the most significant change in reimbursement methods in the past 10 years, it is not the exclusive means by which institutions are paid. **Retrospective payment,** or paying for services already provided, remains a mode by which some third-party payers reimburse hospitals. Most commercial insurers, such as Blue Cross, pay hospitals on the basis of submitted charges, or the prices set by hospitals for the care they provide. A more sophisticated retrospective repayment system is based on cost. In this system, third-party payers take a sum of total hospital costs and then, based on allowable items, reimburse hospitals on a per-patient-day basis.

Federal Cost Control and Its Effect on Physician Payment

Although fee for service remains the dominant method of physician reimbursement in this country, physician reimbursement mechanisms also were changed as a result of federal legislation, primarily under provisions in the Omnibus Budget Reconciliation Acts (OBRAs), especially OBRA 1989 and OBRA 1993.[43–47] Before the enactment of OBRA 1989, physicians were permitted wide discretion in establishing their own prices for each type of service they delivered. Once care was received, patients or their insurers paid the set price.

After OBRA 1989 was enacted, the amount that Medicare reimbursed and the amount that physicians were allowed to charge patients in excess of that amount were restricted to repayments in amounts equal to the "prevailing" fee (also known as "usual and customary rates") and by limiting the maximum payment allowed in communities for each type of physician's service.

Even though indemnity plans offered by private insurance companies continued to reimburse physicians based on the fee-for-service approach, many insurers have followed Medicare's approach by adopting a wide range of methods for establishing scales for covered services, limiting the ability of the physician to establish prices.

The resource-based relative value system (RBRVS) that went into effect in 1992 represents the most recent attempt by the federal government to control physician-related costs. With its introduction, Medicare substantially changed its approach to paying physicians. Based on a national fee schedule, the **RBRVS** assigns cash values to services based on the time, skill, and intensity required to provide them. The relative values are then further adjusted for geographic variations in payment.

The object of this new system was to rebalance reimbursement so that payment for cognitive services would be increased and payment for procedural services decreased relative to prices established in prior years. Unfortunately, evidence suggests that the RBRVS has not been as successful as expected.[9] To date, there is no indication that the commercial insurers are incorporating the RBRVS into their reimbursement methods.

In the private arena, the preferred-provider approach to paying physicians used by PPOs offers a variation on the fee-for-service system. Using this approach, insurers pay physicians discounted amounts for care delivered to enrollees on a service-by-service basis. The discounted payment schedule is usually negotiated between the insurers and the physicians or by physician groups.

Salary and capitation (discussed earlier) are the two other forms of provider reimbursement. The use of salary arrangements as a payment mechanism for health professionals is widespread and needs little explanation. Generally, this arrangement proves satisfactory to both employer and provider. In a salaried arrangement, employers can generally enjoy administrative simplicity, while providers are usually assured a more protected income as compared with those being reimbursed through other arrangements.

The Evolution of Managed Competition: The Need for Change

Managed competition and corporate health care have clearly emerged as key economic strategies guiding health-care restructuring in the United States today. Advocates of managed competition claim that it provides one solution that would contain costs while providing universal coverage without compromising quality. Although there are many possible explanations for the steady rise in health-care costs, advocates of managed competition view the primary evils as a cost-unconscious demand by consumers and perverse incentives to providers created by the fee-for-service third-party insurance system.

According to advocates of managed care and others who have studied health-spending trends, patients and physicians have grown insensitive to the rising cost of health care in this country. On average, insured patients pay very little directly for every dollar spent for hospital care and physicians' services. Most of the expense is borne by either employers or the government.

Because patients feel relatively little financial burden associated with their health-care expenses, they have exerted little pressure on providers to keep costs low. Providers generally had no real incentive to seek and use medical services that would yield the same health-care outcome at reduced cost. Rather, they were and, to a great extent, continue to be rewarded for delivering as many of the most expensive services as possible. Consequently, there has been little competition among providers to produce services efficiently and pass savings on to the consumers. In light of these perceptions, most proposed health-care reform initiatives, regardless of their origin, are directed toward restraining medical inflation by sensitizing consumers and providers to the high cost of health care.

MANAGED COMPETITION AS A SOLUTION

The health-care delivery system built with such little regard for cost is one characterized by Alain Enthoven as the "paradox of excess and deprivation."[48,49] As a strategy for curbing health-care costs, Enthoven, a business school professor at Stanford University, advanced a proposal known as **managed competition.** According to the basic theory of managed competition, groups of purchasers could negotiate with large groups of providers to determine price and some other terms of services in advance of purchase.[50,51] Although managed competition has not been implemented on any large, unified scale, it has attracted the attention and support of a wide range of institutions.

Managed competition has been proposed as a strategy that can solve the problem of skyrocketing health-care costs by restructuring the market to promote cost-conscious consumer choice among health plans. The market, as presented by Enthoven,[49,52] involves three key groups of players:

1. The consumer
2. The health plan
3. The sponsors

Consumers include both the individual and the employer-employee dyad. In managed competition, individuals could choose from, and employers would be required to offer employees, a variety of health plans. Employees would be encouraged to select the most economical plan from among the options offered because managed competition (as originally conceived) limits the tax-free employer contributions to the cost of the lowest-priced plan. Individuals joining more costly plans would not receive extra subsidies, as they currently do, but would have to pay extra cost out of their own pockets. As a result, consumers would be more likely to obtain necessary information to make informed decisions in selecting plans that offer them the most value for their money.

Health plans in managed-competition models are equivalent to accountable health partnerships that integrate financing and delivery of health care. HMOs, PPOs, and IPAs represent several examples of these health plans as they exist today. Although configurations vary, these plans, which integrate providers (physicians, nurses, laboratories, and so forth), insurers, and hospitals, would compete for subscribers and would be required to deliver value for money spent.

The structure of such health plans is significant to the organization's ability to manage a patient's care. Organizations that are able to improve quality while cutting costs would be most successful in attracting and maintaining subscribers. Strategies short of constituting all of the elements of managed competition that are being used by health plans to improve quality while limiting costs include:

- Closed- versus open-panel plans
- Prepaid group practices
- Economic credentialing
- Gatekeeping
- Utilization review
- Resource allocation
- Risk-sharing reimbursement
- Truncated treatment plans

Public sponsors are the third group of players identified as critical in managed competition. Sponsors would be recognized in each state and would act as the final guarantor of health coverage, acting as collective purchasing agents for employment groups of 100 or fewer employees and for the self-employed. State sponsors would be essential for those without employment-based coverage; these public sponsors would subsidize enrollment and contract with private-sector health plans on behalf of potential subscribers. Sponsors would essentially act as brokers for groups of subscribers.

THE CLINTON ADMINISTRATION PLAN AS AN ILLUSTRATION

Caught up in the health-care reform momentum, many legislative, executive, professional, and consumer groups offered their own versions or proposals for health-care reform. Some were confusing, most were complex, and many offered compelling options for consideration. For example, the Physicians for a National Health Program proposed a single-payer government system that supposedly ensured universal coverage under a government-financed system like the Medicare program. The Nursing's Agenda for Health Care Reform, developed by the American Nurses' Association, National League of Nursing, and other nursing organizations, was similar to the plan proposed by the American Medical Association.[54] The "Nursing's Agenda" suggested the adoption of a mandated employer-based insurance system that would continue the current public- and private-financing system. Other plans focused on the provision of basic services and a proposed single-payer model for long-term care services.

Regardless of the origin of the proposed plans, a common thread to many was the reliance on the "pay-or-play" managed-competition approach in one form or another. The plan proposed by the Clinton Administration, the Health Security Act of 1993,[55] is presented here to illustrate how managed competition might be used to strengthen the country's economy by restructuring the delivery of health care. The Clinton plan combined government regulation (managed) and free-market forces (competition) in an attempt to recognize the imperatives of reform from a moral and an economic perspective. This hybrid of managed competition and a single-sponsor health alliance represented a fundamental break from the traditional medical-industrial model under which the American health-care system has operated. According to the Clinton Administration plan, health-insurance cooperatives would have been established and would have contracted with various insurance companies that offered plans meeting federally mandated guidelines, including a package of mandated services or benefits. Under this plan, insurance companies would have competed with each other on price and quality to attract the greatest number of consumers to their plans. Moreover, consumers would have been encouraged to buy the least expensive plan through tax incentives.

Although Clinton's plan was not adopted as a national health plan, managed competition did emerge as an acceptable solution to the current health-care crisis. This occurred, in large part, because managed competition appears to offer significant advantages over the traditional fee-for-service plans. Subsequently, many of the features associated with managed competition have been adopted by both private and public sponsors.

The nation's largest health insurers, almost all of which are publicly held corporations, are all heavily invested in attempts to enlarge their managed-care businesses. The implementation of selected features of managed competition is further evidenced by the growth in the number and type of managed-care organizations in the United States, such as HMOs, PPOs, IPAs, point of service, and others and in the recent explosive increase in enrollment in each of these systems.

Managed Competition and Corporate Health: The Implications for Advanced Practice Nursing

Advanced practice nurses must be prepared for the substantial opportunities and considerable threats that are evolving as managed competition and corporate health continue to emerge as economic strategies guiding health-care reform. For the first time since the beginning of this century, both delivery and receipt of health care are operating on a budget. In addition, the consumer, whether an elderly person selecting from among several health-insurance plans to supplement Medicare coverage or a large corporation's employee benefits administrator deciding between a self-insured health plan or an HMO, is once again in a position to exercise control over what to buy and how much to pay. A more subtle fact is that the APN is currently absent from the competition for these tight health-care dollars.

This change to a value-driven consumer in a cost-conscious environment translates to an opportunity for APNs to be the value-conscious health-care provider. This is an opportunity that should not be squandered. As reiterated by each of the leaders interviewed by Dr. Komnenich, there was in the past—and should be today—the commitment by APNs to promote themselves and the advanced practice role as an essential element in the successful development of managed competition.

As Dr. Komnenich makes clear in Chapter 1, the APNs who brought advanced practice nursing to where it is today did so largely by the dint of their own initiative and by a devotion to excellence. They made their mark and thus made a place for today's APNs by collecting and disseminating data that promoted their value; by refusing to accede to organized nursing's and medicine's efforts to constrain their vision to some preconceived idea about what a nurse should be; and by actively seeking out and seizing opportunities for advancement presented by others outside the profession or occasioned by sociological, political, and/or economic events.

Suggested Exercises

1. As a result of the health-care revolution in America, medical care is evolving into health care. Develop a platform that illuminates the actual and potential effects or consequences of this transformation on advanced practice nursing.

2. Vast opportunities exist for APN intrapreneurs and entrepreneurs in today's competitively managed market. Create a business plan for the new health-care environment that recharacterizes the APN identity, redefines APN role components, and relocates advanced nursing practice arenas.

3. Organize a portfolio that can be presented to prospective markets providing evidence to support the position that APNs are well suited to assume a variety of positions in integrated health-care systems.

4. Debate whether APNs would be better advised to assume complementary (value added) or substitution positions in managed-care markets.

5. Design a master plan for an IPA that consists exclusively of APNs. Identify potential consumer groups to be served as well as insurers to be approached. Discuss strategies for reimbursement.

6. How would you "sell" or market the concept of an APN IPA to selected consumers and prospective insurers? Develop a marketing plan to accomplish that goal.

REFERENCES

1. McCarthy, MC, and Berman, JA: Advanced practice nursing in today's health care market (in review). Journal of Advanced Practice Nursing, in press, 1997.
2. Fox, JC: The role of nursing. Journal of Psychosocial Nursing 31:9, 1993.
3. Caper, P: Managed competition that works. JAMA 269:2524, 1993.
4. Estes, CL, Harrington, C, and Davis, S: The medical-industrial complex. In Harrington, C, and Estes, CL (eds): Health Policy and Nursing: Crisis and Reform in the US Health Care Delivery System. Jones and Bartlett, Boston, 1994.
5. Iglehart, JK: The American health care system: Introduction. N Engl J Med 326:962, 1992.
6. US Department of Commerce, International Trade Administration: Health and Medical Services. Industrial Outlook. US Documents, Washington, DC, 1990.
7. Lu, E: The potential effect of managed competition in health care on provider liability and patient autonomy. Harvard Journal on Legislation 30:517, 1993.

8. Health Care Financing Administration. HHS News. Health Insurance Association of America, Washington, DC, November 18, 1988.

9. Knickman, JR, and Thorpe, KE: Financing for health care. In Kovner, AR (ed): Jonas's Health Care Delivery in the United States, ed 5. Springer, New York, 1995.

10. Binstock, RH: Older Americans and health care reform in the nineties. In Rosenau, PV: Health Care Reform in the Nineties. Sage Publications, Newbury Park, Calif, 1994.

11. Intriligator, MD: A way to achieve national health insurance in the United States: The Medicare expansion proposal. In Rosenau, PV (ed): Health Care Reform in the Nineties. Sage Publications, Newbury Park, Calif, 1994.

12. Baldor, RA: Managed Care Made Simple. Blackwell Science, Cambridge, Mass, 1996.

13. Lichtenstein, R, et al: The national health care cost containment crisis: How school of public health experts view it. Findings 2:11, 1993.

14. Levit, KR, et al: National health care spending: 1989. Health Aff (Millwood) 10:117, 1991.

15. Iglehart, JK: The American health care system: Medicare. N Engl J Med 327:1467, 1992.

16. Levit, KR, et al: National health expenditures. In Harrington, C, and Estes, CL (eds): Health Policy and Nursing: Crisis and Reform in the US Health Care Delivery System. Jones and Bartlett, Boston, 1994.

17. Kronenfeld, JJ: Controversial Issues in Health Care Policy. Sage Publications, Newbury Park, Calif, 1993.

18. Harris, JS: The evolution of the health care crisis. In Harris, JS (ed): Strategic Health Care Management. Jossey-Bass, San Francisco, 1994.

19. Moyer, EM: A revised look at the number of uninsured Americans. In Harrington, C, and Estes, CL (eds): Health Policy and Nursing: Crisis and Reform in the US Health Care Delivery System. Jones and Bartlett, Boston, 1994.

20. Thorpe, KE: Health care cost containment. In Kovner, AR (ed): Jonas's Health Care Delivery in the United States, ed 5. Springer, New York, 1995.

21. Grogan, CM: Federalism and health care reform. In Rosenau, PV (ed): Health Care Reform in the Nineties. Sage Publications, Newbury Park, Calif, 1994.

22. Kaplan, RM: A look at solutions. In Kaplan, RM (ed): The Hippocratic Predicament. Academic Press, San Diego, 1993.

23. State Initiatives in Health Care Reform: Medicaid Waiver Programs: Lessons for the Future or Time-limited Experiments? Robert Wood Johnson Foundation, Alpha Center 6:1, 1994.

24. Gibson, RM, et al: National health expenditures, 1983. Social Security Bulletin 6:2, 1984.

25. Kaplan, RM: The Hippocratic Predicament: Affordability, Access, and Accountability in Medicine. Academic Press, San Diego, 1995.

26. Iglehart, JK: The American health care system: Private insurance. N Engl J Med 326: 1715, 1992.

27. US Office of National Cost Estimates (US ONCE): National health expenditures, 1988. Health Care Financing Review 11:1, 1990.

28. Health Insurance Industry of America: Source Book of Health Insurance Data: 1992. Health Insurance Association of America, Washington, DC, 1992.

29. Blue Cross/Blue Shield Corporate Report. Blue Cross/Blue Shield of Massachusetts, Boston, May 1990.

30. State initiatives in health care reform: New York adopts pure community rating—Other states take incremental approach. Robert Wood Johnson Foundation, Alpha Center 7:1, 1994.

31. Harris, JS: Strategic Health Care Management. Jossey-Bass, San Francisco, 1994.

32. Abramowitz, KS: The Future of Health Care Delivery in the United States. Sanford C Bernstein & Co, New York, 1993.

33. Group Health Association of America: National Directory of HMOs: 1991. Group Health Association of America, Washington, DC, 1991.

34. Iglehart, JK: Health policy report: Physicians and the growth of managed care. N Engl J Med 331:1167, 1994.

35. Morrison, EM, and Luft, HS: Health maintenance organization environments in the 1980s and beyond. In Harrington, C, and Estes, CL (eds): Health Policy and Nursing: Crisis and Reform in the US Health Care Delivery System. Jones and Bartlett, Boston, 1994.

36. Loeppke, RR: Restructuring the American health care system. Managed Care Journal 2:30, 1993.

37. Kassler, J: Bitter Medicine: Greed and Chaos in the American Health Care System. A Birch Lane Press, New York, 1994.

38. Harris, JS: Alliances with managed care. In Harris, JS (ed): Strategic Health Management. Jossey-Bass, San Francisco, 1994.

39. Health Insurance Industry of America: Source Book of Health Insurance Data: 1990. Health Insurance Industry of America, Washington, DC, 1990.

40. Inglehart, JK: The American health care system: Managed care. N Engl J Med 327:742, 1992.

41. Relman, AS: What market values are doing to medicine. In Harrington, C, and Estes, CL (eds): Health Policy and Nursing: Crisis and Reform in the US Health Care Delivery System. Jones and Bartlett, Boston, 1994.

42. Harrington, C: Quality, access, and costs: Public policy and home care. In Harrington, C, and Estes, CL (eds): Health Policy and Nursing: Crisis and Reform in the US Health Care Delivery System. Jones and Bartlett, Boston, 1994.

43. Omnibus Budget Reconciliation Act of 1989, Public Law No. 101–239.

44. Omnibus Budget Reconciliation Act of 1990, Public Law No. 101–508.

45. Omnibus Budget Reconciliation Act of 1987, Public Law No. 100–203.

46. Omnibus Budget Reconciliation Act of 1980, Public Law No. 96–499.

47. Omnibus Budget Reconciliation Act of 1986, Public Law No. 99–509.

48. Enthoven, AC: Health tax policy mismatch. Health Aff (Millwood) 4:5, 1985.

49. Enthoven, AC: Theory and Practice of Managed Competition in Health Care Finance. Amsterdam Publishing, North Holland, 1988.

50. Enthoven, AC, and Kronick, R: A consumer-choice health plan for the 1990s: Universal health insurance in a system designed to promote quality and economy. N Engl J Med 320:29, 1989.

51. Enthoven, AC, and Kronick, R: A consumer-choice health plan for the 1990s: Universal health insurance in a system designed to promote quality and economy. N Engl J Med 320:94, 1989.

52. Enthoven, AC: Health care cost: A moral and economic problem. California Management Review 35:134, 1993.

53. Himmelstein DU, et al: A national health program for the United States. In Harrington, C, and Estes, CL (eds): Health Policy and Nursing: Crisis and Reform in the US Health Care Delivery System. Jones and Bartlett, Boston, 1994.

54. American Nurses' Association: Nursing's agenda for health care reform. In Harrington, C, and Estes, CL (eds): Health Policy and Nursing: Crisis and Reform in the US Health Care Delivery System. Jones and Bartlett, Boston, 1994.

55. Clinton, W.: The President's Health Security Plan. Random House, New York, 1993.

Selected Theories and Models for Advanced Practice Nursing

MICHELLE WALSH, PhD, RN, CPNP
LINDA A. BERNHARD, PhD, RN

Michelle Walsh, PhD, RN, CPNP, is a pediatric nurse practitioner certified by the National Certification Board of Pediatric Nurse Practitioners and Nurses (NCBPNPN). She provides primary care to children of all ages in a busy pediatric practice in Columbus, Ohio. She serves as a clinical preceptor for pediatric nurse practitioner students. Before becoming a nurse practitioner, she taught pediatric nursing, research utilization, and nursing leadership to baccalaureate, master's, and doctoral students. She is the coauthor of *Leadership: The Key to the Professionalization of Nursing.*

Linda A. Bernhard, PhD, RN, is an associate professor of nursing and women's studies at Ohio State University in Columbus, Ohio. Her specialty is women's health. She teaches health promotion in the Primary Care Adult Nurse Practitioner program. She taught nursing leadership for many years and is co-author of *Leadership: The Key to the Professionalization of Nursing.*

4

CHAPTER OUTLINE

THEORIES OF LEADERSHIP
Theory X and Theory Y
Consideration and initiating structure
Path-goal theory
Fiedler's contingency model and cognitive resource theory
Tridimensional leadership-effectiveness model
THEORIES OF TEACHING AND LEARNING
Behaviorist theory
Cognitive theory
Humanistic theory
THEORIES OF CHANGE
The freezing model

Strategies for changing
Change in practice by the advanced practice nurse
MODELS OF HEALTH PROMOTION
Health belief model
Health promotion model
PRECEDE-PROCEED Model
Theory of care-seeking behavior
MODELS OF ADVANCED PRACTICE NURSING
Novice to expert
Advanced nursing practice
Differentiated practice
Comparison of advanced practice models
SUMMARY
SUGGESTED EXERCISES

CHAPTER OBJECTIVES

After completing this chapter, the reader will be able to:

1. Select a theory of leadership appropriate to their area of advanced practice.
2. Compare and contrast types of teaching-learning theories.
3. Explain the research utilization process in the context of planned change.
4. Apply theories of health promotion to all types of advanced nursing practice.
5. Summarize a variety of advanced nursing practice and other related nursing models.

Leadership is a process that is used to move a group toward goal setting and goal achievement.[1] The components of leadership are the leader and group, the theory of leadership, and the organization. Leadership can be used by any nurse but is especially important for advanced practice nurses (APNs). This chapter provides an introduction to the theory component of leadership by describing theories and models that can be used in advanced practice nursing. Theories of leadership will be presented, as well as related theories and models of teaching-learning, change, health promotion, and advanced practice nursing.

Critical thinking and leadership go hand in hand. Critical thinking involves **attitude,** or a frame of mind for viewing issues or problems. Leadership requires a frame of mind to move a group to turn problems into goals and then work to achieve those goals. Critical thinking involves the acquisition of knowledge and skills. Leadership can be learned and includes skills, such as planning change. APNs use leadership skills to promote the health of clients.

Theories of Leadership

THEORY X AND THEORY Y

Assumptions about motivation are the basis for McGregor's[2] theories of leadership. Theory X reflects the traditional view of direction and control, whereas Theory Y includes an integration of individual and organizational goals. McGregor was careful to indicate that X and Y are not opposite but are separate philosophies. Theory X is the basis of managerial theory; Theory Y was operationalized through a strategy commonly referred to as *management by objectives.*

In Theory X, the assumption is that people dislike work and avoid it whenever possible. Because of the dislike of work, people must be controlled and directed to engage in goal-directed activity. Further, according to McGregor,[2] people wish to avoid responsibility and prefer direction to feel secure.

A different view of people is proposed in Theory Y, which states that work is as natural as play. People are self-directed and engage freely in goal-directed activity so long as they are in agreement with the goals. It is the commitment to the goals, as well as goal attainment, that is fulfilling, making external direction unnecessary. Because all individuals have the potential to succeed, the creation of conditions that allow the individual to pursue goals is essential. By creating conditions that enable goal setting, the leader fosters participation and creative problem solving.

CONSIDERATION AND INITIATING STRUCTURE

The two constructs of **consideration** and **initiating structure** were identified through investigations to determine which behaviors used by a leader had a positive influence on group satisfaction and productivity.[3] Consideration encompasses those behaviors of the leader that emphasize concern for the individual or group. Consideration includes trust, respect, warmth, and rapport and thus encourages communication.[4] Initiating structure includes the behaviors of the leader that focus on the task to be accomplished or on the organizational goals. Initiating structure includes defining roles, assigning tasks, planning, and encouraging production.[4]

Researchers found that group productivity is more closely associated with initiating structure, whereas individual satisfaction is more dependent on consideration. However, individuals seem to be more secure when they know what is expected of them; thus, both behaviors are important for success at both individual and organizational levels. Moreover, group cohesiveness is fostered by both consideration and initiating structure.

While reviewers of leadership theory indicate that the most effective leaders use both consideration and initiating structure,[5] the measures and, consequently, the validity of the measurement of these two behaviors has been questioned.[6] Inconsistent findings among the studies led to further investigation of missing variables that could explain effective leader behavior.

PATH-GOAL THEORY

The path-goal theory was an attempt to identify the missing variables by specifying the conditions under which the leader's behavior affects member satisfaction.[7] The degree to which the leader exhibits consideration determines the members' perceptions of available rewards, whereas the degree to which the leader initiates structure determines the members' perceptions of the paths that will ultimately lead them to their goals.[5]

Using the path-goal theory, the leader initiates structure to demonstrate to members how their actions will result in goal attainment. The leader also exhibits consideration by helping to remove barriers, and so makes the path to the goal easier.[8] Both consideration and initiating structure enhance members' motivation and satisfaction to the extent that such leadership behaviors clarify the path to the goal.

FIEDLER'S CONTINGENCY MODEL AND COGNITIVE RESOURCE THEORY

Using similar variables to develop a model of leadership effectiveness, Fiedler[9] created the contingency approach, or contingency theory. Fiedler's model measures leadership effectiveness by examining group productivity. According to Fiedler,[9] leadership is an interpersonal relation in which power and influence are unevenly distributed so that one person is able to direct and control the actions and behaviors of others to a greater extent than they direct and control the leader's (p. 11). In this model the leader has the primary responsibility for completion of the group task.

Because leadership is a relationship based on power and influence, the leader must classify each situation based on the amount of power and influence that the group members allow the leader. In any given situation, the amount of power and influence depend on a combination of three variables that yield a favorable or unfavorable situation for the leader.

The first variable that determines a favorable situation for the leader is the relationship between the leader and group members. The notion that the leader-member relationship is the single most important variable determining the leader's power and influence is well supported in the literature.[10] The degree to which group members accept the leader determines whether leader-member relationships are classified as good or poor.

The second variable is task structure. Routine or predictable tasks are classified as structured, whereas tasks that require analysis of multiple possibilities are classified as unstructured. Finally, the third variable, position power, refers to the leader's place within the organization and the amount of authority given to the leader by virtue of that position. Position power is not a personality characteristic; rather, it measures the leader's status in the organization. Position power is classified as strong or weak.

According to Fiedler,[9] these three variables create eight different situations that can be ranked from "most favorable" to "least favorable." Each possible situation is numbered and termed a *cell*, with cell 1 characterized as the most favorable situation and cell 8 the least favorable.

On the basis of his earliest research, Fiedler[9] predicted that cells 1, 2, and 3 were the very favorable situations and that cell 8 was the least favorable situation. Thus, using a task-centered, controlling behavior would be most effective. Cells 4, 5, 6, and 7 were intermediate situations. Thus, a more effective approach for the leader is a permissive, relationship-centered one (Table 4–1).

Fiedler continued to predict that with cells 1, 2, 3, and 8, the leader should use a more controlling or task-oriented behavior. However, he eventually determined that only cells 4 and 5 represented situations of intermediate or moderate favorableness, requiring a permissive or relationship-oriented approach.[11] Cells 6 and 7 were defined as unfavorable to the leader, and Fiedler predicted that little difference would occur in outcome, whether permissive or controlling behavior was used (Table 4–2). Even though the model is predictive, only two conclusions are specified:

1. Task-oriented leaders will perform best in groups in which the situation is either very favorable or very unfavorable.

2. Relationship-oriented leaders will perform best in groups in which the situation is either of moderate or intermediate favorableness.

TABLE 4–1
Fiedler's Contingency Table, 1967

Cell	Leader-Member Relationship	Task Structure	Position Power	Situation Rating	Preferred Behavior
1	Good	Structured	Strong	Very favorable	Controlling
2	Good	Structured	Weak	Very favorable	Controlling
3	Good	Unstructured	Strong	Very favorable	Controlling
4	Good	Unstructured	Weak	Intermediate favorableness	Permissive
5	Poor	Structured	Strong	Intermediate favorableness	Permissive
6	Poor	Structured	Weak	Intermediate favorableness	Permissive
7	Poor	Unstructured	Strong	Intermediate favorableness	Permissive
8	Poor	Unstructured	Weak	Very favorable	Controlling

Source: From Fiedler, FE: A Theory of Leadership Effectiveness. McGraw-Hill, New York, 1967, p. 142, with permission.

TABLE 4–2
Fiedler's Contingency Table, 1973

Cell	Leader-Member Relationship	Task Structure	Position Power	Situation Rating	Preferred Behavior
1	Good	Structured	Strong	Very favorable	Controlling
2	Good	Structured	Weak	Very favorable	Controlling
3	Good	Unstructured	Strong	Very favorable	Controlling
4	Good	Unstructured	Weak	Moderately favorable	Permissive
5	Poor	Structured	Strong	Moderately favorable	Permissive
6	Poor	Structured	Weak	Unfavorable	
7	Poor	Unstructured	Strong	Unfavorable	
8	Poor	Unstructured	Weak	Unfavorable	Controlling

Source: From Fiedler, FE: The trouble with leadership training is that it doesn't train leaders. *Psychology Today* 6:23, 1973. Reprinted with permission from *Psychology Today* magazine. Copyright 1973. Sussex Publishers, Inc.

Considerable research supports the validity of the contingency model of a leader's effectiveness. Although only three variables are evaluated to determine the favorableness of a situation, these variables are the most significant in a given situation. Nonetheless, the model has been criticized because it fails to explain the underlying processes that result in a leader's effective performance.

Fiedler addressed the limitations of the contingency model by developing the cognitive resource theory.[12] Cognitive resources include the intellectual abilities, technological competencies, and job-relevant knowledge of a leader. Cognitive resources are acquired during formal education and through experience.

Cognitive resource theory is depicted in Fig. 4–1. The cognitive resource theory attends to task accomplishment and the role that the group members play in task accomplishment. Task accomplishment is often the outcome of the leader's effectiveness. The leader's behavior results from both the situation and the leader's personality, as measured by the Least Preferred Coworker Scale.[12]

The most important idea from cognitive resource theory is that the situation is the most important variable. Only under certain conditions do the leader's and the members' abilities contribute positively to group performance.[12]

TRIDIMENSIONAL LEADERSHIP-EFFECTIVENESS MODEL

Hersey and Blanchard[13] used Fiedler's[9,11] early work and the consideration and initiating structure theories to propose another way of viewing leadership. They believed that no single leadership style or behavior could be effective in every situation. Combining the variables of task orientation and relationship orientation with effectiveness, Hersey and Blanchard created the tridimensional leadership-effectiveness model (Fig. 4–2).

In the tridimensional leadership-effectiveness model, the leader's behavior is integrated with situational dimensions. **Leadership style** is defined as the behavior pattern that a leader exhibits when attempting to influence the activities of others as perceived by those others.[13]

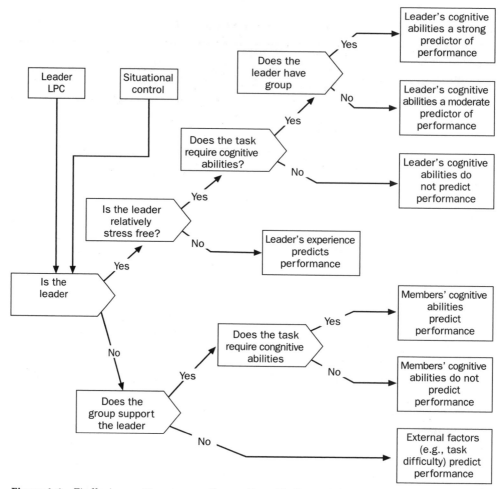

Figure 4–1. Fiedler's cognitive resource theory. (From Fiedler and Garcia,[12] p. 9, with permission.)

According to Hersey and Blanchard,[13] task behaviors include organizing and defining roles of group members and directing activities. Task behaviors focus on production. Relationship behaviors include facilitating, supporting, and maintaining personal relationships through open communication. The four basic leadership styles in the model are combinations of relationship and task behavior. The styles are arranged in quadrant fashion as shown in Fig. 4–2.

In addition to the task and relationship behavioral dimensions, an effectiveness dimension is added. Effectiveness depends on appropriateness to the situation and is conceptualized as a continuum from effective to ineffective. The four basic styles are effective or ineffective depending on their appropriateness for the situation as seen by the group members. Hersey and Blanchard[13] developed an instrument, the Leader Effectiveness and Adaptability Description (LEAD), to be used with their model. The LEAD instrument measures leadership style, style range or flexibility, and style adaptability or effectiveness. Style range and adaptability are particularly important, because the more flexible a leader can

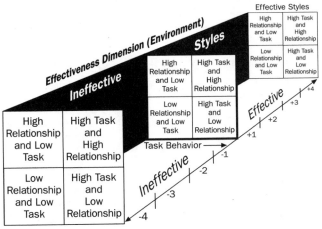

Figure 4–2. Tridimensional leadership effectiveness model. (From Hersey and Blanchard,[13] p. 119, reprinted with permission from Paul Hersey, Escondido, CA: The Center for Leadership Studies. All rights reserved.)

be, the more likely the leader is to be effective in any situation. There are two forms of the LEAD, one for leaders to evaluate themselves (LEAD-self) and a second for group members to rate their perceptions of the leader (LEAD-other).

Certain predictions are possible without using the LEAD instruments. An indication of group members' willingness or motivation in relation to a given task, in addition to their ability or competence, gives an indication of readiness (Fig. 4–3). Four classifications of readiness can be determined[13]:

1. Member is both willing and able to accept this responsibility.

2. Member is willing but unable to accept this responsibility.

3. Member is unwilling but able to accept this responsibility.

4. Member is neither willing nor able to accept this responsibility.

After determining which level of readiness members represent, the leader can select an appropriate style.

Research results demonstrate a curvilinear relationship within the quadrants.[13] The low-relationship, low-task quadrant style is called *delegating;* the high-relationship, low-task quadrant style is *participating;* the high-task, high-relationship quadrant style is called *selling;* and the high-task, low-relationship quadrant style is called *telling.*[13] The relationships between style and readiness are depicted in Fig. 4–3. The telling style is best used with group members who have the lowest level of readiness. Members with the second lowest level of readiness respond better to the selling style. For members in the third level of readiness, participating is the most effective style. Finally, delegating, or allowing a maximum amount of freedom, is most effective for members with the highest level of readiness.[13]

Another prediction that should help the leader become more effective is based on the readiness of the group as reflected in their actual performance.[13] The leader style should shift to the left on the curvilinear line (see Fig. 4–3) when performance in the group increases and should shift to the right when performance declines.

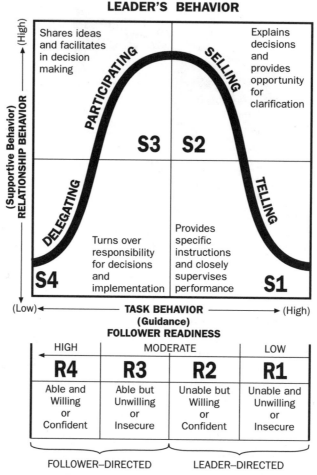

Figure 4–3. Situational leadership model. (From Hersey and Blanchard,[13] p. 171, reprinted with permission from Paul Hersey, Escondido, CA: The Center for Leadership Studies. All rights reserved.)

Theories of Teaching and Learning

Theories of teaching and learning can be summarized according to three views:

1. Behaviorist
2. Cognitive
3. Humanistic

In each of these views, the definition of learning and, consequently, the definition of teaching differ. The APN can use concepts from each view to construct an effective teaching-learning situation in practice.

BEHAVIORIST THEORY

Behaviorist learning theory is based on the belief that there is a direct association between events or ideas.[14] Behaviorists assume that people react to their environments and that behavior can be explained in mechanistic terms.[15]

Learning is defined as a change in performance, including the development of habits or procedures in response to certain conditions, including need arousal, repeated practice, and reinforcement.[14] Learning occurs when an unmet need produces sufficient motivation to satisfy that need. An unmet need causes tension, and the learner's desire to relieve the tension encourages action. The action is the response evoked by teacher-supplied stimuli. Through **conditioning,** or providing rewards for the desired response, the learner's needs are met and the tension is decreased. Need fulfillment accompanying the decrease in tension is also rewarding. If this pattern continues, habits develop through repeated practice.

Teaching is the arrangement of the contingencies of reinforcement.[16] The teacher controls the learning experience, and the learner is acted on by the teacher. The teacher specifies the desired response, and the learner, through trial and error, tries to produce the desired response. The teacher rewards the learner for correct or nearly correct responses.

To put it simply, Skinner[16] noted that we learn by doing, by experience, and by trial and error. What is learned is that responses are emphasized, the situation where the responses occur is important, and consequences result from actions.

COGNITIVE THEORY

Cognitive theory developed as researchers grew to believe that simple reflex arcs, or associations, could not adequately explain learning behavior. Cognitive learning theories are based on the assumption that learners interact with their environments. Learning occurs by focusing on the whole, rather than by studying the parts.

In cognitive theories, learning is considered an interaction between the learner and the environment, mediated by the teacher. Learning is internal; it occurs within the learner as new insights are formed or as cognitive structures are changed.[15] Understanding is the focus of learning, and learners develop a coding system in their mind to store information. Thinking and conceptualizing are the learner's major activities, and the teacher evaluates cognitive development in the learners.

Teaching focuses on the relationships and organization of facts. Teaching involves creating situations that make meaningful learning experience more likely for individual learners.[17] Teachers who understand the cognitive development of their learners and present organized subject matter appropriate to the learners produce learning.

HUMANISTIC THEORY

Humanistic theory is an approach to teaching and learning that involves being human in the process. Teachers and learners trust each other to be competent human beings who both learn through the process of self-discovery. Humanistic theory is a person-centered approach that involves specific values which emphasize the individual and choice, responsibility, and creativity.[18]

Learning in humanistic theory has been called *significant,* or *experiential,* learning. Learning is the process of developing one's full potential. The elements of humanistic learning are[18]:

- The whole person, both feeling and cognition, is involved in learning.
- Learning is learner initiated.

- Learning is pervasive.
- Learning is learner evaluated.
- The essence of learning is meaning.

Learning may include practicing to make a new skill a habit or incorporating a new idea into one's own understanding, so long as the learner is actively involved in the process and not merely acted on by the teacher.

Teaching is the facilitation of learning.[18] The learner as a person, rather than as the subject matter, is the teacher's focus, and the learner is viewed as the one responsible for the learning. The teacher is available to assist the learner but is not necessarily the initiator of the process. Certain qualities of the humanistic teacher, including genuineness, appreciation of the learner, and empathic understanding, are essential to trusting the learner to develop and learn.[18]

Theories of Change

Change is inevitable both in nursing and in society. APNs must be able to accept the changes they face, as well as function as change agents to foster change in individuals and groups. Integration of the theories and models of change into the knowledge base of APNs will facilitate their relationship to change.

THE FREEZING MODEL

Planned change occurs in a three-step process[19]:

1. Unfreezing
2. Moving
3. Refreezing

The freezing theory derives from field theory, a method of analyzing causal relationships. In field theory, change is due to certain forces within the field. Forces are directional entities that work in opposition to each other to maintain a dynamic equilibrium. For every force, there is an opposite force. Positive, or driving, forces indicate the likelihood of moving a system toward a desired goal. Negative, or restraining, forces indicate obstacles that decrease the likelihood of a system moving toward a desired goal.

Three possible situations result from an analysis of the forces within a field:

1. A state of dynamic equilibrium exists when the sum of the driving forces is equal to the sum of the restraining forces.
2. Change occurs in the desired direction when the sum of the driving forces is greater than the sum of the restraining forces.
3. A change in the undesired direction, or away from the desired goal, occurs when the sum of the driving forces is less than the sum of the restraining forces (Fig. 4–4).

Change occurs whenever the forces in a given field are unequal.

Change involves three stages[19]:

1. Unfreezing the present level of equilibrium
2. Moving to a new level of equilibrium
3. Refreezing the new level so that it is relatively permanent

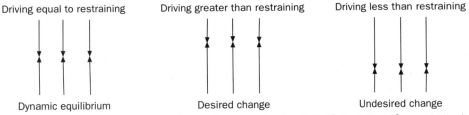

Figure 4–4. Driving and restraining forces. (From Bernhard and Walsh,[1] p. 169, with permission.)

The three stages occur sequentially, with the moving phase dependent on the outcome of the unfreezing phase and with the refreezing phase dependent on the outcome of the moving phase.

Unfreezing   LEWIN'S

During unfreezing, conditions are viewed as stable, or "frozen." Change begins with a felt need, a desired goal that has not been achieved. When one individual shares a felt need with another individual, unfreezing has begun. During the unfreezing phase, the current condition is critically analyzed.

The goal of the unfreezing phase is to clarify the present situation and make persons aware of the need for change by creating dissatisfaction with the situation. The target of change can be attitudes, knowledge, and/or behaviors. A change agent encourages group members to raise questions and explore their feelings and attitudes about present conditions. When group members acknowledge their dissatisfaction with the present situation, they begin to commit themselves to the change process. For change to occur, a plan that maximizes driving forces and minimizes restraining forces is made.

Moving

The goal of the moving phase is to achieve the desired change. The moving phase is also known as the changing phase because it is during this phase that the change is implemented. The moving phase depends on the outcome of the unfreezing phase. If the equilibrium has been upset in a favorable fashion—driving forces exceed restraining forces—then the desired change can occur. Moving ends when the change has been fully implemented, that is, the desired change in knowledge, attitude, or behavior has occurred. When the target has been changed, refreezing can occur.

Refreezing

The goal of the refreezing phase is stabilization of the change. The new knowledge, attitude, or behavior learned during the moving phase must continue to be practiced until it becomes as familiar as the one that preceded it. The change agent can help the group to refreeze by actions that help to legitimate the change, such as providing articles for the group to read about others who have made the same or a similar change.

Refreezing represents the end point in the change process and indicates that the change has been fully accepted and internalized. The change agent knows that refreezing has occurred when group members consistently demonstrate the new attitude or behavior and talk positively about it, their words and actions being congruent. Once it has been determined that refreezing has occurred, the group's performance should be evaluated periodically to confirm that the planned change is indeed refrozen.

STRATEGIES FOR CHANGING

Chin and Benne[20] presented a model of strategies for changing. Strategies are approaches used by the change agent to influence a group to adopt a proposed change. Three strategies, which may be used individually or in combination, include:

1. Empirical-rational
2. Normative-reeducative
3. Power-coercive

The *empirical-rational strategy* is based on the closely related assumptions that human beings are rational and that they follow a pattern of self-interest. From these basic assumptions, it follows that people will change when they understand that a proposed change is rationally justified and is beneficial to them.[20] The empirical-rational strategy is the oldest and most frequently used strategy. It is based on reason and intelligence.

The *normative-reeducative strategy* is a more active strategy. People do what they do because of held norms and commitment to those norms. Norms come from society, culture, religion, and family or from other sources. Change occurs when commitment to some present norm decreases to a point where a new norm can be adopted. Thus, change resulting from the normative-reeducative strategy is a modification of values and attitudes, as well as of behavior.[20]

The normative-reeducative strategy requires direct intervention by a change agent to aid in the unlearning and relearning process. The individual and change agent actively work together to produce the change. Behavioral science techniques, such as consciousness-raising, may be used to help individuals become aware of their values and norms, so that they may change to new ones.[20]

The *power-coercive strategy* requires some type of legitimate power to force compliance with change. Very simply, those with greater power influence and control those with lesser power.[20] The power-coercive strategy may be used by persons in top-level positions of an organization to effect change that they believe is needed. The group affected by the change is forced to comply, without having any input. Because of its approach there are many disadvantages to the power-coercive strategy; however, combined with another strategy, it may be used to promote acceptance by group members.

With any strategy, the change agent must allow time for the group to accept and/or practice the change. Practice time serves as a trial period that allows the group to adjust to and experience the benefits of a new condition. The group is then able to evaluate their new knowledge, attitude, or behavior. When group members see that their new knowledge, attitude, or behavior meets their desired goal, they will be reluctant to return to their former ways of thinking and acting.

When selecting a strategy, change agents must take into account both their relationship with the group and the target of change. Change agents will be most effective when the strategy used is consistent with the overall goals of the planned change and does not jeopardize the relationship with group members.

CHANGE IN PRACTICE BY THE ADVANCED PRACTICE NURSE

In addition to the theories of Lewin[19] and Chin and Benne,[20] the APN should be familiar with the process of research utilization. Research utilization is a planned change process. Research utilization is important to improve clinical practice, providing a link between problem identification and problem solving that incorporates current research-based knowledge.

The research utilization process involves reviewing existing research-based knowledge to determine whether substantive investigations have been conducted that address the practice problem to be solved. Elements of traditional research critique are used in identifying and summarizing the research base. In Stetler's model[21] of research utilization, at least three phases must occur before the decision to use research in practice:

1. Preparation
2. Validation
3. Comparative evaluation

When data are insufficient or when no research base to guide the APN exists, an original research approach may be needed. The research process and the research utilization process are quite similar (Table 4–3). When a sufficiently

TABLE 4–3
**The Research Process Compared with the Research
Utilization Process**

Research ← Interdependent processes →	Research utilization
Purpose: To identify and refine solutions to problems through the generation of new knowledge	*Purpose:* To get the new solutions used for the good of society; to identify need for refinement
Delimit problem.	Identify patient-care problem.
Review related literature.	Identify and assess research-based knowledge
Develop conceptual framework.	to solve problem.
Identify variables.	Design nursing practice innovation and patient outcomes based on research knowledge.
Select design.	Compare patient outcomes produced by innovation with those of existing practice.
Formulate hypothesis.	
Specify population.	Choose patient sample representative of those
Select sample.	in original research.
Develop or select instruments.	Use instruments identified in original research.
Collect data.	Conduct clinical trials.
Analyze data.	Analyze data.
Interpret results.	Decide to adopt, alter, or reject full-scale implementation of innovation.
Communicate findings.	Develop a means to extend (diffuse) the new practice and maintain it over time.

Source: Firlit, S, Kemp, MG, and Walsh, M: Preparing master's students to develop clinical trials to confirm research findings. West J Nurs Res 8:108. Copyright © 1986 by Sage Publications, Inc. Reprinted by permission of Sage Publications, Inc.

strong research base exists, the change or "innovation" can be introduced by the APN. The innovation should first be introduced on a trial basis to allow group modification and acceptance of the innovation. The APN should incorporate a sufficient evaluation plan—often a replication study in one's own setting to determine the effectiveness of the innovation to solve the identified practice problem.

The process of research utilization includes the following phases or steps[22]:

1. Identify the patient care problem.
2. Identify and assess relevant research-based knowledge.
3. Adapt and design a research-based practice innovation.
4. Conduct a trial of the innovation.
5. Decide whether to adopt, modify, or reject the innovation.
6. Develop the means to extend or diffuse the adopted innovation.
7. Develop mechanisms to maintain the innovation over time.

Models of Health Promotion

Health promotion is a goal of all nurses, but for many APNs, it is their principal goal. If the best method for predicting people's participation in health behaviors can be identified, APNs can intervene in the best ways with their clients. These are some of the models and theories that the APN might use for health education, anticipatory guidance, and health promotion.

HEALTH BELIEF MODEL

The health belief model (HBM) was developed in the 1950s to explain people's actions (or lack of actions) regarding preventive health behavior.[23] Through considerable research over the years, the HBM has been clarified and modified, and it is now used to explain or predict people's use of a broad range of health actions.[24]

The underlying assumption of the HBM is that behavior is determined more by a person's perceived reality than by the physical environment. People take actions to screen for or prevent a disease or health problem, but only to the extent that the disease exists in their perception. Further, people must have incentives for action and feel themselves capable before undertaking a given health action.[25] The current HBM is represented in Fig. 4–5. Numerous sociodemographic variables, especially education, are assumed to influence behavior indirectly, through effects on the other components.

Motivation or readiness to act is determined by three components[24]:

1. Threat
2. Outcome expectations
3. Efficacy expectations

Threat is composed of the perceived susceptibility, that is, people's subjective beliefs about their own vulnerability to develop a disease or their ability to accept the diagnosis of a disease, and their perception of the seriousness or severity of

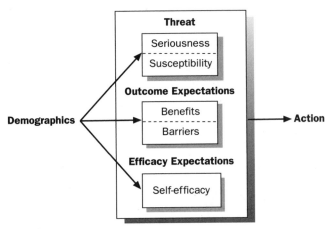

Figure 4–5.   Health belief model.

the disease and the (medical or social) consequences of the disease should it develop.

Outcome expectations are people's perceived barriers to the action minus the benefits of taking the action. Both barriers and benefits are beliefs, rather than objective facts, about the effectiveness of actions. Efficacy expectations are people's convictions about their own ability to perform the necessary health actions.

Cues to action are triggers that may promote action. Cues may be internal, such as physical symptoms, or external, such as the media or discussion with someone who has the disease. Cues to action were included in the original HBM but are no longer considered essential. Nonetheless, some researchers and clinicians believe that cues can have a direct impact on action.

The most common criticism of the HBM is that the relationship between beliefs and behavior has never been established clearly. Many studies have been conducted using the HBM to explain or predict actions as diverse as having a Pap smear, maintaining a diet, and writing a living will. The amount of variance explained differs considerably, suggesting that other factors are involved. Still, until other factors are specifically identified, many researchers and APNs will continue to use the HBM in research and to guide practice.

HEALTH PROMOTION MODEL

In an attempt to define additional variables that might explain preventive health behavior, Pender[26] took the HBM, added a number of cognitive variables, and applied it to nursing practice. As she expanded and clarified her thinking, she created the health promotion model (HPM).[27] Pender views the HPM as an organizing framework for theory development and research and acknowledges that it is continually subject to change.

The current version of the HPM is shown in Fig. 4–6. The HPM shows the great complexity involved in explaining the performance of health behaviors, and the model has increased in complexity as it has developed. Most simply, the model shows that an individual's personal biologic, psychological, and sociocul-

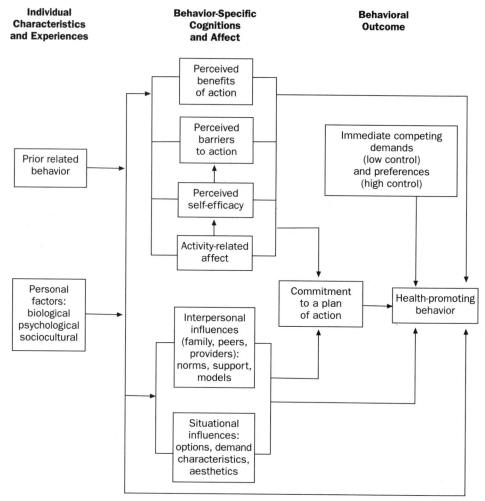

Figure 4–6. Health promotion model. (From Pender,[27] p. 67, with permission.)

tural characteristics, as well as certain behavioral and cognitive processes, are responsible for health behaviors. The boxes and arrows in the model demonstrate that the cognitive processes are interrelated, and that personal characteristics and cognitive processes may, both directly and indirectly, result in health behavior.

New variables were added to this edition of the model. Perhaps the most important new variable is commitment to a plan of action, since researchers have long questioned whether deciding to perform a behavior and actually performing a behavior are the same or different processes. Pender apparently has joined the forces of those who believe that they are unique.

To facilitate their health promotion research, Pender et al.[28] developed the Health-Promoting Lifestyle Profile (HPLP) to be used in research as a predictor variable that represents health action. The original HPLP was used in large numbers of research studies, but it too has been revised recently. The HPLP-II is a 52-item questionnaire that has been analyzed, to include six factors[27]:

1. Health responsibility
2. Physical activity
3. Nutrition
4. Interpersonal relations
5. Spiritual growth
6. Stress management

Together, these factors represent a balanced and positive approach to healthful living and wellness potential.

Both researchers and APNs can use the HPM and the HPLP-II. Researchers may use the HPLP-II as either a dependent or an independent variable. APNs can use the HPM as a framework for thinking about health behavior. They can use results of the HPLP-II to communicate specifically with clients about aspects of their health.

PRECEDE-PROCEED MODEL

The PRECEDE-PROCEED model is used for comprehensive planning in health education and health promotion with individuals and communities.[29,30] The acronym stands for *p*redisposing, *r*einforcing, and *e*nabling *c*auses in *e*ducational *d*iagnosis and *e*valuation (PRECEDE) and *p*olicy, *r*egulatory, and *o*rganizational constructs in *e*ducational and *e*nvironmental *d*evelopment (PROCEED). Although PRECEDE was developed and used before PROCEED was added, both are now integrated into a single model.

The PRECEDE portion of the model is the diagnostic phase that assists the APN in considering the many factors that influence health status and in choosing a highly focused subset of factors as the target for a health intervention.[29,30] The PROCEED phase provides steps for developing policy and for initiating the implementation and evaluation processes of the health intervention.[30]

A unique feature of the model is the concept of "beginning at the end." Instead of planning an intervention that promotes outcomes, the APN looks first at extant outcomes or the quality of life of the designated population or individual. The APN must ask "why" before "how" and, by thinking deductively, identify consequences before seeking causes. As seen in Fig. 4–7, the process is ultimately circular.

In the initial social diagnosis phase, the APN considers the general hopes or problems of the target population by having them engage in a self-assessment, which, in itself, can be an educational process. In phase 2, epidemiological diagnosis, specific health goals or problems that contribute to the issues or problems identified in phase 1 are identified. During phase 3, specific behavioral or environmental factors that could be linked with the problems established as most important in phase 2 are identified. Because these problems will be the focus of the intervention, they must be described as specifically as possible.

Phase 4 is termed the educational and organizational diagnosis. The large number of potential factors that could influence a given health behavior are identified, sorted, and categorized into three classes:

1. Predisposing factors
2. Reinforcing factors
3. Enabling factors

Precede

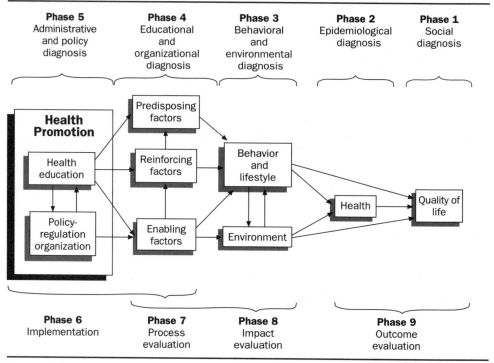

Figure 4–7. PRECEDE-PROCEED model. (From Green and Kreuter,[30] p. 24, with permission.)

Predisposing factors are those attitudes, values, perceptions, and knowledge that foster or inhibit motivation for change. Enabling factors are those skills and resources that make possible behavioral or environmental changes. Barriers to change must also be considered, because some resources (e.g., laws) may either foster or inhibit changes. Reinforcing factors include the rewards and feedback received after adoption of a change. As with enabling factors, there are some reinforcing factors (e.g., weight gain) that can encourage or discourage continuation of a change.

In phase 5, the APN assesses the resources, policies, abilities, and constraints of the situation or organization, then selects the best combination of methods and strategies to be implemented in phase 6. Although various types of evaluation are noted for phases 7 through 9, evaluation is a continuous process throughout the model.

PRECEDE-PROCEED can be used in community, workplace, and medical-care settings. PRECEDE has been used for health education programs of many types and in numerous settings. PRECEDE-PROCEED has been used in programs to decrease blood pressure and to stop smoking. Green and Kreuter[30] suggested that using the whole model makes planning and evaluation of health promotion programs more efficient and effective.

THEORY OF CARE-SEEKING BEHAVIOR

A more recent theory for health promotion is the theory of care-seeking behavior (CSB) developed by Lauver[31] and based on the concepts from Triandis's theory

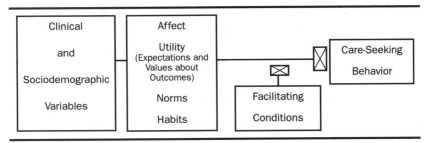

Figure 4–8. Care-seeking behavior model. (From Lauver,[31] p. 281, with permission.)

of behavior. According to the CSB theory, engaging in health-care behavior is a function of the psychosocial variables of affect, utility, norms, and habits, which may be influenced by facilitating conditions (e.g., insurance and having a regular health provider). Clinical and sociodemographic variables, such as the presence of symptoms or age, do not influence behavior directly but may influence the psychosocial variables (Fig. 4–8). *Affect* refers to feelings, *utility* (i.e., expectations and values about outcomes of care) refers to one's own beliefs, *norms* refer to others' beliefs; and *habits* refer to one's usual actions concerning a proposed health behavior.[32]

Empirical research findings from a number of studies support the individual relationships proposed in the CSB theory for secondary prevention, such as cancer screening.[31,32] The CSB theory is similar to HBM and HPM theories, although it uses fewer variables to explain behavior, which can be an advantage for both research and practice if the CSB can be shown to predict behavior. Still, like HBM and HPM, there are very few studies that have examined all of the possible variables and all of the relationships within a single study. If APNs use CSB, HBM, or HPM, their clinical experiences can give support for the theory, which can then be further developed in research.

Models of Advanced Practice Nursing

Models and theories of advanced practice nursing describe primarily who an APN is and/or what an APN does. In comparison to leadership, teaching-learning, and change theories, the models of advanced practice are relatively new and are more descriptive than predictive level theories.

NOVICE TO EXPERT

Benner's novice-to-expert theory[33] may be the most familiar theory of advanced practice nursing. However, what Benner really describes is expert nursing[33] rather than advanced practice nursing. Nonetheless, the expert nurse may very well be an APN.

Benner's theory[33] was based on Dreyfus's model of skill acquisition, in which increments of change occur with increases in skilled performance, based on education and experience. Three kinds of changes occur with increasing levels of proficiency:

1. There is movement from reliance on abstract principles to the use of past concrete experiences as paradigms.

2. Perception of situation changes so that a situation is seen less as a compilation of equally relevant bits and more as a complete whole in which only certain parts are relevant.

3. The person changes from a detached observer to an engaged and involved performer.

Benner identified five levels of performance for nursing:

1. Novice
2. Advanced beginner
3. Competent
4. Proficient
5. Expert

Novices, with no experience in situations in which they are expected to perform, are focused only on rules and are unable to use discretionary judgment. Advanced beginners demonstrate marginally acceptable performance. Advanced beginners have had enough experience to recognize (or to see when pointed out by a mentor or instructor) the recurrent characteristics of a situation, but cannot make those characteristics objective nor differentiate importance among them. Advanced beginners operate on general guidelines or standards of care and are beginning to recognize recurrent patterns in clinical practice.

Competent nurses begin to see their actions in terms of long-range goals or plans. Competent nurses establish plans using considerable conscious, abstract, and analytic consideration of problems. However, their use of plans also limits awareness of the situation because they are focused on the plan rather than on the whole situation. Competent nurses feel a sense of mastery and the ability to cope with and manage the many contingencies of clinical nursing. They become efficient and organized. This level of competence is often viewed as ideal.

Proficient nurses continue to move forward with a vision of what is possible. Proficient nurses perceive situations as wholes rather than as parts, and their performance is guided by maxims, which are developed over time through a deep understanding of the situation. Proficient nurses know what to expect from a given situation, quickly recognize when a situation is different, and know how to modify plans when a situation varies from the expected. They acquire a perspective about the important attributes and characteristics of a situation and use fewer options while developing focus for the most important aspects of situations.

Proficiency marks the transition from competence to expertise.[34] A transformation occurs between the competent nurse and the two higher levels of performance. Proficient (and expert) nurses use past concrete experiences to guide their analyses of present situations in a way that competent nurses do not.

Expert nurses do not rely on analytic principles to connect their understanding of a situation to an appropriate action. Experts use their vast background of experience and intuitive grasp of situations to focus immediately on the accurate range of problems without wasting effort and time on a large range of unlikely possible solutions. Experts see what needs to be accomplished and how to accomplish it. They operate from a deep understanding of situations and often cannot clearly describe the rationale for their actions. What experts can describe with clarity are the goals established and the outcomes achieved.

From the descriptions of nurses about their practices, Benner[33] identified seven domains of nursing practice:

1. The helping role
2. The teaching-coaching function
3. The diagnostic and patient-monitoring function
4. The effective management of rapidly changing situations
5. The administration and monitoring of therapeutic interventions and regimens
6. The monitoring and assuring of quality of health-care practices
7. The implementation of organizational and work-role competencies

In their continuing research and development of the novice-to-expert theory, Benner and her colleagues explore the complexity of clinical judgment and caring practices.[34] A limitation of Benner's work for use by APNs is the fact that the research has been limited to hospital nurses, and particularly critical care nurses. Because the essential content of the model is embedded in clinical examples, the APNs must be able to extrapolate from the examples and to apply the content to their own practices.

ADVANCED NURSING PRACTICE

Calkin[35] described a model of advanced nursing practice, defining advanced practice as that enacted by nurses with master's degrees. Calkin used the 1980 American Nurses' Association definition of nursing: the "diagnosis and treatment of human responses to actual or potential health problems," as the basis for differentiating advanced practice from other levels of practice.

Calkin[35] describes three levels of practice:

1. Novice
2. Expert-by-experience
3. Advanced

Novices, or beginning nurses, can manage only a narrow range of usual or average human responses. Because of the knowledge that they bring to the clinical situation from their educational programs, Calkin suggested that novices have greater knowledge than skill. That is, they are more comfortable with the science of nursing than with the art of nursing.

Experts-by-experience are those nurses who have excelled in their ability to diagnose and treat human responses. They are able to identify and intervene in a much wider range of human responses than novices. Calkin said experts-by-experience may intuit much of their skill and may be unable to explain their actions. Nonetheless, they provide skillful care, having developed skill greater than knowledge.

Advanced practice nurses are those able to manage the fullest range of human responses that is closest to the actual range of potential responses. This ability develops as a result of the specialized knowledge and skills they acquired through education as and experience. They can identify and intervene in the extremes of responses and in unpredictable as well as in predictable situations.

Calkin[35] suggested that APNs use deliberation and reasoning more than intuition when diagnosing and treating. She argued that APNs articulate about nursing, use reasoning to deal with practice innovations, and develop or contribute to newer forms of practice. They do not focus on tasks and skills.

DIFFERENTIATED PRACTICE

Differentiated practice is another approach to describing the differences between levels of nursing practice. Koerner[36] described three levels of practice based on education:

1. Associate degree
2. Baccalaureate degree
3. Master's degree

In her integrated model, competency can be achieved at each level of nursing practice, so long as the differentiated roles are clear.

The associate-degreed nurse provides care for a specified period of time and/or in structured settings with established policies and procedures. The baccalaureate-degreed nurse provides integrated health care from preadmission through postdischarge in structured and unstructured settings and/or in environments that may not have established policies and procedures. The master's-degreed APN provides leadership that promotes holistic patient outcomes, functions in a variety of dynamic settings, and uses independent nursing judgment based on theory, research, and specialized knowledge. Koerner[36] discussed the importance of mutual valuing, partnerships, and collegiality among nurses at all levels and suggested that at each level, the nurse can be an expert. Koerner further suggested that APNs support professional development by focusing on contextual and environmental issues more than the other levels of nurses do, and APNs have more career options.

COMPARISON OF ADVANCED PRACTICE MODELS

Advanced practice models for nursing practice consider two factors:

1. Education
2. Experience

Advanced practice requires a minimum of a master's-degree education. Both Koerner[36] and Calkin[35] base their models on educational preparation and define advanced practice as master's preparation. Advanced practice also requires experience in nursing, beyond that of newly graduated registered nurses, even if the experience is limited to that required for completion of the master's educational program. There is no novice APN.

Advanced practice nursing is not the same as expert nursing practice. Though Calkin[35] equated her expert level with that of Benner,[33] we believe that any nurse at any level can be an expert practitioner, but APNs are distinguished by the master's degree. Benner's model[33] was developed through research with practicing clinical nurses and reveals much about what nursing practice includes. Nurses practicing in any setting for a long enough period may become expert in that role. It is our contention that Benner's model can be applied to any nurse in any kind of practice, regardless of educational level. The level of expertise develops with experience as well as with education.

Leadership is not explicitly described by either Benner[33] or Calkin.[35] It is, however, implicit in Benner's domains of nursing practice, especially those dealing with teaching, managing, monitoring, and organizing. Leadership also is inherent in Calkin's advanced nursing practice, because it is based on deliberative action that requires specialized skill and rationale. Leadership is an explicit part of the role of Koerner's APN. [36] APNs use leadership in all of their actions, by making judgments based on theory, research, and specialized knowledge.

Summary

In each of the leadership, teaching-learning, and change models and theories, assessment of the group members is key to choosing the specific approach or style the APN would use. Assessment of the situation or organization is also necessary, so that the APN can focus on goals appropriate for individuals in that setting. Finally, the relationship between the APN and the group members is critical to achieving any desired goal, such as health promotion.

Suggested Exercises

1. Select one of the theories of leadership presented in this chapter. Specify the variables that you would assess to determine an effective style of leadership to enact in your practice.

2. Construct two teaching-learning plans on the same topic, one plan directed to a professional audience and the other to a client audience. How would these two plans differ with regard to the following:

   a. Intended audience and setting in which teaching would occur

   b. Objectives

   c. Content

   d. Teaching aids

   e. Evaluation

3. Analyze a change that occurred in your organization. Was the change planned or unplanned? Who was the change agent? What strategies were used by the change agent? Evaluate the effectiveness of the strategies and suggest alternatives.

4. Identify a needed change in your organization. What are the driving and restraining forces that will enable or prevent the change? Develop a prospectus for planned change that takes into account the identified forces. Role-play with student colleagues and present your prospectus to them; convince them of the soundness of your plan.

5. Discuss a problem in clinical practice. Plan a course of action to determine if a research base exists that could be used to solve the problem. Propose a clinical trial of the research-based solution.

6. Form into teams. Create a health promotion clinical scenario or describe one in which you were involved. Detail all important factors in one of the health promotion models and describe a plan for implementation. Present your work to your student colleagues and have them critique your interpretation.

7. Analyze the similarities and differences between the Calkin and Benner models. Are these models sequential and of what importance is this? Describe how one might apply the models to your practice situation.

8. Consider how the Calkin and Benner models relate to the concept of leadership described in the introductory chapter. Sketch the parallels among key ideas. Again, how do the models relate to those of change presented in this chapter? Create a comparison chart.

9. Calkin described the APN role and compared it to other levels of nursing practice. A nurse colleague declares to you that "there is little or no difference between you and me in the way you practice and what you can capably perform. Just compare my 15 years of practice and experience to your education and credentials." Respond as Calkin would by identifying major characteristics of advanced nursing practice, and relate Calkin's ideas to the need and justification for your role.

REFERENCES

1. Bernhard, LA, and Walsh, M: Leadership: The Key to the Professionalization of Nursing, ed 3. Mosby, St. Louis, 1995.
2. McGregor, D: The Human Side of Enterprise. McGraw-Hill, New York, 1960.
3. Fleishman, EA: Twenty years of consideration and structure. In Fleishman, EA, and Hunt, JG (eds): Current Developments in the Study of Leadership. Southern Illinois University Press, Carbondale, Ill, 1973.
4. Fleishman, EA, and Harris, EF: Patterns of leadership behavior related to employee grievances and turnover. Personnel Psychology 15:43, 1962.
5. Stogdill, RN: Handbook of Leadership: A Survey of Theory and Research. Free Press, New York, 1974.
6. Korman, AK: "Consideration," "initiating structure," and organizational criteria: A review. Personnel Psychology 19:349, 1966.
7. Evans, MG: The effects of supervisory behavior on the path-goal relationship. Organizational Behavior and Human Performance 5:277, 1970.
8. Davis, K, and Newstrom, JW: Human Behavior at Work: Organizational Behavior, ed 7. McGraw-Hill, New York, 1985.
9. Fiedler, FE: A Theory of Leadership Effectiveness. McGraw-Hill, New York, 1967.
10. Fiedler, FE, and Chemers, MM: Leadership and Effective Management. Scott, Foresman, Glenview, Ill, 1974.
11. Fiedler, FE: The trouble with leadership training is that it doesn't train leaders. Psychology Today 6:23, 1973.
12. Fiedler, FE, and Garcia, JE: New Approaches to Effective Leadership: Cognitive Resources and Organizational Performance. John Wiley & Sons, New York, 1987.
13. Hersey, P, and Blanchard, KH: Management of Organizational Behavior: Utilizing Human Resources, ed 5. Prentice-Hall, Englewood Cliffs, NJ, 1988.
14. Bower, GH, and Hilgard, ER: Theories of Learning, ed 5. Prentice-Hall, Englewood Cliffs, NJ, 1981.
15. Bigge, ML: Learning Theories for Teachers, ed 4. Harper & Row, New York, 1982.
16. Skinner, BF: The Technology of Teaching. Appleton-Century-Crofts, New York, 1968.
17. Cantor, N: The Teaching-Learning Process. Dryden, New York, 1953.
18. Rogers, CR: Freedom to Learn for the 80s. Merrill, Columbus, Ohio, 1983.
19. Lewin, K: Field Theory in Social Science. Harper, New York, 1951.
20. Chin, R, and Benne, KD: General strategies for effecting change in human systems. In Bennis, WG, Benne, KD, and Chin R (eds):

The Planning of Change, ed 4. Holt, Rinehart, and Winston, New York, 1985.

21. Stetler, CB: Refinement of the Stetler / Marram Model for application of research findings to practice. Nurs Outlook 42:15, 1994.

22. Horsley, J, et al: Using Research to Improve Nursing Practice: A Guide. Orlando, Fla, Grune and Stratton, 1983.

23. Rosenstock, IM: Why people use health services. Milbank Memorial Fund Quarterly 44: 94, 1966.

24. Rosenstock, IM: The health belief model: Explaining health behavior through expectancies. In Glanz, K, Lewis, FM, and Riner, BK (eds): Health Behavior and Health Education. Jossey-Bass, San Francisco, 1990.

25. Rosenstock, IM, Strecher, VJ, and Becker, MH: Social learning theory and the Health Belief Model. Health Educ Q 15:175, 1988.

26. Pender, N: A conceptual model for preventive health behavior. Nurs Outlook 23:385, 1975.

27. Pender, NJ: Health Promotion in Nursing Practice, ed 3. Appleton & Lange, Stamford, Conn, 1996.

28. Walker, SN, Sechrist, KR, and Pender, NJ: The health-promoting lifestyle profile: Development and psychometric characteristics. Nurs Res 36:76, 1987.

29. Green, LW, et al: Health Education Planning: A Diagnostic Approach. Mayfield, Palo Alto, Calif, 1980.

30. Green, LW, and Kreuter, MW: Health promotion planning: An educational and environmental approach, ed 2. Mayfield, Mountain View, Calif, 1991.

31. Lauver, D: A theory of care seeking behavior. Image J Nurs Sch 24:281, 1992.

32. Lauver, D: Psychosocial variables, race, and intention to seek care for breast cancer symptoms. Nurs Res 41:236, 1992.

33. Benner, P: From Novice to Expert. Addison-Wesley, Menlo Park, Calif, 1984.

34. Benner, PA, Tanner, CA, and Chesla, CA: Expertise in Nursing Practice. Springer, New York, 1996.

35. Calkin, JD: A model for advanced nursing practice. J Nurs Adm 14:24, 1984.

36. Koerner, J: Differentiated practice: The evolution of professional nursing. J Prof Nurs 8:335, 1992.

Primary Care and Advanced Practice Nursing: Past, Present, and Future

LINDA LINDSEY DAVIS, PhD, RN, ANP
CATHERINE L. GILLISS, DNSc, RN, CS, FAAN

Linda Lindsey Davis, PhD, RN, ANP, is a professor of nursing at the University of Alabama at Birmingham (UAB) and senior scientist in the UAB Center for Aging. Dr. Davis is an adult nurse practitioner and a distinguished practitioner in the US National Academy of Practice (Nursing). Dr. Davis holds a doctorate in nursing from the University of Maryland at Baltimore, a master's of science in nursing from the University of North Carolina at Chapel Hill, and a bachelor's in nursing from Old Dominion University in Norfolk, Virginia. Dr. Davis's work is in primary and long-term health care for families and family caregiving for the aged. Dr. Davis worked with the American Association of Retired Persons and Alabama State Health Department representatives in developing a community-based health-maintenance project for homebound elderly in Birmingham. She currently is the principal investigator for a project entitled Telephone-based Skill Training for Alzheimer's and Related Dementias Caregivers, funded by the UAB Alzheimer's Disease Center.

Catherine L. Gilliss, DNSc, RN, CS, FAAN, is a professor of nursing at the University of California at San Francisco (UCSF), where she chairs the Department of Family Health Care Nursing. Since 1989, she has also coordinated the UCSF's Primary Care Nurse Practitioner Program, the largest graduate primary care nurse practitioner program in the nation. In 1994, the program was recognized by the Pew Health Professions Commission with honorable mention for the Excellence in Primary Care Education Award. In 1995, the program was recognized as the winner of the award in the educational program category. Dr. Gilliss received her undergraduate nursing education at Duke University and has been honored by Duke's School of Nursing as a distinguish alumna. She earned her master's degree in psychiatric–mental health nursing from The Catholic University of America and an adult nurse practitioner certificate from the University of Rochester. She completed her doctoral and postdoctoral work at the UCSF's School of Nursing. In 1993, she was a fellow in the U.S. Public Health Service's Primary Care Policy Fellowship program. Her research interests include families and chronic illness and the development of the primary-care workforce. An elected fellow in the American Academy of Nursing, Dr.

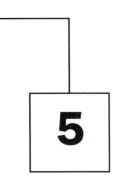

5

Gilliss serves on the boards of several professional societies and journals. She is now the president of the Interdisciplinary Primary Care Fellowship Society, the immediate past president of the National Organization of Nurse Practitioner Faculties, and a regent at the University of Portland (Oregon).

CHAPTER OBJECTIVES

After completing this chapter, the reader will be able to:

1. Analyze socioeconomic and political forces contributing to a renewed interest in the development of primary-care systems in the United States.
2. Synthesize the implications of various health-care manpower projections for emerging primary-care systems in the twenty-first century.
3. Weigh the advantages and disadvantages of using the following methods for evaluating advanced practice nursing in primary-care settings:
   a. Classification of patient encounters
   b. Comparison in standards of care
   c. Documentation of functions of primary care
4. Explore facilitating and inhibiting factors influencing advanced practice nursing in emerging primary-care systems.
5. Articulate a personal philosophy on the nature and scope of advanced practice nursing skills and primary-care services.

Although governmental efforts in the mid-1990s failed to bring about health-care reform, the American health-care system is rapidly implementing many of the proposed changes. While access, quality, and service fragmentation continue to drive the development of alternative health-care delivery models in some areas of the United States, many areas are now responding to insurance-industry-based changes that have restructured the delivery of care. As the twentieth century draws to a close, the focus on reducing the high cost of health care while capturing a profit through managed-care delivery has led to a renewed interest in primary-care systems. This chapter provides an overview of the social, political, and economic issues that have stimulated this resurgent focus on primary care and the factors that will facilitate and inhibit the participation of advanced practice nurses (APNs) in primary-care systems into the next century.

Health Care in the Twentieth Century

In hierarchical health-care systems, **primary care** is the term used to describe basic services on which other, more specialized services are built. Presumably, primary-care systems can handle as much as 99 percent of the health problems in a community.[1] In 1978, the World Health Organization proposed that primary health care, designed to bring accessible, economical care into communities where people live and work, should be a basic component of every country's health-care system.[2] Primary care is considered the necessary foundation for health care in the majority of industrialized nations, with the United States being a notable exception. The U.S. health-care system has been described as a pluralistic, overlapping collection of practitioners providing different aspects of care in a variety of settings.[3] The late twentieth century witnessed a growing dissatisfaction with U.S. health care, described by many as:

- *Disease-focused,* concerned more with the technology of medical diagnosis and treatment of specific diseases, rather than with holistic health care
- *Fragmented,* so that patients and their families receive uncoordinated, episodic treatment from various specialists for their health problems
- *Inaccessible,* in that services and providers are located primarily in urban population centers, creating pockets of unserved or underserved areas in rural towns and inner cities
- *Costly,* in that many people, particularly elderly persons, minorities, and the poor are unable to afford needed health-care services, creating growing numbers of underinsured and uninsured Americans

Health Care in the Twenty-first Century

Because health-care costs under the current system are projected to reach 20 percent of the gross national product by the year 2000, solutions to the problems in the American health-care system are increasingly defined in economic terms.[4] The increasing numbers of individuals, families, and communities enrolled in health-maintenance organizations (HMOs), the cost savings demonstrated by new managed-care models, and the growing competition between large and small, public and private health-care organizations will contribute to making the U.S. health-care system a buyer's market by the twenty-first century. In part, as a result of these and similar situations, changes in the system that will occur during the next decade will include the following[5-9]:

- Downsizing or closure of many hospitals nationwide
- Increased emphasis on disease prevention and health promotion, both for cost savings to the system as well as for quality-of-life benefits to consumers
- Development of health-care partnerships between medical centers and corporate and business entities to deliver the most economical health care for enrolled and prepaid populations
- Utilization of health-outcome data as justification for spending health-care dollars
- Significant expansion of primary care in ambulatory and community-based settings
- Sweeping changes in the education and practice of health professionals to staff these emerging primary-care systems

For more than 30 years, health-care providers, educators, and policy makers in the United States have described primary care as an economical strategy for increasing consumer access to a broad range of holistic and humanistic services. To many, building more primary-care systems in the United States represents a logical solution to longstanding problems that have troubled the American health-care delivery system in the past: unequal access, rising costs, fragmentation, and overemphasis on medical technology.

The Nature of Primary Care

DEFINITIONS OF PRIMARY CARE

Definitions of primary care have evolved over time. White[10] defined primary care as first-contact care. Alpert and Charney[11] added that primary-care medicine involves longitudinal responsibility for a patient, including integration of both health and disease services. In 1978, the Institute of Medicine[12] (IOM) defined primary care as having the functions of improved accessibility, continuity, comprehensiveness, coordination, and accountability. Golden[13] reported that primary care is characterized by long-term, close relationships between practitioner and patient and family, in which the primary-care provider treats common and acute illnesses, with referral to specialists of patients with less frequently occurring and more complex problems. Starfield[14] summarized the four key functions of primary care:

1. *First contacts*, in which services are timely, accessible, and available at the point of entry into the system
2. *Longitudinal*, in that services, organized to focus on the patient and not the illness, are provided to the patient by the same provider over time
3. *Comprehensive*, in that a broad range of services are offered by the provider
4. *Coordinated*, in that a single provider organizes information related to patient referral, procedures, and therapies to improve the continuity and quality of care

More recently, the IOM[15] re-examined early definitions of primary care as a first step toward projecting the future of health care in the United States. The revised IOM definition includes many of the elements originally introduced but added a focus on the family and community contexts in which care should be provided:

> Primary care is the provision of integrated, accessible health care services by clinicians who are accountable for addressing a large majority of personal health care needs, developing a sustained partnership with patients, and practicing in the context of family and community. (p. 16)

CONTENT OF PRIMARY CARE

Based on the most recently published IOM definition, a number of assumptions can be made about the nature of primary care. Integrated primary care must include consideration of the total person—body and mind—as well as the context in which care occurs. Accessible care must be personalized according to the needs of individuals within their communities. The majority of primary care includes both episodic and ongoing services. A sustained partnership between primary-care provider and patient over the life cycle implies the provider's need for knowledge about biomedical health problems, social sciences (including personal, interpersonal, and larger social systems), and the way to work successfully with other providers in interdisciplinary practice teams. Given the socioeconomic and political contexts in which primary care is practiced today, providers also need to understand expected and desired outcomes of care based on normative evidence and the particular client's situation. The sophistication required to accomplish these expectations cannot be overestimated.

GENERALIST VERSUS SPECIALIST CARE

The most recent IOM definition of primary care suggests that there are significant distinctions to be made between generalist and specialist care. Primary care involves the delivery of health-care services by generalist practitioners, with referral of patients to specialists for complex health problems. Table 5–1 shows examples of generalist services delivered by primary care providers. The characteristics, processes, and goals of generalist and specialist care are not the same. The goal of specialty practice is to cure or treat a specific problem, disease, or illness. The goal of generalist care is health promotion, prevention of disease or illness, and amelioration of symptoms.[13] Table 5–2 compares generalist with specialist care.

According to Starfield,[14] the nature of hospital-based education and practice makes it difficult for specialists to provide the key components of primary care described earlier. First-contact primary care typically occurs early in the natural history of a health problem, when evolving signs and symptoms cannot easily be tied to a specific disease or illness. In addition, because many of the presenting problems seen in primary-care settings can be traced to stressful personal, familial, or environmental factors, counseling and affective support often are the major treatment components. Hospital-based training and practice do not provide experiences and necessary skills for managing the physical, psychological, or social problems that commonly are presented in primary-care settings (e.g., individual patient problems such as stress reaction, vague anxiety and confusion, family turmoil relating to marital conflict or adolescent crises, alcohol or other

TABLE 5–1
Examples of Primary Care Services

- Preventive care and screening
- Health and nutrition education and counseling
- History taking
- Physical examination
- Diagnostic testing
- Prescription and management of drug therapy
- Prenatal care and delivery of normal pregnancies
- Well-baby care
- Diagnosis and treatment of common health problems and minor injuries
- Diagnosis and treatment of chronic conditions
- Minor surgery
- Coordination of services and referral for specialty care when needed

Source: Adapted from The Alliance for Health Reform: *A Primary Care Primer*, The Alliance for Health Reform, Washington, DC, 1993, p 14, with permission.

substance abuse, divorce or death or dying of a family member). Because of the time spent in developing and implementing successful interventions for managing these and similar primary-care problems, specialist providers often have less time to see specialty patients and less time to stay current on new knowledge and discoveries in their specialties. Finally, primary-care delivery is difficult for a specialist because few specialists have the educational preparation, background experiences, or skills to perform the time-consuming but necessary function of coordinating services provided by others.

EVALUATION OF PRIMARY CARE

There are numerous approaches to evaluating clinical services. Three methods that have potential for documenting the nature and scope of advanced nursing practice in primary-care systems are:

1. Classification of patient encounters
2. Comparison in standards of care
3. Documentation of functions of primary care

TABLE 5–2
Specialist Versus Generalist Services

Service Characteristic	Specialist Care	Generalist Care
Nature of service	**Scope of services:** management of specific, complex problems	**Scope of services:** management of varied problems, needs
Focus of service	Problem-focused, short-term, episodic service for diagnosis and treatment of specific problem	Patient-focused, long-term, continuous delivery of services
Role of service provider	Direct-care provider	Direct-care provider, plus plan and coordinate service delivery provided by others

A brief description of the three methods and an example of a recent study using each method demonstrate their usefulness for evaluating advanced nursing practice in primary-care settings.

Classification of Patient Encounters

Patient encounters are classified according to whether visits are first encounters, encounters for continuing care by the same provider, encounters for ongoing, nonspecialized services, or encounters for consultation and referral to a specialist. Alternatively, visits are classified according to whether they are primarily for health screening or prevention, for health promotion, for management of a specific illness (acute or chronic), or for referrals to specialized services not available in the primary-care setting.

Most of the information on patient encounters in primary-care settings comes from data collected through the periodic National Ambulatory Care Survey.[16] The NACS is an ongoing survey of community-based physicians stratified by specialty and by geographic regions in the United States. Conducted annually since 1990, the survey data continue to demonstrate that the majority of visits to U.S. physicians by individuals in all age groups is for management of specific symptoms, the most common being that of colds. Screening or preventive services rank below symptom management as the common reason for patient encounters with a primary-care physician.[16] The NACS's exclusive focus on physicians does not permit characterization of patient encounters with nonphysician providers. A more widely defined focus would be useful in classifying APN encounters with patients in primary-care settings.

Classification of encounters provides a typology of service needs and of services delivered. Classification of the purposes of patient encounters allows providers and administrators to identify individual and family services needs within a target population. Classification of patient encounters according to the predominant focus of each encounter also enables evaluators in multidisciplinary settings to determine which member of the multidisciplinary team is providing those services. By classifying the encounter, evaluators are able to determine whether physicians are providing most of the illness-management services and/or whether nurse practitioners (NPs) are providing most of the health-screening procedures.

This method also enables evaluators to analyze the nature of service referrals. For example, the evaluator may wish to know whether providers are referring emotional or social problems outside the primary-care setting, even though competent care providers are available in that setting. Finally, a frequency count of the types of services offered can assist in determining whether staff continuing education is needed. However, classification of patient encounters by service need and service frequency does not assess quality of care.

Comparison in Standards of Care

With the standards-of-care method, patient encounters are analyzed to determine whether they meet commonly accepted standards for quality of care, such as the appropriate use of diagnostic tests, the accurate recognition of the patient problems, selection and implementation of an acceptable regimen for treatment, documentation of plans for patient education, and follow-up care. Given the current emphasis on patient outcome data, this evaluation method enables evaluators to compare *actual* patient outcomes with *expected* patient outcomes.

A good example of a study of compliance with commonly accepted standards of care in primary-care practice may be found in the work of Avorn, Everitt, and Baker.[17] These investigators compared 501 practicing physicians and 298 practicing NPs in their approach to a patient presenting with epigastric pain. Using a case vignette of a patient presenting with a history of aspirin, coffee, cigarette, and alcohol use plus severe psychological stress and the negative results of an endoscopy, the investigators compared the reported treatment decisions of the two types of providers. An analysis of the reported practices of the two provider groups indicated that nearly half of the physician sample recommended immediate treatment of the hypothetical patient with medication, whereas only 20 percent of the NPs recommended immediate medication as the desirable action. Investigators found that the physician sample more often omitted the standard practice of collecting an adequate medical history. In contrast, the NP group more often recommended a more extensive medical history before making a treatment choice and, when making treatment choices, more frequently began with nonpharmacologic interventions. These findings led investigators to conclude that the medical providers were less likely to comply with standard history-taking procedures. While this study relied on the responses of two types of providers regarding their actual practice activities, the results indicate a significant difference in physician and NP practice activities. This method has great potential for further exploration of APN adherence to quality-of-care standards.

Comparing practice activities against commonly accepted standards for care is a useful assessment of the quality of patient care. Evaluation of compliance with quality-of-care studies also is useful to identify continuing education needs among providers. The Avorn, Everitt, and Baker study[17] recommended enhanced physician continuing education about the importance of extensive history taking before initiating a treatment regimen.

The standards-of-care method would be particularly useful for documenting the quality of care delivered by APNs in primary-care settings. However, this evaluation method does not document whether desirable primary-care functions, as described earlier, are present in the practices of providers.

Documentation of Functions of Primary Care

Documentation of functions of primary care assesses whether selected primary-care characteristics are present in the care delivered. For example, patient encounters might be analyzed and given a score based on whether the encounters are longitudinal, comprehensive, and coordinated. As managed-care models continue to proliferate, evaluation studies that document the existence of functions believed to demonstrate the advantages of primary care will likely become more commonplace. An example of a study of how provider characteristics can influence care delivery demonstrates the potential of this method for documenting the advantages of advanced nursing practice in primary care.

As part of a larger study of medical outcomes in the United States, Safran, Tarlov, and Rogers[18] documented primary-care characteristics in the care provided to 1208 patients by physicians. The physicians practiced in either traditional fee-for-service care plans or were employed by HMOs or independent practice associations (IPAs). Patients with one of four conditions—hypertension, diabetes, congestive heart failure, or recent myocardial infarction—were asked to complete a series of questionnaires about whether the care they received over a 2-year period had the characteristics of:

- Accountability (interpersonal and technical)
- Accessibility (financial and organizational)
- Continuity and comprehensiveness
- Coordination

TABLE 5–3
Three Approaches to Evaluating Primary-Care Services

Method	Purpose of Evaluation	Examples of Evaluation Data	Strengths/Limitations of Methods
Classification of patient encounters	Determine the nature and scope of services provided.	Classification of patient visits according to a purpose, such as screening, management of disease, or consultation	• Helpful for determining needs of target population • Useful for determining staffing needs • Useful for staff continuing education • Not useful in assessing quality of services provided
Comparison on standards of care	Compare services provided against accepted standards for quality of care.	Comparison of encounter against known standards of care for problem, such as: • Problem identification • Use of diagnostic tests • Treatment regimen • Patient education	• Useful in assessing quality of specific services • Useful for staff continuing education • Not helpful in considering the unique characteristics of primary care
Documentation of functions of primary care	Document the presence or absence of functional characteristics of high-quality primary care.	• Use of setting for first contact • Length of relationship with one care provider for longitudinality • Documentation of results of referrals in patient records for coordination • Evidence that a variety of patient problems are managed for comprehensiveness	• Useful in assessing whether key primary-care functions are present in patient encounters • Not useful in assessing quality of care

Patients who received care through the HMO or IPA model reported greater financial accessibility and better coordination of care. However, those patients who received care through a traditional fee-for-service (private practice) model reported greater continuity and better organizational access and provider accountability. Investigators concluded from these mixed findings that the orientation of individual practitioners influences the characteristic nature of the services provided.

The documented-characteristics evaluation method can also be used to identify the presence of other functions considered to be exemplary of high-quality primary care (e.g., the family-centered nature of a patient encounter, the use of existing community-based resources for referrals, and so forth). This method also would be useful in determining whether advanced practice in primary-care settings demonstrates the desired function of primary-care contacts. Table 5–3 outlines the three different approaches to evaluation of primary care. Because each of these common approaches to primary-care evaluation has both strengths and limitations, some combination of the three likely would provide the best assessment of the nature, scope, and quality of care and of the unique characteristics of advanced nursing practice in primary-care settings.

Primary-Care Providers in the Twenty-first Century

The rapid and successful growth of managed-care plans in the last decade has stimulated considerable discussion about who will provide care in the emerging health-care delivery systems. Successful efforts in building a primary health-care delivery system, to a great extent, depend on the number and types of health-care generalists needed for delivery of services; the availability and ideal mix of providers; and the incentives, benefits of, and barriers to practice.

PHYSICIANS AS PRIMARY-CARE PROVIDERS

Although there is general agreement that by the year 2000, 50 percent of practicing physicians should be primary-care generalists (i.e., practitioners in family practice, internal medicine, or pediatrics), contemporary medical practice continues to focus largely on specialty care. Despite forecasts of major changes in medical education and practice, the number of physicians seeking to enter specialty practice continues to increase and the number choosing generalist practice continues to decline.[19] Yet the need for new medical specialists is considered to be limited. Unless major changes occur in physician education and practice, it is estimated that by the year 2000, the number of medical specialists in the United States will exceed the demand for specialty services by more than 60 percent.[20] There are two competing predictions about the supply of primary-care physicians for the next decade: either that there will be a *deficit* of primary-care physicians or that there will be an *adequate supply* of primary-care physicians.

The Physician Supply Deficit Prediction

Critics have identified several organizational factors that discourage the rapid shift of medical education and practice from hospital-based specialty care to community-based, generalist care. First, as secondary and tertiary settings, hospitals and health science centers provide the necessary technological support for medical-specialist education and practice. Second, existing mechanisms for medical-student education funding continue to favor specialty practice. The majority of medical-student education occurs traditionally in hospitals, with more than 80 percent of the cost of medical-resident training covered by the provision of inpatient clinical services. Last, because primary-care residencies typically generate less clinical revenue than specialty residencies, many teaching hospitals have been reluctant to reduce specialty residencies in exchange for an increase in the number of generalist-care residencies.[21]

Efforts to increase the number of medical primary care providers in the United States have concentrated on providing incentives for medical schools to establish more family-practice training and residency programs and to encourage more new physicians to choose the generalist practice option.[11,14,19] Despite incentives that favor medical-school applicants with a stated interest in generalist practice, which increases medical students' exposure to primary-care and generalist practice by way of more community-based education and residency training, and despite offering student loan forgiveness for those choosing primary care, the number of new graduates entering specialty practice has remained constant.[22] Levinsky[23] speculated that primary-care practice will continue to be unattractive to physicians for several reasons:

- *Lack of financial incentives,* because the annual income of generalist physicians is typically 40 to 60 percent less than that of specialists

- *Reduced satisfaction with the physician-patient relationship,* which many physicians relate to the loss of practice autonomy as physicians become employees of managed-care practices

- *The large number of "unsatisfying" patients seen in primary-care settings* (i.e., elderly, poor, HIV-positive, and substance-abuse patients and others for whom medical treatment options are limited and long-term, successful medical outcomes are unlikely)

The Adequate Physician Supply Prediction

More optimistic forecasters predict that the same market issues catalyzing change in the health-care system during last decade will ultimately bring about the necessary refocusing of medical education and practice. Iglehart[24] has noted that, as academic health science centers find themselves increasingly in competition with HMOs and other providers of comprehensive services, attempts to recast medical-education and service-delivery programs into community-based models will accelerate. The resulting adjustment in medical education and practice will produce the necessary numbers of generalist (primary-care) physicians well into the twenty-first century. These two competing predictions—for a deficit of primary-care physicians and an adequate supply of primary-care physicians—complicate drawing conclusions about the supply of primary-care physicians for the next decade.

PHYSICIAN ASSISTANTS IN PRIMARY CARE

Since the passage of Medicare and Medicaid laws in the 1960s, federal efforts in primary care have focused on increasing the numbers of both nonphysician and physician generalists. Early efforts to build a cadre of primary-care providers in the United States took place in the 1960s, when physician shortage and maldistribution stimulated the development of various nonphysician primary-care provider programs, primarily to provide physician substitutes for rural and underserved areas.

The Physician Assistant (PA) program at Duke University and the Medex programs at the University of Washington and University of Utah are early examples of nonphysician provider education programs. The first PA program opened at Duke University under the direction of Eugene Stead, MD. Interestingly, Stead had originally planned to develop this role in conjunction with his nursing colleague, Thelma Ingeles. However, the nursing community reacted strongly against the development of a nursing role that appeared to take on medical tasks. Consequently, Stead initiated this first PA program by drawing from the large pool of military corpsmen returning from the Vietnam War. By 1992, there were over 24,000 PAs in the United States, 56 percent of whom practiced in ambulatory- and primary-care settings and 31 percent of whom practiced in communities of 50,000 or fewer residents.[25] The content of PA practice, as described by Jones and Cawley,[26] includes evaluation, monitoring, diagnostic testing, therapy, counseling, and referral. The scope of PA practice is regulated under state medical-practice acts, and thus, the activities of PAs in primary-care practice vary from state to state. However, PAs are generally licensed as dependent to physicians, in contrast to NPs whose practices are more independent.

The majority of PA programs in the United States are based in medical schools or have strong relationships with medical schools. Numerous studies have documented the PA's ability to provide medical services with a high level of patient satisfaction.[27] PAs are reported to see patient populations similar to those of physicians and are considered capable of providing approximately 75 percent of physician-specific services.[28] Regan and Harbert[29] reported that depending on their particular use in a practice, a PA can reduce overhead and increase the financial productivity of a physician by a total of $72,077 to $332,200 annually.

ADVANCED PRACTICE NURSES AS PRIMARY CARE PROVIDERS

To date, APNs in primary-care settings have practiced as NPs or certified nurse midwives (CNMs). The introduction of the NP occurred simultaneously with that of the PA. Conceived as a primary-care generalist, the NP role (initially called a pediatric associate) was originally developed by Loretta Ford, PhD, a nurse, and Henry Silver, a pediatrician, both practicing in Colorado.[30] The role developed over time and extended into adult health, family health, and gerontological health.

In 1992, there were almost 30,000 NPs and 5000 CNMs in the United States.[31] Today, more than 200 graduate nursing programs prepare NPs for a variety of specialist roles. The greatest numbers of programs offer preparation for family NPs (78 percent), followed by pediatric NPs (35 percent), geriatric NPs (28 percent), adult NPs (27 percent), and obstetric-gynecological women's health NPs (26 percent). Enrollment in such programs has increased significantly and new post-master's programs are now being offered in more than 125 institutions.

According to the National Organization of Nurse Practitioner Faculties (NONPF),[32] NPs are educated to practice independently and interdependently in collaborative practice arrangements. As primary-care generalists, NPs employ a population-based perspective to care for individuals, families, and communities. Clinical decision making, based on critical thinking, is essential to the work of the NP, who must synthesize theoretical, scientific, clinical, and practical knowledge to diagnose and manage actual and potential health problems. Central to the role of the NP is the promotion and maintenance of health. NPs have major roles in health promotion, disease prevention, service coordination, and acute and chronic disease monitoring.[33] Although NPs are expected to use short-term encounters to address the restoration of health, long-term contact and teaching encounters are viewed as more meaningful opportunities to contribute to the long-term health of the patient. Strategies of NP care include patient advocacy, therapy and health education, counseling, service coordination, and treatment evaluation. According to NONPF, NP practice is not setting specific, but rather, is focused on the primary-care needs of patients, wherever they may occur.[32] More recently, NPs have begun to move into acute-care settings, taking the place of medical residents in hospital.[34,35]

Research on Advanced Nursing Practice

An extensive body of literature is available documenting the effectiveness of APNs (in particular NPs). Three reviews of APN practice in primary care are considered definitive. The first, a study commissioned by the U.S. Congress and conducted by the Office of Technology Assessment (OTA),[36] reviewed the published reports of NP practice. The OTA study findings demonstrated that NP care is of *equal* quality to that of physicians in the areas of history taking, diagnosing of minor, acute illnesses, and managing stable, chronic diseases and *superior* in the areas of communication and preventive care.[36]

In the second literature synthesis, Crosby, Ventura, and Feldman[37] reviewed 248 published reports on NP practice from the period 1963 to 1983. The review included 187 reports judged to be methodologically sound and summarized findings in relation to NP utilization, delivery of patient-care services, short-term patient outcomes, and long-term patient outcomes. On the basis of their analysis of the reports, Crosby, Ventura, and Feldman concluded that NPs:

- Work primarily in ambulatory settings and physicians' offices
- Perform a range of services, including both physician-substitute services (history taking, physical and diagnostic examinations, and management of chronic illnesses) as well as complementary services (patient teaching and counseling) comparable or superior to that of other providers
- Have positive, short-term patient outcomes (patient knowledge, compliance, return for health-maintenance and follow-up visits) equal to, or better than, those of other providers

(Long-term patient outcomes were described in only 14 percent of the reports and, therefore, were not analyzed.)

Brown and Grimes[38] provided a synopsis of both NP and CNM practice. The strength of their report is found in its use of rigorous statistical techniques that combined the probability values (P values) and arrived at standard mean differences across statistical comparison studies of APN providers (experimenting groups) and physicians (control group). To be included in the review, the report had to describe:

- Practice in American or Canadian settings
- An intervention provided by an NP-CNM or an NP-CNM-physician team
- Data on a control group of patients managed by a physician
- Outcomes related to process of care, clinical (patient) outcomes, or utilization and cost effectiveness
- Use of a traditional research design (i.e., experimental, quasi-experimental, or ex post facto)
- Statistical data sufficient to compare the experimental and control groups

More than 900 reports were reviewed and 38 NP and 15 CNM studies met the methodological requirements for inclusion. From the review of the 38 NP studies, the investigators concluded that NPs[38]:

- Provide more health promotion care and ordered more diagnostic tests than the physician group
- Have comparable scores on patient knowledge but higher scores than their physician counterparts on patient compliance, functional outcomes, resolution of pathologic conditions, and satisfaction with care
- Spend more time with patients and have lower laboratory costs and fewer hospitalizations than their physician counterparts

While costs per NP visit were lower, the investigators noted this finding was confounded by salary differentials between NPs and physicians. Though small, effect sizes demonstrated statistically significant findings indicating that for the variables listed, NP care was comparable or better than physician care.

Certified nurse midwives, individuals educated in both nursing and midwifery, are considered to be well-qualified primary-care providers for women and newborns.[39] In the CNM studies reported by Brown and Grimes,[38] only those in which CNMs and physicians had patients with comparable risks were compared. These nine studies demonstrated that CNMs[38]:

- Used less analgesia and intravenous fluids and performed less fetal monitoring, episiotomies, and forceps deliveries
- Induced labor less frequently than physicians
- Had patients who more often delivered in sites other than delivery rooms (process of care)
- Had infant outcomes (incidence of low birth weight, fetal distress, 1-minute Apgar scores, and neonatal mortality) comparable to their physician counterparts (clinical outcomes)
- Had shorter hospital lengths of stay and more postpartum visits than their physician counterparts

CNMs and physicians differed most in the process-of-care variables, reflecting the midwives' tendency to provide less technology-oriented care.

Critics of these three reports cite lack of control for differences in the complexity of patients managed by physicians and NPs-CNMs. However, Brown and Grimes,[38] who selected for analysis only those randomized clinical trials where patient complexity was comparable for NPs and physicians, still found results indicating that NP-CNM care is comparable or superior to that of physicians.

Nurse practitioners can provide 80 to 90 percent of the services provided by physicians. Because the cost of educating NPs and CNMs is approximately 20 to

25 percent less than the cost of educating physicians, these two types of APNs are considered economical sources for primary-care providers in the next century.[36] Recent reports have suggested that managed-care organizations are using APNs and PAs to control costs and that roughly two-thirds of all sampled groups reported employment of APNs and PAs.[40]

Policy Issues Influencing Advanced Practice in Emerging Primary-Care Systems

BARRIERS TO ADVANCED PRACTICE IN PRIMARY CARE

Given that NP and CNM outcomes are comparable to physician outcomes, the lower health-care education and delivery costs associated with APNs should result in more APNs in primary-care settings. Yet professional barriers continue to influence APN practice. Despite the increased number of nurses completing programs preparing them for primary-care practice, the number of APNs actively involved in practice is far smaller. Safriet[4] identified three major barriers to advanced nursing practice in primary-care settings:

1. Regulation of advanced nursing practice
2. Prescriptive authority for APNs
3. Reimbursement for APNs' services

Regulation of Advanced Nursing Practice

Every state has licensing laws designed to protect the public. State practice acts govern the nature and scope of the practices of physicians, nurses, and other health professionals. Physicians were the first practitioners to receive legislative approval for their practice activities, and state medical-practice acts are all-encompassing in reserving to physicians the legal right to diagnose, prescribe, treat, and cure health problems. Because medical-practice acts deny these functions to anyone not licensed as a physician, other health professionals seeking to perform these functions are compelled to negotiate changes in their own practice acts to include diagnosis, prescriptive, and curative functions. Progress by APNs to achieve legislative authority in the 50 states and District of Columbia to perform these functions has been slow, spanning more than three decades.

Prescriptive Authority for Advanced Practice Nurses

The ability to prescribe drugs and therapeutic agents is a second requisite for comprehensive primary care. Numerous strategies have been used by APNs to prescribe medications in primary-care settings, even in the absence of legal authority. These include choosing a medication for a patient and then having a physician write and sign a prescription for that medication; using a physician's name to call in a prescription to a pharmacy; cosigning (with a physician) a prescription; and using written protocols to allow the nurse to prescribe medications with the type and dosage determined by formulary. Although these strategies have enabled APNs to manage medication regimens, they often result in APNs being hidden providers of this important primary-care service.

Reimbursement for Advanced Practice Nurses' Services

Perhaps the greatest barrier to advanced nursing practice in primary-care settings has been the uneven success nurses have experienced in receiving reimbursement for their services. Because reimbursement decisions rest with states (where third-party insurers are regulated), the issue of reimbursement for APNs' services depends on individual state statutes. Where state statutes permit reimbursement for APNs' services, Medicaid- and Medicare-approved nurse provider rates range from 60 to 100 percent of what physicians are paid for the same services.[41] Progress on resolving these three barriers to primary practice by APNs has been slow. Using economic projection techniques, Nichols[42] estimated that barriers to practice preventing APNs from providing the full range of services that they are educated to provide cost the nation $9 billion annually. Table 5–4 shows individual states that, as of 1995, granted unrestricted practice or prescriptive authority to APNs.

In a study of practice barriers among a sample of practicing California NPs,[43] those reporting the greatest barriers were NPs whose practices addressed the needs of unserved populations (prisons, psychiatric patients, rural communities), thus documenting the fact that advanced nursing practice barriers continue to limit access for those groups who can least afford denial of primary health care. Removal of practice barriers is necessary if APNs are to be major providers of primary care in the future. In a 1994 report, the Pew Health Professions Commission[44] specifically called for removal of barriers to the expansion of NP practice. In its 1995 report, the commission called for changes in the health professions regulatory system to permit standardized regulation, where appropriate, to support optimal access to a competent workforce.[45]

THE MIX OF PROVIDERS FOR PRIMARY-CARE SYSTEMS

Health care over the life span requires services ranging from health promotion and disease prevention to management of chronic or life-threatening illness, to end-stage, palliative care. This broad range of services cannot likely be delivered by a single health professional. Thus, a major issue for future primary health-care systems is creating an ideal mix of interdisciplinary service providers to provide the broadest range of needed services with the greatest economy.

The value of interdisciplinary provider teams is often praised in the literature.[46-48] According to the Pew Commission,[46] interdisciplinary collaborative practice is necessary for integrated clinical care. It requires providers conversant in team concepts who can respectfully engage in open communication with other team members. Practice situations that favor collaborative teamwork are those characterized by situational complexity requiring more than one set of skills, clinical knowledge too great for one clinician to possess, and team members willing to sacrifice some degree of autonomy in order to achieve the best quality of care.

Despite the philosophical support for team practice, there is little literature on organizing the most efficient and effective team of health-care clinicians. At least three factors will likely influence the mix of team providers for emerging primary-care systems:

1. The needs of the target population
2. The provider's skills and services
3. Incentives for interdisciplinary practice teams

TABLE 5–4

Summary of Advanced Practice Nurse Legislation: Legal Authority for Scope of Practice and Prescriptive Authority

STATES WITH APN TITLE PROTECTION AND THE BOARD OF NURSING AS SOLE AUTHORITY IN SCOPE OF PRACTICE WITH NO REQUIREMENTS FOR PHYSICIAN COLLABORATION OR SUPERVISION
CO, CT, DC, DE, HI, IA, IN, KS, MI, MT, NH, NM, OK, OR, RI, TX, UT, VT, WA, WY
STATES WITH APN TITLE PROTECTION AND THE BOARD OF NURSING AS SOLE AUTHORITY IN SCOPE OF PRACTICE, BUT SCOPE OF PRACTICE HAS A REQUIREMENT FOR PHYSICIAN COLLABORATION OR SUPERVISION
AL, AR, AZ, CA, FL, GA, HI, KY, LA, ME, MD, MO, MS, NJ, NY, NV, SC, WY
STATES WITH APN TITLE PROTECTION BUT THE SCOPE OF PRACTICE IS AUTHORIZED BY THE BOARD OF NURSING AND THE BOARD OF MEDICINE
ID, NC, NE, PA, SD, VA
STATES WITHOUT APN TITLE PROTECTION WHERE APNS FUNCTION UNDER A BROAD NURSE-PRACTICE ACT
IL, MN, OH, TN
STATES WITH CURRENT LAWS OR STATUTES THAT INCLUDE CNSS WITHIN THE APN CATEGORY
CO, CT, DC, DE, FL,[†] GA,[†] HI, IA, IN, KS, KY, LA, MA,[†] MD,[†] MI, MN,[†] MO, MT, ND, NH,[†] NJ, NM, NV,[†] OK, SC, SD, TN, TX, UT, VA, VT, WA, WI, WV, WY
STATES WHERE NPS CAN PRESCRIBE (INCLUDING CONTROLLED SUBSTANCES) INDEPENDENT OF ANY REQUIRED PHYSICIAN INVOLVEMENT IN PRESCRIPTION WRITING
AK, AZ, DC, IA, MT, NM, OR, VT, WA (schedule V), WI, WY
STATES WHERE NPS CAN PRESCRIBE (INCLUDING CONTROLLED SUBSTANCES) WITH SOME DEGREE OF PHYSICIAN INVOLVEMENT OR DELEGATION OF PRESCRIPTION WRITING
CO, CT, DE, GA, IN, MA, MD, ME, MN, MO, MS,[†] NE, NC, ND, NH, NY, PA, RI, SC,[‡] SD, UT, WV
STATES WHERE NPS CAN PRESCRIBE (EXCLUDING CONTROLLED SUBSTANCES) WITH SOME DEGREE OF PHYSICIAN INVOLVEMENT OR DELEGATION OF PRESCRIPTION WRITING
AR,[†] CA, FL, HI, ID, KS, KY, LA,[†] MI, NJ, NV, OH,[†] TN, TX,[†] VA
STATES WHERE NPS HAVE DISPENSING AUTHORITY
AK, AZ, CT, LA,[†] MD,[†] MS,[†] MT, NH, NV, OR, TN,[†] TX,[†] WI
STATES WHERE NPS HAVE NO STATUTORY PRESCRIBING AUTHORITY
AL, IL, OK

*States so marked indicate that CNSs are the exception.
†States so marked address only psychiatric–mental health CNSs.
‡States so marked are in narrowly specified situations.
(Note that Washington, DC, is counted as a state in the table.)
Source: Pearson, L: Annual update of how each state stands on legislative issues affecting advanced nursing practice. Nurse Practitioner 20:14,16, 1995, with permission.

The Needs of the Target Population

The characteristics of the target population to be served by a primary-care system is a decisive factor in developing a mix of providers. For example, communities with a high proportion of families with school-age children will need a group of primary-care providers with a set of skills and services different from those of communities with a large proportion of retired senior citizens. Primary-care systems that serve homeless people would need to have providers with skills in managing chronic and infectious diseases and in finding and using social services. Farm communities would require a primary-care system of providers skilled in accident prevention and management and controlling occupational toxic exposures. The skill base and expertise of providers in a primary-care setting must vary depending on the target population's needs.

The Provider's Skills and Services

There are three approaches to multidisciplinary service delivery that have implications for APNs who seek to practice in primary-care systems. Under a **provider-substitution** model, all providers in the setting offer the same set of services. Thus, APNs, physicians, and PAs in the setting offer the same diagnostic, disease prevention, health promotion, and disease management services.

With a **supplemental** model, multidisciplinary providers offer a core set of services, with each team member also offering supplemental services. Under this model, all APNs, physicians, and PAs in a setting might provide first-contact services (taking a health history, performing diagnostic tests, and identifying the priority health problem). However only the physician would manage patients diagnosed with chronic illnesses. The PA would manage acute illnesses and trauma, and the APN would provide disease prevention and/or health promotion services.

Finally, in a **complementary** model, providers in a setting offer only those services for which they are uniquely prepared by education, experience, or legal statute. Using the complementary model for primary-care services, the PA might do all initial, first-contact patient encounters, the physician might see patients with illnesses, and the APN might provide health-screening and disease prevention programs for individuals and families.

The decision to use a substitute, supplemental, or complementary model of provider practice in a setting will influence recruiting and employment decisions. Under a substitution model, the decision to employ APNs, physicians, PAs, or other service providers would be influenced *only* by the availability and costs of employing those different types of providers. If there is an adequate and economical supply of physician generalists during the next decade, exclusive focus on a physician substitution model may have negative connotations for APNs who want to work in primary-care settings.

Under the provider supplement model, each provider offers the same core set of services plus a skill-specific service. However, in a system increasingly concerned with costs, the connotation that any provider's services are *supplemental* in nature could have negative implications for APNs, unless the need for and cost justification of those services is successfully marketed to consumers. Settings driven by economical concerns may elect not to offer supplemental services.

Exclusive emphasis on *complementary* services, such as those offered by physicians or by APNs, increases the risk of fragmentation of services in a system already criticized for lack of service articulation. However, if complementary interdisciplinary practice is thoughtfully implemented, it can result in each provider offering those services for which they are qualified. Complementary interdependent team practice has great promise for primary-care settings.

Because the broad range of needed primary-care services cannot likely be provided by a single professional, the manner in which primary-care systems conceptualize and implement service delivery has great implications for new APNs who will enter practice in the next decade. Table 5–5 summarizes advantages and disadvantages of each method of skill and services division among providers. While proponents of emerging primary-care systems emphasize the need for collaboration and service coordination, little attention has been given to mechanisms for articulating the services of multidisciplinary providers. Given the forecasts of a crowded health-care system, APNs must be clear when marketing their services whether their skills and services substitute, supplement, or complement those services offered by other providers.

Incentives for Interdisciplinary Practice Teams

Gatekeeping, patient ownership, and control of service delivery by selected professionals have been identified as deterrents to the delivery of economical primary-care services. Efforts to limit patient access to the services of other providers are often seen in the "turf battles" regularly played out between medical specialists and generalists, between physicians and nurses, and between nurses and PAs. In its recent recommendations for the future education of all

TABLE 5–5

Advantages and Disadvantages of Substitutive, Supplemental, and Complementary Service Delivery in Primary Care

Provider Services	Potential Advantages	Potential Disadvantages
Substitutive: multidisciplinary providers who offer the same services	▪ Standardization of services offered ▪ Reimbursement tied to *services*, not to discipline of provider	▪ Provider competition ▪ Little or no collaborative, interdependent team practice
Supplemental: multidisciplinary providers who offer a *core* set of services, plus additional, or supplemental, services	▪ Standardization of core set of services offered ▪ Utilization of unique practice strengths of multidisciplinary providers for supplemental services	▪ Services of some providers considered supplemental "extras" ▪ Collaborative, interdependent team practice around supplemental services only
Complementary: multidisciplinary providers, who offer different services	▪ Utilization of interdependent collaborative practice to offer coordinated, comprehensive services ▪ Utilization of unique practice strengths of multidisciplinary providers	▪ Potential fragmentation in service delivery ▪ Lack of service coordination

health professionals, the Pew Commission[45] concluded that future health-care systems must have practitioners who are able to work effectively as team members in settings that emphasize "integrated services."

However, current organizational and service reimbursement characteristics serve as strong disincentives to the development of interdisciplinary teams. Academic health centers, considered by many health policy planners to represent the best hope for the practice education of future primary care providers, continue to emphasize separate education of physicians, nurses, pharmacists, and other health professionals.[49] Health-care delivery models continue to emphasize the compartmentalization of services, organized around the single provider-patient encounter. Existing reimbursement patterns continue to factor reimbursement of a single provider without considering the unique skills and services of different providers, or the specific health needs of individuals and families.[50]

Because existing professional education models continue to favor one-on-one provider-patient relationships, the development of productive interdisciplinary team practices for primary care will require the redesign of health-professional education as well as service delivery and reimbursement models. A novel approach to changing the behavior of practicing clinicians is one proposed by an economist, Scheffler.[48] He suggests that financial incentives be offered to primary-care teams who will work together to enhance the quality of care. Changes in reimbursement patterns that promote team-practice reimbursement must occur as well. To offset the educational elitism of health professionals, the Pew Commission[45] recently published a sample curriculum guide for interdisciplinary education for primary care and a reference guide to assist educators in accomplishing this goal.

Summary

High-quality health-care systems are those that provide accessible, economical, and effective services to specific target populations. Spiraling health-care costs and consumer dissatisfaction with unequal access and fragmented services have generated renewed interest in primary-care systems and primary-care providers. The most recent IOM definition of primary care manifests the wide-ranging expectation that the primary-care system of the future must be staffed by generalists who are capable of providing comprehensive, holistic care that addresses a wide range of individual and family health problems. Because no single provider can be expected to possess the knowledge and skills to address the complete range of episodic and chronic health problems commonly experienced across the life span, multidisciplinary team practice will be a necessity. Whether future primary-care system will achieve their expected goals of first-contact, longitudinal, and coordinated and comprehensive care will depend, to a great extent, on whether multidisciplinary practice teams successfully collaborate in balancing substitutive, supplemental, and complementary services for target populations. The purpose of this chapter has been to explore the social, political, and economic issues that will facilitate or inhibit the participation of APNs in these types of primary-care practice endeavors.

Suggested Exercises

1. How might nurses work to amend state nurse-practice acts to allow APNs to better meet the primary-care needs of underserved and unserved populations groups in the United States?

2. Which model of practice do you believe offers the greatest opportunity for APNs in primary-care settings: the physician-substitute model? the physician-supplement model? or the physician-complement model? Justify your answer.

3. What do you believe is the ideal provider mix for a multidisciplinary practice team in primary care?

4. Discuss incentives for developing and supporting multidisciplinary practice teams in primary care.

5. How might health policy planners ensure an adequate supply of primary-care providers for the next decade?

REFERENCES

1. Starfield, B: Roles and functions of non-physician practitioners in primary care. In Clawson, D, and Osterwels, M (eds): The Role of Physician Assistants and Nurse Practitioners in Primary Care. Association of Academic Health Centers, Washington, DC, 1993.
2. World Health Organization: Primary Health Care. Geneva, Switzerland, 1978.
3. Franks, P, Nutting, P, and Clancy, C: Health care reform, primary care, and the need for research. Acad Med 270:1449, 1993.
4. Safriet, B: Health care dollars and regulatory sense: The role of advanced practice nursing. Yale Journal of Regulation 9:417, 1992.
5. American Nurses' Association: Nursing's Agenda for Health Care Reform. American Nurses' Association, Washington, DC, 1991.
6. Pew Health Professions Commission: Healthy America: Practitioners for 2005. Pew Health Professions Commission, San Francisco, 1991.
7. Council on Graduate Medical Education: Third Report: Improving Access to Health Care through Physician Workforce Reform: Directions for the 21st Century. US Department of Health and Human Services: Washington, DC, 1992.
8. Public Health Service: Health Professions Report. US Department of Health and Human Services, Washington, DC, 1993.
9. The Alliance for Health Reform: A Primary Care Primer. The Alliance for Health Reform, Washington, DC, 1993.
10. White, K: Primary medical care for families. N Engl J Med 277:847, 1967.
11. Alpert, J, and Charney, E: The Education of Physicians for Primary Care. US Department of Health, Education and Welfare, Public Health Service, Health Resources Administration, Rockville, Md, 1973. HRA publication 74–3113.
12. Institute of Medicine: Report of a Study: A Manpower Policy for Primary Health Care. National Academy of Science, Washington, DC, May 1978.
13. Golden, A: A definition of primary care for educational purposes. In Golden, A, Carlson, D, and Hagan, J (eds): The Art of Teaching Primary Care. Springer, New York, 1982.
14. Starfield, B: Primary Care: Concept, Evaluation and Policy. Oxford University Press, New York, 1992.
15. Institute of Medicine: Defining Primary Care: An Interim Report. Washington, DC, National Academy Press, 1994.
16. Schappert, S: National Ambulatory Care Survey: 1991 Summary. National Center for Health Statistics, Vital and Health Statistics, Hyattsville, Md, 1994.
17. Avorn, J, Everitt, D, and Baker, M: The neglected medical history and therapeutic choices for abdominal pain. Arch Intern Med 151:694, 1991.
18. Safran, D, Tarlov, A, and Rogers, W: Primary care performance in fee-for-service and prepaid health care systems. JAMA 271:1579, 1994.
19. Rivo, M, and Satcher, D: Improving access to health care through physician workforce reform. JAMA 270:1074, 1993.

20. Weiner, J: Forecasting the effects of health reform on US physician workforce requirement. JAMA 272:222, 1994.
21. Barnett, P, and Midtling, J: Public policy and the supply of primary care physicians. JAMA 262:2864, 1989.
22. Kassebaum, D, Szenas, P, and Ruffin, A: The declining interest of medical school graduates in generalist specialties: Students abandonment of earlier inclinations. Acad Med 68:278, 1993.
23. Levinsky, N: Recruiting for primary care. N Engl J Med 328:656, 1993.
24. Iglehart, J: Health policy report: II. Rapid changes for academic medical centers. N Engl J Med 332:407, 1995.
25. Fowkes, V: Meeting the needs of the underserved: The roles of physician assistant are nurse practitioners. In Clawson, D, and Osterweis, M (eds): The role of physician assistants and nurse practitioners in primary care. Association of Academic Health Centers, Washington, DC, 1993.
26. Jones, P, and Cawley, J: Physician assistants and health system reform: Clinical capabilities, practice activities, and potential roles. JAMA 272:725, 1994.
27. Hooker, R: The role of physician assistants and nurse practitioners in a managed organization. In Clawson, D, and Osterweis, M (eds): The Role of Physician Assistants and Nurse Practitioners in Primary Care. Association of Academic Health Centers, Washington, DC, 1993.
28. Cawley, J: Physician assistants in the health care workforce. In Clawson, D, and Osterweis, M (eds): The role of physician assistants and nurse practitioners in primary care. Association of Academic Health Centers, Washington, DC, 1993.
29. Regan, D, and Harbert, K: Measuring the financial productivity of physician assistants. Medical Group Management Journal, November/December 1991, p 46.
30. Ford, L: Practice perspectives in primary care, nursing. In Miller, R (ed): Primary Health Care: More than Medicine. Prentice-Hall, Englewood Cliffs, NJ, 1983.
31. American Association of Colleges of Nursing: 1994–1995 Special Report on Masters and Post-Masters Nurse Practitioners Programs, Faculty Clinical Practice, Faculty Age Profiles, and Undergraduate Curriculum Expansion in Baccalaureate and Graduate Programs in Nursing. December 1995, p 8.
32. National Organization of Nurse Practitioner Faculties: Curriculum Guidelines and Program Standards for Nurse Practitioner Education. Washington, DC, National Organization of Nurse Practitioner Faculties, 1995.
33. Booth, R: Leadership challenges for nurse practitioner faculty. Keynote address presented at the Twentieth Annual Conference of the National Organization of Nurse Practitioner Faculties, Portland, Ore, 1994.
34. Genet, C, et al: Nurse practitioners in a teaching hospital. Nurse Pract 20:47, 1995.
35. Goskel, D, Harrison, C, Morrison, R, and Miller, S: Description of a nurse practitioner inpatient service in a public teaching hospital. J Gen Intern Med 8:29, 1993.
36. Congress and Office of Technology Assessment: Nurse Practitioners, Physician Assistants and Certified Nurse Midwives: A Policy Analysis. US Government Printing Office, Washington, DC, 1986. OTA-HCS publication 37.
37. Crosby, F, Ventura, M, and Feldman, M: Future research recommendations for establishing NP effectiveness. Nurse Pract 12:75, 1987.
38. Brown, S, and Grimes, D: Executive Summary: A Meta-analysis of Process of Care, Clinical Outcomes and Cost-Effectiveness of Nurses in Primary Care Roles: Nurse Practitioners and Nurse-Midwives. University of Texas, Houston, 1992.
39. American College of Nurse-Midwives: Position Statement. American College of Nurse-Midwives, Washington, DC, 1992.
40. Dial, T, Palsbo, S, Bergsten, C, Gabel, J, and Weiner, J: Clinical Staffing in Staff- and Group-Model HMOs. Health Aff (Millwood) 14:168, 1995.
41. Pearson, L: Annual update of how each state stands on legislative issues affecting advanced nursing practice. Nurse Pract 20:13, 1995.
42. Nichols, L: Estimating costs of underusing advanced practice nurses. Nursing Economics 10:343, 1992.
43. Anderson, A, Gilliss, C, and Yoder, L: Practice environment for nurse practitioners in California: Identifying barriers. West J Med 165(3):209, 1996.
44. Pew Health Professions Commission: Nurse practitioners: Doubling the graduates by the year 2000. In Commission Policy Papers. Pew Health Professions Commission, San Francisco, 1994.
45. Pew Health Professions Commission: Critical Challenges: Revitalizing the Health Professions for the Twenty-first Century. San Francisco, Calif. Pew Health Professions Commission, 1995.
46. Pew Health Professions Commission: Interdisciplinary Collaborative Teams in Primary Care: A Model Curriculum and Resource Guide. The UCSF Center for the Health Professions, San Francisco, 1995.
47. Baldwin, D: The Role of Interdisciplinary Education and Teamwork in Primary Care and Health Care Reform. Department of Health and Human Services, Public Health Service, Bureau of Health Professions, Office of Research and Planning, Rockville, Md, 1994.

48. Scheffler, R: Life in the kaleidoscope: The impact of managed care on the US health care work force and a new model for the delivery of primary care. In Institute of Medicine (Donaldson, M, Yordy, K, Lohr, K, and Vanselow, N, eds): Primary Care: America's Health in a New Era. National Academy Press, Washington, DC, 1996, pp 312–340.

49. Low, D: Commentary. In Larson, P, Osterweis, M, and Rubin, E (eds): Health Workforce Issues in the 21st Century. Association of Academic Health Centers, Washington, DC, 1994.

50. Pestronk, R, Oxman, G, Gilliss, C, Dempster, J, Badgett, J, Garnett, E, Parham, D, and Toro-Alphonso, J: Managed outcomes. Journal of the American Academy of Nurse Practitioners, 63:121, 1994.

CHAPTER 6

Formulation and Approval of Credentialing and Clinical Privileges

Formulation and Approval of Credentialing and Clinical Privileges

JOAN M. STANLEY, PhD, CRNP

GERALDINE "POLLY" BEDNASH, PhD, RN, FAAN

Joan M. Stanley, PhD, CRNP, was appointed director of education policy of the American Association of Colleges of Nursing in 1994. She has served as member of the association's Task Force of Essentials of Master's Education for Advanced Practice Nurses and currently serves as a staff member on its Task Force on Essentials of Baccalaureate Nursing Education. She has also served as the association's representative to a number of advanced practice nursing projects, including the American Nurses' Association's Task Force on the Scope and Standards for Advanced Practice Nursing, the National Council of State Boards of Nursing Advisory Committee for the Family Nurse Practitioner Pharmacology Curriculum Project, and the National League of Nursing–National Organization of Nurse Practitioner Faculties' Task Force on Evaluation Criteria for Nurse Practitioner Program Approval. Since 1991, Dr. Stanley has served as project director for two contracts awarded to the American Association of Colleges of Nursing by the National Health Service Corps and has recently been appointed to the Technical Advisory Group on the Evaluation of the Effectiveness of the National Health Service Corps. Dr. Stanley is editor of *Nurse Practitioner World News*. She also maintains a practice as an adult nurse practitioner at the University of Maryland Hospital Faculty Practice Office. Before joining the American Association of Colleges of Nursing, Dr. Stanley was assistant professor at the School of Nursing at the University of Maryland and associate director of Primary Care Nursing Services at the University of Maryland Hospital. Dr. Stanley received her bachelor's of science in nursing from Duke University and her master's of science in nursing and doctorate from the University of Maryland.

Geraldine "Polly" Bednash, PhD, RN, FAAN, was appointed executive director of the American Association of Colleges of Nursing in December 1989. Dr. Bednash oversees the educational, research, governmental affairs, data bank, publications, and other programs of the only national organization dedicated exclusively to furthering nursing education in America's universities and 4-year colleges. Since 1986, Dr. Bednash has headed the association's legislative and regulatory advocacy programs as director of government affairs. In that post, Dr. Bednash has directed the association's efforts to secure strong federal support for nursing education and nursing research, has coordinated new initiatives

6

with federal agencies and major foundations, and has coauthored the association's landmark study of the financial costs to students and to clinical agencies of baccalaureate and graduate nursing education, among other responsibilities. Dr. Bednash currently serves as vice president for nursing of the Health Professions Education Council of the Association of Academic Health Centers and is a member of the editorial boards of several leading nursing publications, including *Nursing Economic$*. Her publications and research presentations cover a range of critical issues in nursing education, nursing research, clinical practice, and legislative policy. Before joining the American Association of Colleges of Nursing, Dr. Bednash was assistant professor at the School of Nursing at George Mason University and a Robert Wood Johnson Nurse Faculty Fellow in Primary Care at the University of Maryland. Her experience includes developing resource policy for the Geriatric Research, Evaluation, and Clinical Centers of the Veterans Administration and serving as nurse practitioner and consultant to the family-practice residency program at DeWitt Army Hospital at Fort Belvoir, Virginia, and as an Army Nurse Corps staff nurse in Vung Tau, Vietnam. Dr. Bednash received her bachelor's of science in nursing from Texas Women's University, her master's of science in nursing from the Catholic University of America, and her doctorate from the University of Maryland. She is a fellow of the American Academy of Nursing and a member of Sigma Theta Tau.

CHAPTER OBJECTIVES

After completing this chapter, the reader will be able to:

1. Analyze the differences between certification and licensure and the manner in which each is used in the regulation of advanced practice.
2. Engage in a dialogue regarding the meaning and rationale for second licensure for advanced practice nurses (APNs).
3. Compare and contrast the scopes of practice for each of the four traditional APN roles authorized by the nurse-practice act in the state in which an APN intends to practice, including barriers to practice.
4. Seek clinical privileges at a health care-institution, which may or may not include membership on the medical staff of that institution, in a knowledgeable way.

Licensure, certification, and clinical privileges are all interwoven components of advanced nursing practice. The first two—licensure and certification—are the gates through which the clinician must successfully pass to be granted both the authority and the recognition for practice. The third—clinical privileges—can be an obstacle or a pathway for extending practice and functioning as a comprehensive clinical provider. Unfortunately, gaining either of the first two does not always automatically provide APNs with the authority to acquire clinical privileges to practice in nursing homes, hospitals, clinics, and a variety of other settings. However, APNs must be well versed in how to acquire these professional standings or to challenge barriers placed in their way.

Regulation: Professional and Public

The regulation of professional practice is accomplished in a variety of ways. Licensure, certification, and professional standards of practice represent variations on the regulation of practice. Each is structured on the basis of different value sets to control safety and quality in practice. Standards of practice are internally directed and professionally controlled entities. Professions such as nursing, medicine, law, or others engage in thoughtful deliberation regarding the standards that represent their efforts to self-regulate.[1] Professional self-regulation provides accountability to the society served by the profession and acknowledges that the profession will engage in efforts to protect the public from either unscrupulous or unsafe practice. Professional nursing organizations such as the American Nurses' Association, the American College of Nurse-Midwives (ACNM), the American Association of Nurse Anesthetists (AANA), and others establish professional standards of practice through their collective members. These professional standards may be used as a mechanism for judging the practice of individual APNs and may also serve as a measure of quality of practice in legal assessments of a clinician's capabilities.

External regulation can occur through licensure or certification of the individual practitioner. Licensure is a publicly controlled operation in which the state or governing authority sets minimum standards for safe practice. The individual must meet these standards in order to be granted the privilege of practicing in a particular jurisdiction.[1] Licensure is a public function that has been delegated to the states and territories by the Constitution. Unlike licensure, certification is voluntarily sought by the professional. The professional agrees that certification has value and engages in a process of testing to establish that the standards developed by the certifying body, usually a nongovernmental and professionally monitored organization, have been met. In contrast to licensure, which validates the clinician's minimum level of competence, certification is a mechanism to document that the clinician has achieved a higher level of competence and perhaps specialization.[2]

For APNs, public regulation and professional certification have become intertwined as employers and regulators increasingly seek APNs to deliver safe, appropriate, and cost-effective care. Professional certification and licensure are receiving a great deal of scrutiny as policy makers, regulators, professional associations, and employers attempt to bring some order to the confusing array of regulations affecting advanced practice nursing. This chapter will capture the system in this period of rapid change.

CURRENT ISSUES IN REGULATION

The regulation of advanced practice nursing has undergone significant upheaval in recent years. A number of factors have led policy makers to question the appropriateness or adequacy of the current systems of regulation for APNs. These include regulatory barriers to practice, difficulties with interstate mobility, the lack of uniformity in public regulation of APNs, and the increased use of telecommunications as a mechanism for delivering care. In addition, the dramatic changes in the health-care delivery system have caused policy makers to carefully scrutinize the regulation of all health professionals. A number of commissions or advisory bodies have engaged in review of the entire spectrum of licensure and certification activities for health professionals.[3–5] The Pew Health Professions Commission report, *Reforming Health Care Workforce Regulation: Policy Considerations for the 21st Century*,[6] represents the most recent overview of regulation in all the health professions. This report raises a number of regulatory issues that have affected, and will continue to affect, advanced practice in nursing.

The Pew Report is the result of a year-long review by a commission task force of current public regulation systems and their usefulness for protecting the public. The commission task force has made 10 recommendations for reform of current regulatory systems (Table 6–1) and has strongly urged the implementation of these to produce standardized, accountable, flexible, effective, and efficient regulatory structures. The Pew commissioners and others have reviewed the complex array of issues affecting access to health care and have identified a growing concern that the regulation of professional practice often decreases access to health care rather than protects it. Regulations very often serve professional interests and are used to draw regulatory lines around practice domains and to limit the care activities in which professionals can "legally" engage.

The Pew report provides an important backdrop to policy discussions regarding the current evolution of health-care delivery. The report makes clear that the regulation of practice should be based on demonstrated competencies, not on the ability of one clinical group to draw territorial lines around a domain and proclaim dominance. This recommendation has been most widely supported by APNs, who have had limits placed on their practice that were either politically or professionally motivated, rather than factually based.

TABLE 6–1
Reforming Health-Care Workforce Regulation: Policy Considerations for the Twenty-first Century

STATEMENT OF RECOMMENDATIONS

1. States should use standardized and understandable language for health professions' regulation and its functions to describe them clearly for consumers, provider organizations, businesses, and the professions.
2. States should standardize entry-to-practice requirements and limit them to competence assessments for health professions to facilitate the physical and professional mobility of the health professions.
3. States should base practice acts on demonstrated initial and continuing competence. This process must allow and expect different professions to share overlapping scopes of practice. States should explore pathways to allow all professionals to provide services to the full extent of their current knowledge, training, experience, and skills.
4. States should redesign health professional boards and their functions to reflect the interdisciplinary and public accountability demands of the changing health-care delivery system.
5. Boards should educate consumers to assist them in obtaining the information necessary to make decisions about practitioners and to improve the board's public accountability.
6. Boards should cooperate with other public and private organizations in collecting data on regulated health professions to support effective workforce planning.
7. States should require each board to develop, implement, and evaluate continuing competency requirements to ensure the continuing competence of regulated health-care professionals.
8. States should maintain a fair, cost-effective, and uniform disciplinary process to exclude incompetent practitioners to protect and promote the public's health.
9. States should develop evaluation tools that assess the objectives, successes, and shortcomings of their regulatory systems and bodies to best protect and promote the public's health.
10. States should understand the links, overlaps, and conflicts between their health-care workforce regulatory systems and other systems that affect the education, regulation, and practice of health-care practitioners and work to develop partnerships to streamline regulatory structures and processes.

The Pew commissioners appropriately cited current changes in the health-care system as they raised questions regarding the appropriateness or utility of regulatory structures that limit access to, or the use of, a variety of health-care providers, including APNs. The growth of large corporate structures for the delivery and management of health-care services, such as integrated networks, has created an interest in reconceptualizing how care is delivered and who is capable of delivering it. The massive restructuring of the health-care environment that has emerged out of the federal government's failure to engineer a reformed health-care system has been characterized as the "industrialization of health care."[7]

These re-engineered, or "industrialized," health-care systems are often are large corporate, multisystem, and multifacility entities that span many types of delivery sites and geographic boundaries. "Bottom-line" concerns drive much of their decision making and shape their utilization of health-care professionals. These systems have been most welcoming of APNs based on their "fit" with the goals of integrated networks. Much of their interest in using APNs has been based on the APN's ability to substitute for more costly providers such as physicians. There is also a growing awareness that APNs are safe, competent, and cost-effective providers of health-care services who have been able to operate within an appropriate independent practice domain. Finally, a growing body of research has documented the different, and enhanced, outcomes achieved by APNs: more cost-effective interventions, higher patient satisfaction, increased compliance with therapeutic regimens, just to name a few. Increasingly, these enhanced outcomes have caused policy makers and employers to question the logic or appropriateness of regulatory policies that limit the practice of APNs.[8–10]

REGULATION OF ADVANCED NURSING PRACTICE: VARIETY AND CONFUSION

Large multifaceted health-care organizations have created practice domains that stretch beyond state boundaries, which usually defined practice regulation. This expansion, in turn, has created interest in greater mobility among APNs and in greater consistency in the requirements for public regulatory oversight. Against this backdrop, however, the APN practices in a regulatory environment that varies widely, is sometimes conflicting, and often is very limiting.

Unlike the uniform standard for licensing of entry-level nurse clinicians, APNs face a panoply of state requirements for licensure. Each state or territory of the United States maintains some form of regulatory oversight over APNs. In 16 states, APNs are granted a second license for practice.[11] In the remaining states, APNs are granted some form of state authority to practice in the advanced role entitled "recognition" or "certification."[12] Unfortunately, state regulatory initiatives for APNs lack any evidence of consistency in the form of titling, practice privileges, or prescriptive authority.[13] APNs are licensed, certified, or recognized by state boards of nursing. In addition, the types of APNs who are authorized for advanced practice or recognized by the state regulatory boards also vary across the states.

In almost all states, NPs have achieved statutory recognition and some form of state authority to write prescriptions.[14] Certified registered nurse anesthetists (CRNA) and certified nurse midwives (CNMs) receive this recognition in almost all states. Forty states recognize clinical nurse specialists (CNSs) as APNs, although frequently state laws or regulations limit their prescriptive authority. In addition, in many states, the CNS is recognized only in particular areas of specialization (e.g., psychiatric–mental health nursing or pediatrics) or is not recognized as an APN. A recent analysis of state regulatory environments, *The Scope of Practice and Reimbursement for Advanced Practice Registered Nurses: A State by State Analysis*,[13] conducted by the George Washington University Intergovernmental Health Policy Institute, concluded:

> The lack of standardization among states' scopes of practice provisions for [advanced practice registered nurses] APRNs causes confusions for APRNs, other health care providers, insurance companies and consumers, and inhibits national unity among APRNs. (p. 3)

A major criticism of APN regulation has been the great array of titles that are recognized by states. Pearson[14] provides an annual update of the recognized state authorities, prescriptive limitations, and titles. The array of titles (and acronyms) reported as recognized by state regulations has created tremendous confusion for employers, other health professionals, policy makers, and APNs.

Safriet[15] was harshly critical of this inconsistent titling as a source of both confusion and loss of potential support by regulators seeking to limit practice by a clinician group.

Safriet's work on the confusing array of regulatory authorities and their sometimes illogical word choices has provided many groups, both nursing and nonnursing, with a clearer picture of the failure of public regulation. Safriet noted that these often illogical regulatory structures most often are based on a concept of advanced practice nursing as a purely substitutive professional role that is secondary to the presence of physician practice. This limitation is not based on fact or experience and fails to take into account the large body of research documenting the efficacy of advanced practice nursing.

Safriet's work has been instrumental in affecting a great deal of change in public regulatory structures, as evidenced by the increasing number of states that have expanded APNs' authority to practice and prescribe. Moreover, the work of Sekscenski et al.,[16] reviewing the effect of state regulation on the availability of advanced practice clinicians, has documented that restrictive regulatory environments are negatively correlated with the presence of APNs. These researchers noted that those states with the most restrictive regulatory structures have the lowest per capita densities of APNs.

Sekscenski et al. noted that mobility of APNs is severely hindered by the lack of consistency in practice regulation. This inconsistency inhibits intrasystem mobility in the emerging large corporate health-care structures. Integrated networks can span state lines in their scope-of-care responsibilities. However, neighboring states can have markedly different regulating policies for the practice of APNs. Therefore, some discussion has occurred about whether the emerging large, corporate-based, integrated networks should assume some of the authority or responsibility for licensing APNs and other health professionals.

These proposals, which represent a reconceptualization of past proposals to institute a system of institutional licensure, take note of the fact that the growing expansion of health corporations makes corporate oversight attractive to employers. In this newer conceptualization, licensure would not be located institutionally but would be system based. The obvious benefit is the ability to locate professionals across a wide variety of systems without the hindrances associated with the confusing array of state licensure or certification procedures. In addition, proponents of corporate-controlled regulation of APNs and other health professionals note that such a licensure procedure would provide organizations with more flexibility in the use of APNs, thus, overcoming the artificial or inappropriate barriers to their full utilization. Moreover, the "brave new world" of cyberspace has created new modes of care delivery, such as computer- and video-transmitted patient-care experiences, that can create uncertainty about where care is being delivered and who has authority for oversight of the professional's authority to practice. Some employers argue that if oversight of practice was organizationally based, the issue of practice location would not be limited by state boundaries.

The nursing profession historically has been vocally and visibly opposed to the notion of institutional licensure for professional nurses. Opponents of this approach to the regulation of APNs contend that quality of care could be hindered by the use of inadequately prepared clinicians who are educated by the corporation and are authorized to practice in a system that is more concerned with cost than quality. Questions also arise as to the ability of these corporate structures to engage in the expensive process of testing and evaluation necessary to assure competence for advanced practice.[17]

NEED FOR UNIFORMITY IN THE ADVANCED PRACTICE LICENSURE PROCESS

The growing concerns regarding the confusing array of advanced practice licensure mechanisms, titles, or authorities have created interest in a national approach to the regulation of APNs that would mimic the process used by the National Council Licensure Examination (NCLEX) for the regulation of entry-level licensure. To be granted initial licensure to practice, all nurses must successfully pass the NCLEX examination, which is developed and administered by the National Council of State Boards of Nursing (NCSBN). The NCSBN, a national membership organization that represents individual state or territorial boards of nursing, has engaged in a variety of efforts that have brought more urgency to the issue of advanced practice regulation. In 1993, the NCSBN House of Delegates approved a position statement mandating that all APNs be granted a second license for practice and that APNs be required to hold a master's degree to be eligible for this license. The position statement noted that second licensure already existed in a number of states, that APN practice was markedly different from that authorized through the registered nurse (RN) licensure process, and thus, that advanced practice required a new regulatory mechanism.

The second-licensure issue was opposed by a number of nursing organizations, including a variety of specialty certifying organizations and the American Association of Colleges of Nursing. These groups argued that the use of two levels of licensure was both confusing and unnecessary and that the existing use of professional certification was adequate to assure the skills and competence of APNs. The NCSBN also cited inconsistent requirements and the limitations to mobility that resulted from these inconsistencies as significant factors in the development of the second-licensure proposal. Most nursing organizations, however, did not oppose the proposed graduate degree requirement also included in the 1993 NCSBN position statement and experienced some conflict that second-licensure and graduate degree requirements were tied to the same proposal.

As previously noted, all states and territories engage in some formal recognition of advanced nursing practice. The second-licensure proposal was an attempt to bring uniformity to titling and educational requirements. The NCSBN House of Delegates adopted this position at its 1993 meeting.[18] However, because all states grant some type of practice recognition equivalent to the pure definition of licensure, the requirement that this additional recognition be termed a "license" to practice would not expand states' authority to regulate, a right already granted to the states through the Tenth Amendment of the Constitution.

The NCSBN's proposal to require a master's degree as eligibility to practice as an APN has received mixed support. In states where the state regulatory bodies have set target dates for meeting this requirement, extensions of these deadlines have been granted in the face of opposition to this higher standard. However, the master's-degree requirement may become irrelevant, because increasing numbers of certifying examinations require the master's degree as a prerequisite to sitting for the examinations.

Despite the NCSBN's passage of the second-licensure proposal, nursing regulators increasingly are questioning their ability to assure the competence of recently graduated APNs. States frequently recognize education and training as a valid means of documenting qualifications. If the education or training requirements closely match the state's requirements for practice, then these documented qualifications can be accepted by the state. In many states, the regulatory agencies governing advanced nursing practice have agreed to accept proof of successful completion of professional certification by the APN as validation of eligibility to practice in the advanced practice role. In many instances, the certification criteria defined by the professional organization match those identified by the state for practice within the state. Professional certification is accepted without further evaluation or duplication as one means of documenting qualification to practice within the state.

Professional certification, as defined by the American Nurses Credentialing Center (ANCC), is the process by which an organization, based on predetermined standards, validates an RN's qualifications, knowledge, and practice in a defined functional or clinical area of nursing. Professional certification is reserved for those nurses who have met the requirements for clinical or functional practice in a specialized field, have pursued education beyond basic nursing preparation, and have received the endorsement of their peers. On satisfying these criteria, nurses are eligible to take certification examinations based on nationally recognized standards of nursing practice that demonstrate special knowledge and skills surpassing those required for state licensure.[19]

The use of professional certification as evidence for validation of public authority to practice intermingles the domains of professional certification and public regulation. The credentialing organization, separate and distinct from the professional membership or specialty organization, bases its credentialing examination on the standards and scope-of-practice definition set by the membership of the professional practice organization. After an in-depth job analysis, a test development committee, composed of individuals who by their education and experience are recognized as experts in the specific area of practice, identifies relevant content, areas of focus, and the professional competencies to be measured. Next, examination questions are solicited from nurses certified in the specialty area and other experts throughout the country. The submitted questions undergo rigorous review, critique, and rating for accuracy and relevancy by a psychometrician. The panel of experts or test development committee then selects a representative sample of the questions for inclusion on the certifying examination.

Many professions also require practical tests and oral reviews to supplement written examinations in determining a candidate's qualifications for certification. Although written examinations are the most frequently used form of evaluation, 47 percent of certification organizations use only written examinations, and an additional 28 percent use written examinations in combination with practical tests and/or oral reviews. While the means of testing depends on the occupation or profession, written examinations can effectively evaluate knowledge: Manual or verbal skills for a particular profession often must be demonstrated through a practical test or oral presentation. Approximately 25 percent of certification programs use a practical test, and 11 percent use an oral review.[20]

The great variety among the states in the use of national certifying examinations as a precursor to state recognition has generated controversy. Recently, NCSBN member boards have raised concerns regarding the psychometric properties of the testing mechanisms used by certifying bodies and have questioned state boards' abilities to assure the competence of an individual to serve in the expanded APN role by reliance on privately controlled and developed certification examinations (see the following discussion of certification examinations and requirements for certification). Other critics of state reliance on professional certification processes point to inconsistencies in the criteria for APNs' certification as a weakness. Educational requirements, graduate degree requirements, and precertification practice requirements vary among certifying organizations. In many instances, some organizations reportedly have applied varying degrees of scrutiny to the educational credentials of certification applicants and have allowed some applicants to waive such requirements. NCSBN member boards continue to express concerns about public regulatory oversight of APNs and its ability to assure that the competence of APNs to serve in expanded roles by reliance on certification examinations.

In 1994, the NCSBN House of Delegates endorsed a proposal to investigate the potential for development of a national testing mechanism for one group of APNs—nurse practitioners (NPs). The NCSBN staff was charged with developing a statement of core competencies for NP practice and with investigation of the "legal, political, and fiscal implications of development of a national exam for practice as a NP"[21] (p. 1). Although this effort focused specifically on NP practice, there was widespread understanding that the concerns for regulation of advanced practice extended to concerns about the preparation of clinical nurse specialists (CNSs) for advanced practice. As this issue has evolved, the relationship between public regulation and private credentialing has become more widely understood. See Table 6–2 for information on the American Board of Nursing Specialties.

Because NCSBN delegates began their work by focusing on NP practice, a variety of groups that certify NPs have engaged in discussions and exchanges regarding the continuing linkage of public regulation and specialty certification. At the 1995 NCSBN House of Delegates meeting, the NCSBN Board agreed to table efforts to develop a national licensure examination for NP regulation in favor of further discussions with the four major NP certifying bodies.[22] However, the House of Delegates empowered the NCSBN staff to begin the construction of a national examination in the event the discussions were not deemed productive. In March 1996, a breakdown in discussions between the certification organizations and the NCSBN resulted in the decision by the NCSBN board to begin analysis of NP practice for the potential development of a series of licensing examinations for nine types of NPs. The NCSBN has circulated a request for proposals to licensure examination experts as the first step in this process.

A variety of other concerns has been expressed regarding the regulation of APNs. Remaining current in both skills and knowledge and the method by which such continuing competence is evidenced are at issue. Moreover, the development of new specialties in advanced practice for which certification examinations do not yet exist has created unintended barriers to practice in states that require national certification for practice authority. Continuing discussions of these issues are driven by concerns for protecting the public and for allowing

TABLE 6–2
American Board of Nursing Specialties

The American Board of Nursing Specialties (ABNS) is the peer review body in nursing that oversees development of national professional certification processes. The ABNS, established in 1991, was the result of a 3-year project funded by the Macy Foundation to bring uniformity to professional certification in nursing and to ensure that certification was a mechanism for enhancing the quality of care delivered. The goals of the ABNS are:

1. To set standards for the formal recognition of professional nursing specialty certification programs
2. To establish policies and procedures for the review and approval of certification programs
3. To recognize specialty nursing certification that meets ABNS standards
4. To maintain procedures for review and approval of certification programs
5. To educate the public about certified professional nursing care

The ABNS has established 12 standards that must be met in order for a certification program to be recognized by the ABNS. Individuals who successfully complete professional certification exams from an organization that is ABNS recognized are considered "board certified." The following 15 organizations have been recognized by the ABNS:

1. American Board of Occupational Health Nurses, Inc.
2. ANCC Board on Community Nursing Practice
3. ANCC Board on Gerontological Nursing Practice
4. ANCC Board on Maternal-Child Nursing Practice
5. ANCC Board on Medical-Surgical Nursing Practice
6. ANCC Board on Nursing Administration
7. ANCC Board on Nursing Continuing Education and Staff Development
8. ANCC Board on Primary Care in Adult and Family Practice Nursing
9. ANCC Board on Psychiatric and Mental Health Nursing
10. Council on Certification of Nurse Anesthetists
11. National Certification Board: Perioperative Nursing, Inc.
12. Nephrology Nursing Certification Board
13. Oncology Nursing Certification Board
14. Orthopaedic Nurse Certification Board
15. Rehabilitation Nurses Certification Board

For information on ABNS standards, contact:

President
American Board of Nursing Specialties
660 Maryland Avenue, Suite 100 West
Washington, DC 20024-2571
202-554-2054

APNs to function to their fullest capacity. These issues bear watching in each state. In any event, it appears certain that the regulation process will change dramatically in the near future as regulators work to develop uniform standards that are transferable and defensible.

Professional Certification for Advanced Practice Nurses

Seven professional organizations offer certification for APNs: four for NPs, one for CNSs, one for nurse midwives, and one for nurse anesthetists. (A list of the professional organizations and specialties certified is shown in Table 6–3.) Some

TABLE 6–3
**Professional Organizations That Certify
Advanced Practice Nurses**

Certifying Body	Areas of Certification
American Academy of Nurse Practitioners	Adult NP
	Family NP
ANCC	Acute care NP*
	Adult NP
	Family NP
	Gerontological NP
	Pediatric NP
	School NP
	Community health CNS
	Gerontological CNS
	Home health CNS
	Medical-surgical CNS
	Adult psychiatric and mental health CNS
	Child and adolescent psychiatric and mental health CNS
American College Nurse-Midwives	Certified nurse midwife
American Association of Nurse Anesthetists	Certified registered nurse anesthetists
National Certification Corporation for the Obstetric, Gynecologic and Neonatal NP Nursing Specialties	Neonatal NP
	Women's health
Oncology Nursing Certification Corporation	Advanced oncology nursing for NPs and CNSs
National Certification Board of Pediatric NPs and Nurses	Pediatric NPs

*NP is jointly credentialed by ANCC and American Association of Critical Care Nurses Certification Corporation.

variation in philosophy, criteria, and requirements exists among the certifying organizations, particularly those that certify NPs. The most obvious difference is the requirement for a master's or higher degree in nursing.

Except for the National Certification Corporation for the Obstetric, Gynecologic and Neonatal Nursing Specialties (NCC) and the Oncology Nursing Certification Corporation (ONCC), all of the organizations that certify NPs require a master's or higher degree for certification examination eligibility. The NCC has convened representatives of all women's health NP and education organizations to examine this issue and to develop and implement a plan that will lay the foundation for a move to requiring a master's degree for certification. A consensus statement issued in September 1995 by all of the organizations focused on women's health and related NPs. The statement recognized the existence of a national movement from certificate to graduate education for NPs and the need to identify and support mechanisms to provide an orderly transition of women's health care NP education from certificate to graduate education.[23]

In its certification materials, the American Academy of Nurse Practitioners (AANP)[24] states that "certification is offered to graduates of approved Master's level adult and family NP programs" (p. 1). The AANP goes on to state that NPs who have not graduated from approved master's-level adult and family NP programs that meet the same criteria as a master's-degree programs may petition the Certification Board for permission to sit for the examinations.

The ONCC,[25] which offers certification for both NPs and CNSs in advanced nursing oncology, allows NPs without a master's degree in nursing to apply for certification if they have completed an NP program, hold a baccalaureate degree in nursing, and meet the practice requirements. After the year 2000, all new candidates for advanced oncology nursing certification must hold a master's degree or higher in nursing.

The ACNM, the only body that certifies nurse midwives, requires graduation from an accredited program. ACNM currently accredits certificate, graduate, and precertificate nurse midwifery education programs. In addition, ACNM recently has decided to accredit nonnurse midwifery programs. To date, no nonnurse program has applied for accreditation; however, the programs being examined for possible accreditation through this process are a combination of physician assistant and midwifery programs, several of which are already in existence. No formal decision has been made by ACNM whether graduates of these programs will be required to sit for the same certification examination as the nurse midwifery graduates.

The AANA offers certification for nurse anesthetists. To be eligible for the certification examination, the individual must be a graduate of a nurse anesthesia program accredited by the Council on Accreditation of Nurse Anesthesia Educational Programs of AANA. Under AANA standards adopted in November 1994, a master's or higher degree will be required by January 1998. Not all nurse anesthesia programs are located in schools of nursing, and therefore, a number of programs may offer a nonnursing master's degree.

The following four sections provide overviews and comparisons of the certification requirements for each of the advanced practice nursing specialties. Requirements for certification are revised regularly. For more detailed and current information regarding eligibility requirements for certification or recertification in each of the specialty practice areas, the APN should contact the named professional organization. For an updated list and addresses of the specialty certification boards and state boards of nursing, the APN can consult the annual January issue of the *American Journal of Nursing*.[26]

NURSE PRACTITIONER CERTIFICATION

Four professional organizations offer NP certification programs: the AANP, the ANCC, the NCC, and the National Certification Board of Pediatric Nurse Practitioners and Nurses (NCBNPN). Certification is offered in a number of specialties: acute-care NP, adult NP, family NP, gerontological NP, neonatal NP, pediatric NP, school NP, women's health care NP, and advanced oncology nursing. The newest NP certification program is the acute care NP certification examination. This examination is administered by the ANCC. However, credentialing of the individual is by both the American Association of Critical Care Nurses Certification Corporation and the ANCC. The ONCC offers certification in advanced nursing oncology for both NPs and CNSs. The same examination is used for both NPs and CNSs; therefore, the process does not test for separate role capabilities. For this reason, state boards of nursing do not recognize this examination as evidence of an individual's capabilities to practice in the NP role.

As mentioned previously, three of the five certifying organizations require a master's degree or higher in order for an individual to sit for the certification examination. The NCC, which certifies neonatal and women's health care NPs, is moving toward a master's degree requirement. The ONCC, which offers certification for advanced oncology nurses, will require all new candidates for NP certification to hold a master's degree by the year 2000.

Another significant difference in the requirements among the various NP certification authorities is the requirement of clinical practice in the area of specialization. Mandatory clinical practice requirements before taking the examination exist for only three of the NP certifications: ANCC certification as a pediatric NP, NCC certification as a neonatal NP, and NCC certification as a women's health care NP. ANCC's requirement of a minimum of 600 practice hours as a pediatric nurse practitioner can be satisfied within a formal pediatric NP program. Certification as an acute care NP has one option for clinical practice in the advanced practice specialty in lieu of educational preparation in an acute care NP program, which will be available only through the year 2000. This option allows an individual to have graduated from an adult NP master's degree in nursing program or a formal postgraduate adult NP program but must also have a minimum of 500 hours of practice within the past 2 years in an advanced practice role, providing direct services to patients who are acutely or critically ill, after completing the NP program. The requirement for postgraduate practice provides a source of obvious conflict if the graduate must practice before receiving public authority to practice while being unable to be certified without such practice. This catch-22 has intensified the debate regarding a second licensing examination for APNs administered by NCSBN.

Before the collaborative development of the Acute Care Nurse Practitioner Certification Examination by the American Association of Critical Care Nurses Certification Corporation and ANCC in 1995, NPs prepared in acute care did not have a mechanism for obtaining national certification, creating a barrier to practice in those states that had enacted legislation requiring national certification by a professional organization for NP practice. Some NPs did choose and were allowed to take the adult certification examinations, although these examinations are primarily geared toward individuals prepared in the area of adult primary care. The creation of the acute care NP certification examination has obviated this barrier.

Recertification requirements also vary among the five professional certifying organizations, with lengths of certification terms ranging from 5 to 6 years. The most common requirements for recertification include either re-examination or documentation of a specified number of hours in direct patient care in one's area of specialization and a specified number of hours of continuing education. A number of states now require the individual to have a specified number of continuing education hours annually in pharmacology to maintain one's prescriptive privileges. The adequacy of continuing education requirements in assuring practitioner competence has been seriously questioned, however, by the 1995 Pew report titled *Reforming Health Care Workforce Regulation.*

The NCBNPN provides two options for maintaining one's certification as a pediatric NP. An individual can take a scored self-assessment learning exercise, an independent-study educational tool, each year, or earn a specified number of continuing education credits. The self-assessment activity must be completed, however, in at least two of the years in the 6-year recertification cycle.[27]

CLINICAL NURSE SPECIALIST CERTIFICATION

Clinical nurse specialist certification is offered by both the ANCC and the ONCC. The ANCC areas of CNS certification include medical-surgical nursing, gerontological nursing, community health nursing, home health nursing, adult psychiatric and mental health nursing, and child and adolescent psychiatric and mental health nursing. The ONCC offers only advanced oncology nursing certification. To become certified in any of these specialty areas, the candidate must have a master's degree or higher in nursing.

Each of these certification programs requires that candidates have a minimum number of hours in direct patient care in their areas of specialization. ANCC certification as an adult or child and adolescent psychiatric and mental health CNS requires not only documentation of a specified number of hours in direct patient care but also a minimum number of hours of consultation and supervision by a nurse who is ANCC certified or eligible for certification as a CNS in psychiatric and mental health nursing.[19]

The American Association of Critical Care Nurses Certification Corporation offers certification programs in adult, neonatal, and pediatric critical-care nursing. To qualify for any of these examinations, an individual must hold a current RN's license and document a specified number of clinical practice hours in direct care of the critically ill patient.[28] Before the collaborative development of the Acute Care Nurse Practitioner Certification Examination by the American Association of Critical Care Nurses Certification Corporation and the ANCC in 1995, a number of CNSs in critical-care specialties opted to sit for one of the American Association of Critical Care Nurses Certification Corporation's certification examinations. Because the American Association of Critical Care Nurses Certification Corporation's certification examinations do not require advanced nursing education, the American Association of Critical Care Nurses Certification Corporation is not included in those organizations that certify CNSs.

NURSE MIDWIFE CERTIFICATION

The ACNM Certification Council is the only professional organization that offers certification for nurse midwives. To be eligible for the national certification examination, the individual must hold a current RN's license to practice in the United States and must document satisfactory completion of a nurse midwifery program that is either accredited or preaccredited by the ACNM Division of Accreditation.[29] Core competencies for basic nurse midwifery are clearly delineated by ACNM for each of the components of nurse midwifery care: preconception, antepartum, intrapartum, postpartum, neonatal, and family planning and gynecological care.[30]

NURSE ANESTHETIST CERTIFICATION

Professional certification for nurse anesthetists is offered solely by the Council on Certification of Nurse Anesthetists, an arm of AANA. To be eligible to take the certification examination for registered nurse anesthetists, candidates must hold a current and unrestricted RN license in the states in which they practice and must have completed a nurse anesthesia educational program accredited by the Council on Accreditation of Nurse Anesthesia Educational Programs.[31] In its requirements for program accreditation, the Council on Accreditation of Nurse Anesthesia Programs delineates the number and type of patient experiences required for graduation. In addition, the number of required experiences and specific types and methods of anesthesia are also defined.[32]

Clinical Privileges

Though not yet the norm, it is becoming more commonplace for APNs in all specialty areas of practice to apply for, and be granted, full clinical privileges at one or more health-care institutions. APNs must have access to a variety of health-care settings to provide the full range of comprehensive health-care services within the scope of their practice and to allow the consumer a full choice of high-quality, cost-effective health-care services. Traditionally, privileges to practice in a given health-care institution have been reserved for members of the institution's medical staff, and admission to this group has been closely guarded. Past battles waged by APNs and other health professionals to obtain hospital or clinical privileges have laid the groundwork for today's APN practice. As the number and diversity of APN specialties increase and as the move toward an integrated health-care delivery system gains momentum, more APNs will seek privileges to practice in all types of health-care settings, from acute care to community based.

PRACTICE SETTINGS

The number of APNs who currently hold clinical privileges at a health-care institution is not known. However, general information on practice settings and arrangements in which APNs in the various specialties are located is available.

In 1994, according to the ACNM,[33] 1101 (30 percent) CNMs listed a hospital as their primary employer. Only 269 (7 percent) said they were in a private CNM practice. A complete breakdown of CNM employment settings is shown in Table 6–4. Also, in 1994, 93 percent of all births attended by CNMs occurred in a hospital, 21 percent occurred in a birthing center, and 5 percent occurred in the home.

According to 1995 demographic data published by the AANA,[34] 10,358 (40.4 percent) of all certified registered nurse anesthetists (CRNAs) were institutionally employed (Table 6–5). More than 11 percent were self-employed or part of a CRNA group practice, and another 25 percent were practicing in a joint nurse anesthetist/anesthesiologist (CRNA/MDA) group practice. Of those in a joint CRNA/MDA practice, only 0.8 percent were partners or joint partners.

As a group, CNSs and NPs are more diverse in their practice settings and scopes of practice. Data regarding the practice arrangements of CNSs and NPs are minimal; however, some inferences can be drawn based on known data. In

TABLE 6–4
Primary Employers of Certified Nurse Midwives, 1994 (*N* = 3670)

Employer	Number (Percentage)
Hospital	1101 (30%)
Physician's office	795 (22%)
Educational institution	354 (10%)
HMO	307 (8%)
Private CNM practice	269 (7%)

Source: Data from American College of Nurse-Midwives: 1994 database.

TABLE 6–5
Certified Registered Nurse Anesthetist Employment Arrangements

Employment Arrangement	N	%
Institutionally employed	10,358	40
Physician employed	1,134	4.4
Government employed	906	3.5
Self-employed	2,995	11.7
Joint CRNA/MDA group	6,423	25
Retired	1,084	4.2
Unemployed	49	0.2
No response	2,703	10.5
Total members	25,652	100

Source: American Association of Nurse Anesthetists: Demographic Information for All CRNA Members, Excluding Students. American Association of Nurse Anesthetists, Chicago, 1995, p. 1.

TABLE 6–6
Financial and Practice Arrangements for Certified Nurse Practitioners

Total	Total NP in Sample 1,378	NP Estimated Total 21,892	NP Estimated Percent 100
FINANCIAL ARRANGEMENTS			
Fixed salary	1,089	17,139	78.3
Practice receipts fee-for-service only	45	753	3.4
Fixed salary plus additional monies based on the number of patients seen (fee for service)	52	885	4
Fixed salary and potential to generate additional benefits other than direct monetary reimbursement	153	2,455	11.2
Unknown	39	660	3
PRACTICE ARRANGEMENT			
Do not work with physician or a psychologist	33	398	1.8
Physician or psychologist available for consultation for a fee paid by NP	29	466	2.1
Physician or a psychologist is available on site a majority of the time	785	12,370	56.5
Physician or a psychologist is available by telecommunication	170	2,600	11.9

Source: Department of Health and Human Services: Survey of Certified Nurse Practitioners and CNSs: December 1992. Department of Health and Human Services, Bureau of Health Professions, Health Resources Services Administration, Division of Nursing, Rockville, Md, 1994, pp. 41–42.

1992, the estimated number of NPs not working with a physician or a psychologist was 398 (1.8 percent), implying that this small percentage of NPs were in independent practice. An additional estimated 466 NPs (2.1 percent) were in a practice arrangement in which the NP paid a consultant's fee to a physician or psychologist. Only an estimated 3.4 percent of NPs were not on a salary and received only fee-for-service practice receipts. The numbers and percentages of NPs by financial and practice arrangements are shown in Table 6–6. The estimated percentage of CNSs who did not work with a physician or a psychologist was 18.4 percent. An estimated 8.6 percent of CNSs paid a consultation fee to a physician or psychologist. An estimated 27.8 percent of all CNSs received fee-for-service practice receipts only. However, this number decreased to only 2.3 percent, however, when psychiatric–mental health CNSs were removed from the sample.[35] The complete breakdown of CNS practice sites and financial arrangements is shown in Table 6–7.

TABLE 6–7
**Financial and Practice Arrangements of Certified
Clinical Nurse Specialists**

Total	Total CNS in Sample 502	Estimated Total 5,868	NP Estimated Percent 100
FINANCIAL ARRANGEMENTS			
Fixed salary	342	3,640	62
Practice receipts fee-for-service only	112	1,632	27.8
Fixed salary plus additional monies based on the number of patients seen (fee for service)	9	130	2.2
Fixed salary and potential to generate additional benefits other than direct monetary reimbursement	27	304	5.2
Unknown	12	162	2.8
PRACTICE ARRANGEMENT			
Do not work with physician or a psychologist	101	1,080	18.4
Physician or psychologist available for consultation for a fee paid by CNS	37	503	8.6
Physician or a psychologist is available on site a majority of the time	246	2,835	48.3
Physician or a psychologist is available by telecommunication	59	774	13.2

Source: Department of Health and Human Services: Survey of Certified Nurse Practitioners and CNSs: December 1992. Department of Health and Human Services, Bureau of Health Professions, Health Resources Services Administration, Division of Nursing, Rockville, Md, 1994, pp.43–44.

Traditionally, most NPs have been employed in ambulatory- or outpatient-care settings. Surprisingly, according to the US Department of Health and Human Services study on certified NPs and CNSs, CNSs were also employed predominantly in ambulatory-care settings. However, for each of the specialty CNS and NP groups, the predominant employment site varied. More than 94 percent of all neonatal NPs were employed in inpatient hospital-based settings. The second highest percentage of specialty NPs employed in inpatient hospital-based practices were adult NPs (11.5 percent). More than one-third of gerontology NPs were employed in a nursing home or an extended-care facility (34.3 percent).[35] Medical-surgical CNSs constituted the largest group of CNSs employed in an inpatient hospital-based setting (62.9 percent). However, only 22 percent of adult psychiatric CNSs were employed in inpatient hospital-based settings.

The number of APNs in all specialty areas involved in independent practice is increasing slowly. Potentially, each of these practitioners is in a position to obtain financially rewarding institutional or clinical privileges. In addition, all APNs, whether they are practicing in an independent practice setting or not, are responsible for the comprehensive health care of clients. The ability of APNs to deliver comprehensive care is compromised by their inability to coordinate and provide services to these clients when their conditions warrant admission to a health-care institution. The financial and quality-of-care benefits associated with the possession of clinical privileges are becoming increasingly evident.

DEFINITION OF CLINICAL PRIVILEGES

Clinical privileges are permission to provide medical or other patient care services in the granting institution, within well-defined limits, based on the individual's professional license and his or her experience, competence, ability, and judgment.
   JOINT COMMISSION ON ACCREDITATION OF HOSPITALS, 1995 ACCREDITATION MANUAL FOR HOSPITALS,[36] p. 55

Today's health-care system includes many diverse types of delivery settings. The term *clinical privileges* is synonymous with the term *hospital privileges*, except that clinical privileges denotes the additional ability to practice at any health-care delivery institution where formal practice privileges are required. This section focuses on clinical privileges in long-term care and acute-care settings. Clinical privileges granted to an individual practitioner must be delineated or specifically defined by the medical staff of the institution and set forth in institutional bylaws. Thus, the scope of privileges or type of services permitted may vary from institution to institution.

The Joint Commission on Accreditation of Healthcare Organizations (JCAHO) first revised its medical-staff standards in 1983 to allow hospitals to extend clinical privileges to nonmedical practitioners. This change in policy was spurred by antitrust case law, changes in reimbursement laws, an increased emphasis on cost control, expanded numbers and types of providers, and an increased spirit of competition.[37] The 1984 JCAHO standards stipulated that medical staff must include physicians but also allowed hospitals to grant medical-staff membership to other licensed practitioners permitted by law and the hospital to independently provide patient-care services.[38] At that time, nursing organizations were concerned that the wording of these standards would restrict the ability of APNs to obtain clinical privileges where state nurse-practice acts required APNs to practice under the supervision of a physician.

The revised 1995 JCAHO accreditation standards state[36]:

> There is a single organized medical staff that has overall responsibility for the quality of the professional services provided by individuals with clinical privileges, as well as the responsibility of accounting therefore to the governing body. (p. 55)

The medical staff includes fully licensed physicians and may include other licensed individuals permitted by law and by the hospital to provide patient-care services independently in the hospital. Other individuals permitted to provide patient-care services independently are further defined as[36]

> any individual who is permitted by law and by the hospital to provide patient care services without direction or supervision, within the scope of his or her license and in accordance with individually granted clinical privileges. Clinical privileges are based on criteria established by the hospital. (p. 55)

The JCAHO accreditation standards allow, but do not require, hospitals or other health-care institutions to grant clinical privileges to other licensed providers. If the hospital admits a practitioner to its medical staff, it also must grant the practitioner delineated clinical privileges.[39] Section MS 2.2 of the JCAHO Standards[36] stipulates that

> all individuals who are permitted by law and by the hospital to provide patient care services independently in the hospital have delineated clinical privileges, whether or not they are medical staff members. (p. 398)

Delineation of privileges is defined as an "accurate, detailed, and specific description of the clinical privileges granted"[36] (p. 398). The intent of this section is to allow hospitals to delineate clinical privileges for individuals who may be permitted to provide patient care independently but

> might not be members of the medical staff because of limitations on medical staff membership under applicable law or regulation or because of hospital choice. (p. 398)

Since the revision of the JCAHO accreditation standards to allow hospitals to grant clinical privileges to "other independently licensed" providers, many institutions have created a separate category of clinical privileges to encompass nonphysician providers. Such terms as *affiliate* or *allied health staff* are some of the more commonly used terms to denote nonphysician staff membership and privileges.

MEDICAL-STAFF VERSUS AFFILIATE-STAFF PRIVILEGES

The granting of affiliate staff privileges generally does not grant the APN full standing on the institution's medical staff. The most common difference between full medical- and affiliate-staff privileges is that APNs are not allowed to admit and discharge patients under their own name. Affiliate- or allied-staff membership also does not include medical-staff voting privileges. Another difference that may exist is that an affiliate-staff member might not be allowed to serve on any of the medical-staff committees that make recommendations to the institution's governing board regarding rules and regulations by which the medical staff operates.

Many hospitals that have created an affiliate-staff category have also delineated specific circumstances under which the practitioner who is granted affiliate-staff status may practice and specific functions that may be performed. These criteria and functions often are more restrictive than the scope of practice allowed by state law. Although it may be seen as self-serving and protective of the medical staff, an institution's board of governors is permitted to establish rules and procedures that maintain and protect the quality of care delivered to patients at that institution. As noted previously, the JCAHO accreditation standards[36] state that

> the medical staff has overall responsibility for the quality of the professional services provided by individuals with clinical privileges. (p. 55)

In addition[36]:

> Medical staff membership and delineated clinical privileges are granted by the governing body, based on medical staff recommendation, in accordance with the bylaws, rules and regulations, and policies of the medical staff and of the hospital. (p. 55)

REASONS FOR OBTAINING CLINICAL PRIVILEGES

A number of benefits to possessing clinical privileges have been cited in the literature.[37,38,40] These include:

- The ability to continue to provide and direct the care received by a patient if admission to a health-care institution is necessary
- The ability to ensure that the patient is discharged back to one's care
- The ability to observe or assist in a patient's surgery
- The ability to review and write in the patient's chart without permission
- The ability to obtain reimbursement from third-party payers for visits made to patients
- The ability to oversee the care received by a patient, including the referral to specialists for consultation
- A means of demonstrating one's credentials and competencies or a way of obtaining a "stamp of approval" from the health-care profession at large
- Preferred provider organizations (PPO) or managed-care companies may use hospital privileges as a means of measuring a provider's competence or as a method of quality assurance for the PPO
- A means of gaining recognition as a legitimate health-care professional in a competitive health-care market
- A way to maintain an ongoing relationship with a patient, including serving as a patient advocate
- A way to increase one's knowledge of, and ability to discuss, a patient's potential hospital experiences

- A means of keeping one's skills and knowledge of technology and procedures current
- The ability to become involved in setting the rules and regulations governing practices at the health-care institution
- The ability to more fully market one's services to the consumer
- The ability to maintain one's self-esteem
- The ability to meet physicians' and consumers' demands for services provided by APNs

Along with the benefits of obtaining clinical privileges, the APNs must be willing to assume the increased accountability and responsibility for the services they provide to patients. APNs must participate fully in the decision-making processes involved in providing care to patients and in ensuring that appropriate coverage is provided 24 hours a day. APNs are liable for their own actions just as physicians or institutions are liable for negligent actions involving the care of patients. In addition, APNs may be held liable for not referring a patient with a problem beyond their level of competence. With full medical-staff membership and privileges comes the ability and responsibility to serve on one or more medical-staff committees. Not only does this provide the practitioner with the ability to participate more fully in the decision-making and policy-making processes of the institution; it also requires a significant amount of time away from one's other professional and personal commitments.

FACTORS GOVERNING THE ABILITY TO OBTAIN CLINICAL PRIVILEGES

An APN's ability to obtain clinical privileges at an institution is governed by three entities:

1. State law and regulations
2. JCAHO accreditation standards
3. Institutional policy and medical-staff bylaws

State Law and Regulations

State law and regulations define the scope of advanced practice nursing within the particular state. Clinical privileges granted to an APN must be in accordance with these state laws and regulations. The number of states that have enacted laws allowing the independent practice of APNs has increased dramatically, and additional state boards of nursing and advanced practice nursing groups are considering similar legislation. All but two states, Illinois and Ohio, have enacted legislation that allow APNs to prescribe to some degree. Fifteen states allow NPs to prescribe medication, including controlled substances, independent of any physician involvement.[14]

Only two states, Oregon and Florida, have enacted legislation that specifically refers to APNs' obtaining hospital privileges.[13] In most states, hospital admitting privileges for APNs are not regulated and are granted at the discretion of the hospitals. Many hospitals will grant privileges to APNs only if their collaborating physicians have staff privileges at the hospital. In 1983, the District of Columbia enacted legislation that prohibited hospitals or any other health-care facility from denying clinical privileges or medical-staff membership for qualified CRNAs, CNMs, certified NPs, podiatrists, or psychologists. This legislation was expanded in 1985 to include CNSs.

Joint Commission on Accreditation of Healthcare Organizations' Standards

The second factor limiting APNs' ability to obtain clinical privileges is the standards for institutional accreditation established by JCAHO. As noted previously, JCAHO revised its medical-staff standards in 1983, effective 1984, to allow accredited hospitals to grant clinical privileges to nonphysician providers. Current JCAHO accreditation standards allow the granting of privileges to include both independent and dependent practit.ioners.

Institutional Bylaws and Policy

The state nurse-practice acts under which APNs practice determine the scope of practice and the degree of dependence or independence with which they may practice. The governing board of an institution, under bylaws approved by the medical staff, grants membership to the medical staff of the institution. The board also must delineate the specific functions that may be performed by individual practitioners if allowed to provide patient-care services independently in the institution, whether or not they are members of the medical staff. Even when federal case law, state law, and accreditation standards stipulate that APNs may obtain clinical privileges at a health-care institution, the individual institution may determine the specific credentials deemed acceptable and the specific clinical privileges allowed. The privileges delineated by the institution may be more restrictive than those allowed under state nurse-practice acts.

PROCESS OF OBTAINING CLINICAL PRIVILEGES

Obtaining clinical privileges involves two separate processes:
1. Credentialing and admittance to the medical staff
2. Delineating of specific clinical privileges

The mechanisms for appointment or reappointment and the granting or renewal of clinical privileges must be fully documented in the bylaws of the institution, which are approved and revised regularly by the medical-staff membership. Copies of the bylaws and application materials usually are available from the medical-staff office. In some institutions, the APN must also apply in a separate process to the nursing-service office. At an institution that has two categories of medical-staff membership, full and affiliate, separate applications and processes may have been adopted.

When applying for clinical privileges at an institution in which there are two types of staff membership, APNs must be aware of the differences in the processes and in the privileges granted to the practitioner. If an affiliate-staff category exists but does not allow the practitioner to admit patients under one's own name or requires physician supervision and signatures for all procedures, the APNs must decide whether functioning under these restrictions will meet their practice needs. Having an affiliate-staff category does not preclude an APN from applying for full medical-staff membership. Many health-care institutions have not had an APN apply for full medical-staff membership and privileges.

Whether separate procedures for physicians and nonphysicians exist, an application must be completed and references obtained. Generally the credentialing processes and application require that the individual document all professional licenses held, graduate or professional education, employment record, and malpractice coverage. If applying for affiliate-staff membership, some institutions require a less vigorous scrutiny of an individual's past employment record, such as only the past 5 years.

Generally, the practitioner's application for membership on the medical staff must pass through several committees, each one making a recommendation to a higher-level committee. The first committee may be a department committee or may be a hospital-wide credentials committee composed of representatives of each of the departments. The credentials committee may include a representative of the nursing department and hospital administration. For affiliate-staff membership, some institutions have established credentialing committees composed of peers or representatives of the affiliate staff. A recommendation is made by the credentials committee to the subsequent level and so forth until reaching the institution's board of directors or some other board officially charged with making a final decision.

The application can be disapproved at any step of the process. A negative recommendation can be overturned by a higher-level committee, but this rarely occurs unless a strong legal or political rationale exists for doing so. JCAHO standards[36] specify that a review mechanism must exist and clearly state

> that [it] includes a fair hearing and appeal process, for addressing adverse decisions for the applicant regarding medical staff appointment, or reappointment and granting of initial or renewed/revised clinical privileges. (p. 58)

Once a practitioner is granted membership on the medical or affiliate staff, an application for specific clinical privileges must be made. Each department or division in the institution has its own privilege designation form. Sample guidelines and privilege delineation forms for the various medical specialties have been created by the American Medication Association. Privilege delineation forms include detailed listings of procedures and clinical conditions that the practitioner is requesting permission to perform and treat in that institution. The procedures and conditions may be divided according to specific body systems. The situation and degree of supervision under which specific procedures may be performed and clinical conditions treated are also delineated in writing. For example, a practitioner may be required to perform a specific procedure under the supervision of a more experienced practitioner until a certain level of competence is demonstrated or a consultation may be required for certain clinical conditions or types of patients.

Bylaws of an institution may specify under what conditions and degree of supervision an APN may practice. Some institutions grant admitting privileges but require that admissions be made under a physician's name. JCAHO standards[36] specify that

> when nonphysician members of the medical staff are granted privileges to admit patients to inpatient services, provision is made for prompt medical evaluation of these patients by a qualified physician. (p. 59)

A "qualified physician" is defined as

a doctor of medicine or doctor of osteopathy who . . . is granted clinical privileges by the institution. (p. 59)

APPEAL FOR DENIAL OF CLINICAL PRIVILEGES

Denial of medical-staff membership and privileges to an individual APN may be due to inadequate credentials or because the institution does not want that type of provider practicing in the institution despite adequate credentials. An institution has the responsibility and right to deny medical-staff membership and privileges to any practitioner if there is inadequate documentation of competence, if there is evidence of prior incident of disciplinary action, and/or if references do not support the granting of clinical privileges. If an application is disapproved, the appeals process documented in the bylaws must be followed. If privileges have been awarded previously to APNs in a given specialty, it is very difficult to prove that privileges were denied due to discrimination.

In attempting to reverse an adverse decision by an institution's board, the appeals process must be followed carefully and exhausted before turning to alternative actions. An alternative mechanism that may be tried is to wait a reasonable amount of time and reapply. Changes in the health-care arena are occurring, and political pressure may be brought to bear on an institution. Alliances with medical and other health professional colleagues and consumers must be sought. Opponents of granting medical-staff membership to APNs may retire or leave the institution. As consumers become more attuned to, and involved in, health-care issues, state legislatures are becoming more willing to enact laws that broaden the scope of advanced nursing practice. This movement will pave the way for increasingly independent practice and the increased use of APNs to provide comprehensive health-care services across all health-care delivery sites.

Legal action, particularly if taken as an individual practitioner, is a lengthy and extremely costly process in terms of both financial and emotional resources. In many instances, the entire appeals process has extended over 13 years. In some instances, decisions have been made in a more timely fashion but generally involve an out-of-court settlement. If legal action is deemed necessary, several courses of action are available; these are most appropriately determined and explained by legal counsel.

FEDERAL TRADE COMMISSION

The Federal Trade Commission (FTC) has the ability to investigate a complaint made by an APN or group of nurses regarding anticompetitive practices of an institution. Although the FTC has refused to hear numerous cases regarding discrimination against APNs, there is some evidence of its willingness to mediate well-documented instances of discrimination. On January 28, 1988, the FTC issued a consent agreement involving a group of nurse midwives and the medical staff of the Memorial Medical Center in Savannah, Georgia. The complaint brought by the nurse midwives alleged that in 1983, the hospital medical staff's credentials committee voted to allow a nurse midwife to perform deliveries at the medical center in the presence of a physician, as authorized under Georgia law. Shortly thereafter, members of the medical staff protested and threatened to shift their patient admissions to another hospital. One month later, the committee reversed itself and denied the nurse midwife hospital privileges, without stating any reasonable basis for the decision. Under the consent agreement, the medical staff agreed not to deny or restrict hospital privileges for any nurse midwife, unless the staff was able to provide a reasonable basis for believing that such restriction would serve the interest of the hospital in providing health-care services.[41]

Although not directly related to the acquisition of clinical privileges, in a still-pending case the New York State Nurses Association (NYSNA), after several years of not being able to settle the problem amicably, filed a complaint from NPs in Rochester, New York, with the New York State Attorney General's Office, which forwarded it to the FTC. The NPs claimed that the Rochester Community Individual Practice Association, the major provider in the area's managed-care market, had unlawfully restricted their practice by its refusal to reimburse APNs for certain types of patient visits unless directly supervised by physicians. The NYSNA alleged that this restriction is contrary to New York State law and results in additional and unnecessary expense to the patient's visit.[42]

ANTITRUST RULINGS

Legal action in response to the denial of medical-staff membership and clinical privileges may also be sought in federal court, alleging violation of the Sherman Antitrust Act. Though extremely expensive and lengthy, such legal recourse has been successfully taken in several cases involving APNs.

As early as 1976, health-care providers were subject to federal antitrust laws. In *Hospital Building Company v Trustees of Rex Hospital*, 428 US 738 (1976), the US Supreme Court held that health care is a commercial business operated for economic benefit and thus subject to the Sherman Antitrust Act.[43] The act[44] prohibits conspiracies "in restraint of trade or commerce among the several states" (Section 1) and prohibits monopolizing "any part of the trade or commerce among the several states" (Section 2). Many health-care practitioners have asserted that a hospital's refusal to permit them to practice at the hospital was illegal under one or both of these provisions of the Sherman Antitrust Act. Health-care practitioners who have been denied privileges because of exclusivity contracts or because they were members of certain professions, including nursing, have also brought suit against hospitals under the Sherman Antitrust Act.[45] Most states have also enacted similar antitrust legislation and may be a viable alternative to action at the federal level.

For a case to be brought under the Sherman Antitrust Act, two preliminary criteria must be satisfied. First, it must be shown that the case or controversy involves interstate trade or commerce. In some cases, the required nexus between the identified conduct and interstate commerce has been implied from facts showing that some patients have come from out of state, that equipment used is purchased from out of state, that the hospital or institution has out-of-state shareholders, and/or that insurance payments have come from out-of-state companies. In other, more restrictive cases, the court has ruled that to qualify under the Sherman Antitrust Act, the practitioner's business or the denial of access to the practitioner must directly affect or involve interstate commerce.[46]

The second criterion that must be proved is that there has been a conspiracy in restraint of trade. The effect of the conspiratorial action must have the effect of restraining competition in a relevant or defined market. The conspiracy may involve little more than a joint understanding or action. For example in the case of

Bhan v NME Hospitals, the court noted that their five hospitals operated within the area indicated that the defendant hospital's policy of not allowing nurse anesthetists to practice was not a restraint of trade.[46] However, in *Oltz v St Peter's Hospital,* a decision was obtained in favor of the nurse anesthetist where the defendant hospital was the only hospital equipped to do general surgery in the area.[46]

In the *Bhan v NME Hospitals* case, several precedents relevant to advanced nursing practice and antitrust case law were established. Mr. Bhan, a CRNA, had worked for one of the NME hospitals on a fee-for-service basis for several years. Under a contract with the hospital, he and an anesthesiologist had provided all of the hospital's anesthesia services until the time that the hospital hired a second anesthesiologist. At that time, Bhan's anesthesiologist associate urged the hospital to drop Bhan from the staff and to rely on himself and the other anesthesiologist, and the hospital followed this recommendation. Mr. Bhan claimed that the all-anesthesiologist policy was adopted as part of a conspiracy to eliminate competition. The federal trial court dismissed the lawsuit on the grounds that nurses and doctors do not compete, because in California, CRNAs were not authorized to write orders and were required to work under a supervising physician. The US District Court of Appeals reversed this decision, stating that although the legal restrictions on CRNAs create a functional distinction between them and anesthesiologists, such restrictions did not preclude their reasonable interchangeability. In effect, the court held that nurses have standing to sue under the antitrust laws when they are excluded from practicing as the result of anticompetitive arrangements between hospitals and physicians.[47]

In the *Oltz v St Peters Community Hospital* case, a federal trial court and the federal court of appeals agreed that the hospital had conspired with anesthesiologists to restrain the nurse anesthetist's practice. Mr. Oltz was an independent contractor providing anesthesia services, primarily for obstetric cases. The facts demonstrated that Mr. Oltz was popular with the obstetricians, who preferred his services over those of the anesthesiologists. When the hospital decided to organize an anesthesia department, Mr. Oltz's contract was terminated. The contract was reinstated when the hospital received correspondence from Oltz's attorney and the state attorney general's office. Subsequently, three of the hospital's four anesthesiologists threatened to quit if Oltz's services were retained, and so his contract was once again terminated. After Oltz's departure, each anesthesiologist received a 40 to 50 percent salary increase. A monetary pretrial settlement was negotiated with the anesthesiologists, and Oltz proceeded successfully in obtaining a jury verdict against the hospital. This is one of the only cases in which a health-care provider has been able to prove that the installation of an exclusive contract violated the Sherman Act and caused economic damages.[43]

In a case involving a nurse midwife, *Nurse Midwifery Associates v Hibbett,*[48] the nurse midwives attempted to invoke the Sherman Antitrust Act and the Tennessee state antitrust laws to prohibit the defendants (three hospitals, one pediatrician, three obstetricians, and an insurance carrier) from denying staff privileges to nurse midwives. The nurse midwives alleged that the defendants' denial of privileges had put them out of business. One of the obstetricians, Hibbett, was also a member of the board of trustees of the insurance company. The court denied the claim against one hospital and the insurance company for various reasons, the most important being that the nurses failed to prove a conspiracy by these defendants. The court did decide that the claims against two of the hospitals and Hibbett warranted a trial. After 13 years, an out-of-court settlement was reached.

The description of antitrust rulings presented here should be considered illustrative cases, rather than a comprehensive discussion of case law. The reader should be familiar with the concepts referred to in antitrust rulings as they relate to APNs. Any decision to enter into an antitrust legal case should be made only after lengthy discussion with qualified legal counsel.

Summary

Regulation of advanced nursing practice is in a state of rapid flux. A number of factors, such as the increased numbers of APNs in the various practice specialties, changes in the health-care delivery system, increased consumer involvement in health care, and public demand for accountability by health-care providers for high-quality, cost-effective care, have, and will continue to have, a significant impact on the regulation of advanced practice nursing. APNs must assume a leadership role not only in the delivery of health-care services but also in the professional and public regulation of nursing practice. To assume such a role, APNs must be able to understand and articulate the authorized scope of their practice. The ability to understand the interrelationships among the processes used by the public and the profession to regulate advanced nursing practice and to respond appropriately to these processes is crucial.

Suggested Exercises

1. Review the statutory and regulatory standards for advanced nursing practice in the state in which you expect to practice after graduation. Determine the correct state regulatory agency, and then make a request for the state authority-to-practice guidelines.

2. Identify the advanced practice nursing certifying corporation that administers the examination most relevant to the your expected area of practice on graduation and request information regarding the standards for practice, the process of application for certification, and the process for renewal of certification.

3. Acquire a copy of the Pew Health Professions report on licensure and regulation and compare that report's recommendations to the standards for regulation in the state in which the you will practice on graduation.

4. Obtain a copy of the bylaws of a hospital to determine the process used to delineate and grant clinical privileges. Based on the hospital's bylaws, determine whether an APN is eligible for membership on the medical staff.

5. Contact the National Council of State Boards of Nursing and identify the current status of licensure and recognition reforms.

6. Review the journal *Nurse Practitioner*'s annual update on licensure and prescriptive privileges and identify changes that have occurred from the previous year.

REFERENCES

1. American Nurses' Association: Nursing's Social Policy Statement. American Nurses' Association, Washington, DC, 1995.
2. Malson, LP: Credentialing in Nursing: Contemporary Developments and Trends. American Nurses' Association, Kansas City, Mo, 1989, p1.
3. Cox, C, and Foster, S: The Costs and Benefits of Occupational Regulation. Bureau of the Federal Trade Commission, Washington, DC, 1990.
4. Friedland, B, and Valachovic, R: The regulation of dental licensing: The dark ages? Am J Law Med 17:249, 1991.
5. Maine Health Professions Regulation Taskforce: Toward a More Rational State Licensure System for Maine's Health Professionals: A Report to the Governor and Maine Legislature. Medical Care Development, Maine Health Professions Regulation Task Force, Augusta, Maine, 1995.
6. Pew Health Professions Commission: Reforming Health Care Workforce Regulation: Policy Considerations for the 21st Century. Pew Health Professions Commission, San Francisco, 1995.
7. Starr, P: The Social Transformation of American Medicine. Basic Books, New York, 1982.
8. Burl, JB, and Bonner, A: Demonstration of the cost-effectiveness of a NP/physician team in long-term care facilities. HMO Practice 8(4):157, 1994.
9. Frampton, J, and Wall, S: Exploring the use of NPs and PAs in primary care. HMO Practice 8(4):164, 1994.
10. Schultz, JM, Liptak, GS, and Fioravanti, J: Nurse practitioners' effectiveness in NICU. Nursing Management 25(10):50, 1994.
11. National Council of State Boards of Nursing: What regulation of advanced nursing practice can offer health care reform. Issues 14(3):4, 1993.
12. King, CS: Second licensure. Advanced Practice Nursing Quarterly 1(1):7, 1995.
13. Henderson, T, Fox-Grage, W, and Lewis, S: Scope of Practice and Reimbursement for Advanced Practice Registered Nurses: A State-by-State Analysis. Intergovernmental Health Policy Project, Washington, DC, 1995.
14. Pearson, L: Annual update of how each state stands on legislative issues affecting advanced nursing practice. Nurse Pract 21:10, 1996.
15. Safriet, BJ: Health care dollars and regulatory sense: The role of advanced practice nursing. Yale Journal on Regulation 9(2), 1992.
16. Sekscenski, E et al: State practice environments and the supply of physician assistants, NPs, and certified nurse-midwives. N Engl J Med 331: 1266, 1994.
17. American Nurses' Association: Institutional Licensure: An Historical Perspective. House of Directors Action Report. American Nurses' Association, Washington, DC, 1995.
18. National Council of State Boards of Nursing: What regulation of advanced practice can offer health care reform. Issues 14(3):4, 1993.
19. American Nurses Certification Corporation: 1996 Certification Catalog. American Nurses Certification Corporation, Washington, DC, 1995.
20. National Certification Corporation: Certification Committee Newsletter. National Certification Corporation, Chevy Chase, Md, 1995.
21. National Council of State Boards of Nursing: Press Release: National Council Delegates Conclude 1994 Meeting. National Council of State Boards of Nursing, Chicago, Ill, 1994.
22. National Council of State Boards of Nursing: 1994 Annual meeting of the National Council sets organization's course for coming year. Issues 16(3):1, 1995.
23. Association of Women's Health Organizations and Neonatal Nurses, National Association of Nurses in Reproductive Health, and Planned Parenthood Federation of America: Consensus Statement on Women's Health Care Nurse Practitioner Education. Washington, DC, pp 19–35, September 15, 1995.
24. American Academy of Nurse Practitioners: National competency-based certification examinations for adult and family nurse practitioners. American Academy of Nurse Practitioners, Austin, Tex, 1996.
25. Oncology Nursing Certification Corporation. Oncology Nursing Certification Corporation Test Bulletin. Oncology Nursing Certification Corporation, Pittsburgh, Pa, 1996.
26. Your Guide to Certification & How to Get a License: Career Guide 1996. Am J Nurs, 1996.
27. National Certification Board of Pediatric Nurse Practitioners and Nurses: Pediatric Nurse Practitioner Certification and Certification Maintenance Programs. National Certification Board of Pediatric Nurse Practitioners, Cherry Hill, NJ, 1995.
28. American Association of Critical Care Nursing Certification Corporation: Certification Renewal Handbook. American Association of Critical Care Nursing Certification Corporation, Aliso Viejo, Calif, 1996.
29. American College of Nurse-Midwives Certification Council: Statement on "Eligibility Requirements for Application to Take the National Certification Examination." American College of Nurse-Midwives Education Committee, Washington, DC, February, 1994.
30. American College of Nurse-Midwives Education Committee: ACNM Core Competencies for Basic Nurse-Midwifery Practice. American College of Nurse-Midwives Education Committee, Washington, DC, 1992.
31. Council on Certification of Nurse Anesthetists. 1996 Candidate Handbook. Council on Certification of Nurse Anesthetists, Park Ridge, Ill, 1996.

32. Council on Accreditation of Nurse Anesthesia Education Programs. Standards for Accreditation of Nurse Anesthesia Educational Programs. Council on Accreditation of Nurse Anesthesia Education Programs, Park Ridge, Ill, 1994.

33. American College of Nurse-Midwives: 1994 database.

34. American Association of Nurse Anesthetists: Demographic Information for All CRNA Members, Excluding Students. Chicago, Ill., 1995.

35. Department of Health and Human Services: Survey of Certified Nurse Practitioners and Clinical Nurse Specialists: December 1992. Department of Health and Human Services, Public Health Service, Health Resources and Services Administration, Bureau of Health Professions, Division of Nursing, Rockville, Md, 1994.

36. Joint Commission on Accreditation of Healthcare Organizations: 1995 Accreditation Manual for Hospitals, Vols 1 and 2, 1992. Joint Commission on Accreditation of Healthcare Organizations, Oakbrook Terrace, Ill, 1994.

37. Rose, M: Laying siege to hospital privileges. Am J Nurs, 84:613, May 1984.

38. Stevens, JE: The question of hospital privileges for allied health professionals. Quality Review Bulletin 10(1):17, 1984.

39. Miles, J: Antitrust implications of allied health practitioner privilege decisions and hospital-physician exclusive contracts. The Medical Staff Counselor 2(1):19, 1988.

40. Smithing, RT, and Wiley, M: Hospital privileges: Who needs them? Journal of the American Academy of Nurse Practitioners 1(4): 150, 1989.

41. American College of Nurse-Midwives: Hospital staff settling charges they illegally denied hospital privileges to nurse-midwife. J Nurse-Midwifery 33:152, 1988.

42. Savage, K: NP rights in the balance. NP News 4(1):3, 1996.

43. Cushing, M: Safeguarding the spirit of competition. Am J Nurs 89:1035, 1989.

44. Sherman Act, 15 USC 1 & 2.

45. Blumenreich, GA: Anesthesia Advantage, Inc. vs. Metz. Journal of the American Association of Nurse Anesthetists 58(5): 335, 1990.

46. Blumenreich, GA: Antitrust protection against a hospital's denial of access. Journal of the American Association of Nurse Anesthetists 56(5):383, 1988.

47. American Association of Nurse Anesthetists: News Release: U.S. Ninth Circuit Court of Appeals Backs Nurse Anesthetists. American Association of Nurse Anesthetists, Chicago, Ill., 1985.

48. *Nurse Midwifery Associates v Hibbett*, 918 F2d 605 (6th Cir 1990).

Reimbursement for Expanded Professional Nursing Practice Services

MICHAEL J. KREMER, DNSc, CRNA
MARGARET FAUT-CALLAHAN, DNSc, CRNA, FAAN

Michael J. Kremer, DNSc, CRNA, received his doctoral degree from the Rush University College of Nursing. His master's of science in nursing is from Seattle Pacific University, Seattle, Washington. He received his nurse-anesthesia education at the University of Illinois in Springfield, Illinois, and undergraduate psychology and nursing degrees from Northern Illinois University in DeKalb, Illinois. He is a faculty preceptor in the Rush University Nurse Anesthesia Program. He has been active in all areas of clinical anesthesia and is formerly chief nurse anesthetist at the University of Washington Medical Center. He is active in elected and appointed local, state, and national professional organization activities. Mr. Kremer has authored multiple articles in peer-reviewed journals and four textbook chapters.

Margaret Faut-Callahan, DNSc, CRNA, FAAN, received her master's and doctoral degrees at the Rush University College of Nursing and attended Loyola University in Chicago, Illinois, for her undergraduate education. She is currently a professor and director of the Nurse Anesthesia Program at the Rush University College of Nursing. Dr. Faut-Callahan has also served Rush-Presbyterian-St. Luke's Medical Center in Chicago as associate chairperson for operating room and surgical nursing. She was an early advocate for the academic affiliation of nurse anesthesia educational programs with colleges of nursing. Her curricular innovations have included front loading of didactic content in the nurse anesthesia program and inclusion of pain content in this curriculum. Dr. Faut-Callahan advises numerous certified registered nurse anesthetist doctoral students in the only nurse anesthesia–focused doctorate in nursing science program nationally. She has served local, state, and national organizations in leadership capacities, including chairing the Foundation of the American Association of Nurse Anesthetists, serving as the association's regional director, and acting as a chair reviewer for the Council on Accreditation of Nurse Anesthesia Programs. Dr. Faut-Callahan is the first advanced practice nurse to sit on the Illinois Department of Professional Regulation's Committee on Nursing.

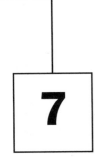

7

CHAPTER OUTLINE

THE ECONOMIC SYSTEM
CRITERIA FOR AN ECONOMIC SYSTEM IN
 RELATION TO HEALTH CARE
TYPES OF ECONOMIC SYSTEMS
MARKET COMPETITION
DISEQUILIBRIUM
SUPPLIER-INDUCED DEMAND
THE EFFECTS OF CHANGES IN PRICE,
 SUPPLY, AND DEMAND FOR HEALTH
 CARE
COST CONSIDERATIONS IN PROVISION OF
 CARE AND REIMBURSEMENT FOR
 PHYSICIANS AND ADVANCED PRAC-
 TICE NURSES
Price of services

Access issues
Health-care plans and health-insurance
 policies
Competition
Antitrust issues
KEY TERMS IN FINANCING AND REIM-
 BURSEMENT
Fee for service versus capitation
Copayment, coinsurance, and deductibles
Adverse selection
Community rating
Experience rating
Global budgeting
SUMMARY
SUGGESTED EXERCISES

CHAPTER OBJECTIVES

After completing this chapter, the reader will be able to:
   1. Discuss the components of a traditional economic system.
   2. Describe the criteria for an economic system in relation to health care.
   3. Note the effect of changes in price, supply, and demand for health care.
   4. Become familiar with cost considerations in the provision of health care by, and re-
      imbursement for, both physicians and advanced practice nurses.
   5. Demonstrate conversance with key terms in finance and reimbursement.

An important policy shift in health care that emerged during the 1980s was the adoption of traditional market forces in an attempt to achieve greater efficiency in the production of health-care services. A reliance on regulatory control of health-care financing, such as the certificate of need system implemented in the 1970s, failed to contain health-care costs. Regulatory control was advocated ostensibly from a quality standpoint, but providers, professionals, and insurers favored only the weakest mechanisms to ensure quality while supporting regulations that advanced their economic self-interests and enabled them to create monopolistic positions in their respective health-care markets.[1] The monopolies created determined the type and amount of health care provided and obtained regulatory barriers to protect professionals from others seeking to enter markets over which they had control. Buerhaus[2] posited that if health care had been governed less by regulations and more by traditional market forces, the genesis of monopolistic forces would have been stifled. In that case, market forces would have predominated, and professionals would have been forced to compete on the basis of price, quality, and the extent to which they provided services that were responsive to the preferences of consumers. This chapter discusses these economic trends as well as the components of the economic system.

The Economic System

The economic system consists of the network of institutions, laws, and rules created by society to answer the following universal economic questions:

- What goods and services shall be produced?
- How shall they be produced?
- For whom shall they be produced?

Every society needs an economic system because human, natural, and man-made resources are scarce relative to human wants, because the resources have alternative uses, and because there is a multiplicity of competing wants. Thus, decisions must be made regarding the use of these resources in production and the distribution of the resulting output among the members of society.[3] As health-care costs have increased to approximately 14 percent of the US gross national product, it has become clear that difficult decisions must be made regarding allocation of health-care resources. Some relevant questions that are raised in this regard include:

- Who will receive health-care services?
- By whom will these services be provided?
- At what cost will these services be provided?

Criteria for an Economic System in Relation to Health Care

Given the scarcity of resources and the existence of competing goals, the economic system with respect to health care should result in:

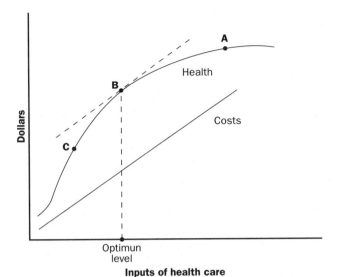

Figure 7–1   Determination of optimum level of health-care utilization.

1. An optimum amount of resources devoted to health care
2. The combination of these resources in an optimal way
3. An optimal allocation of resources between current provision of health care and investment in future health care through research, education, and similar efforts
4. The general rule for reaching such optima is "equality at the margin"[3] (p. 13).

For instance, the first criterion would be met if the last dollar's worth of resources devoted to health care increased human satisfaction by exactly the same amount as the last dollar's worth devoted to other goods.[3] The contrast between this view of a social optimum and the notion of optimal care as used in health care needs to be discussed. The relation between health and health-care inputs can usually be described by a curve that may rise at an increasing rate at first, but then decreases and eventually levels off or declines. Optimal care could be defined as Point A, where no further increment in health is possible. The social optimum, however, requires that inputs of resources not exceed the point at which the value of an additional increment to health is exactly equal to the cost of inputs required to obtain that increment, or Point B. At Point C, where the ratio of benefits to costs is at a maximum, additional inputs still add more to benefits than to costs (Fig. 7–1).

Types of Economic Systems

Economists have identified three "pure types" of economic systems:

1. Traditional
2. Centrally directed
3. Market price

Every actual economy is a blend of types, but their relative importance varies. Primitive and feudal societies relied on basic economic decisions that were made by one person or a small group of people; the former Soviet Union is an example of such a system. The United States, Canada, and most countries of Western Europe have relied on a market system for the past century or two.[3]

A market system consists of a collection of decision-making units called *households* and another collection called *firms.* The households own all the productive resources in the society. They make these resources available to firms, who transform them into goods and services that are then distributed back to the households. The flow of resources and of goods and services is facilitated by a counterflow of money.[3]

In a market system, as shown in Fig. 7–2, the exchanges of resources and of goods and services for money take place in markets where prices and quantities are determined. These prices are the signals or controls that trigger changes in behavior as required by changes in technology or preferences. The market system is sometimes referred to as the *price* system.[3]

In the markets for resources, the households are the suppliers and the firms provide the demand. In the markets for goods and services, the firms are the suppliers and the households are the sources of demand. In each market, the interaction between demand and supply determines the quantities and prices of the various resources and the goods and services. Figure 7–3 demonstrates a typical market. The income of each household depends on the quantity and quality of resources available to it and the prices of those resources; the amount of household incomes determines its share of the total flow of goods and services. The household is assumed to spend its income in such a way as to maximize its utility, or satisfaction. It does this by following the principle of equality at the margin; that is, it adjusts its purchases so that marginal utility, or the satisfaction added by the last unit purchased of each commodity, is proportional to its price.[3]

It is assumed that firms attempt to maximize **profits,** or the difference between what they must pay the households for the use of resources and what they get from them for the goods and services they produce. To maximize profits, they too must follow the equality-at-the-margin rule, adjusting their use of different types of resources so that the marginal products (the addition to output obtained from one additional unit of input) are proportional to price.[3]

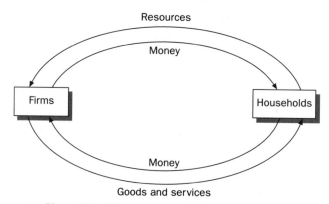

Figure 7–2 Elementary model of a market system.

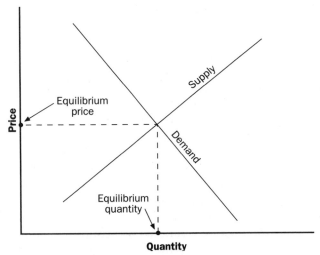

Figure 7–3   A typical market.

The essence of a competitive market is that:

- There are many well-informed buyers and sellers, no one of whom is large enough to influence price.
- The buyers and sellers act independently (that is, without collusion).
- There is free entry for other buyers and sellers not currently in the market.

The US economy departs in many respects from the competitive market model; this departure is particularly noticeable in the health-care sector. Most health-care markets depart substantially from competitive conditions, sometimes inevitably and sometimes as a result of deliberate public or private policy.[3]

Market Competition

In a competitive industry, firms have strong economic incentives to minimize the costs of producing their products and services so they can be priced competitively and sold in the marketplace. To minimize production costs, firms must be innovative in their use of capital and labor, endeavoring to find the least costly number and combination of resources to produce their goods. Because consumers consider both price and quality of goods and services when making purchases, firms attempt to improve the quality of their products without causing significant price increases. Firms conduct market research to determine consumer preferences and initiate promotional activities to inform the public on the price and quality of their products, as well as to differentiate their products from those of competitors.[2]

In a competitive marketplace, consumers are given a variety of choices in the goods and services they may purchase. Influenced by their level of income, their tastes and preferences, and the amount of information available on the product, consumers consider the trade-off between price and quality and purchase those items that are most satisfying. Those in control of supply and demand in competitive markets are in touch with each other; however, satisfying the consumer is the only way that firms can sell their products and earn profits.[2]

Much of the health-care system has been built on what Enthoven[4] called "cost-*un*conscious" demand. The lack of sensitivity to the price of health care has occurred for several reasons. Current tax law permits the exclusion of employer-paid health-insurance premiums from the taxable income of employees. This has led to the purchase of more health-insurance coverage than would be the case if employees bought the insurance directly using after-tax income. This tax policy has resulted in an overconsumption of health care because employees are not conscious of the price of services they consume, and providers, who know that an insurance company will pay for the services, have no economic incentive to restrain the cost of providing a treatment or the amount of care provided.[5] So long as the patient and provider are insensitive to price and are spared from fiscal accountability for their actions, patients will continue to demand more health care than they may require, and providers will supply that care. Under this system, neither party has economic incentives to consider the costs or benefits of consuming additional amounts of health care, but behave as if more is better.

Employers have also fostered cost-unconsciousness by constructing their health-insurance offerings so that the employee who chooses the lowest-priced health plan is not permitted to keep any of the savings.[4] The prevalence of employers subsidizing the more costly fee-for-service third-party payer system against cost-minimizing health-maintenance organizations (HMOs) and competitive health-care plans removed incentives for employees to shop around and select the least costly health-insurance plan. This practice stymied price competition among health-care plans, because lower-cost plans cannot

> take business away from the next-lowest priced plan by cutting the price paid to the people actually making the choice.[2] (p. 369)

It was thought that employers persisted with this irrational strategy because, in addition to the perverse incentives to purchase fee-for-service plans inherent in the tax treatment of employer-paid health-insurance premiums, unions have historically insisted that their members have 100 percent comprehensive health coverage. Employers were reluctant to use their considerable purchasing power to stimulate price competition among health-care plans.[2]

A major economic force having an impact on health-care delivery and its cost was the increasing cost of health care to employers in the late 1980s and beyond. The cost of health care to employers undermined the ability of industry to be price competitive in a global marketplace. Employers have become motivated to adopt reforms demanding health services that stimulate greater price competition among health-care plans and other supply-side providers. It is in the best interest of the nursing profession to become involved in research and management efforts seeking to find solutions to some of these supply, demand, and cost problems in health care and to prepare for a far more competitive health-care system.[2]

One recent example of public economic policy having an impact on reimbursement in health care are the new Medicare payment policies affecting physicians. In 1996, the federal government was expected to complete the 4-year phase-in of the resource-based relative value scale (RBRVS), its payment system for physicians under part B of the Medicare program. Although the program seems to be accomplishing one of its primary objectives—to transfer payments away from tests and procedures and apply them toward evaluation and management services—physicians are experiencing a number of dissatisfactions with the program. The Physician Payment Review Commission (PPRC), which monitors the implementation of the fee schedule, has expressed concern that low Medicare RBRVS payments may negatively affect the access of beneficiaries to physicians. Other investigators[6,7] have shown that low Medicaid fees hamper access to office-based physicians and encourage the use of hospital outpatient departments and emergency services, both of which only reinforce PPRC concerns about the link between physician payments and decreased access to care. Should federal budget-deficit pressures result in prolonging inadequate RBRVS payments (approximately 75 percent of Medicare physician payments are financed using general tax dollars) and should physicians respond by reducing the medical care provided to an increasing number of Medicare beneficiaries, then additional demand for APNs could develop.[8]

The potential economic consequences of the pricing decisions of an advanced nursing practice, including the anticipated effects on physicians and consumers, are discussed later in this chapter. To adequately describe these consequences, it is necessary to first discuss key economic terms and concepts that underpin the relationship between price and the firm's demand, amount of total revenues, profitability, and economic responses by physicians or consumers.[8]

Disequilibrium

One disturbing characteristic of some health-care markets is the failure of price to reach a level of **equilibrium,** or the level at which the quantity demanded and the quantity supplied are equal.[3] Most recently, payers have provided greater incentives for primary- versus specialty-care services, leading to an economic disincentive for the use of services such as surgery and anesthesia. A relative oversupply of surgeons and anesthesia providers can then be said to exist due to this decreased demand for their services. The persistence of a price disequilibrium is a clear indication that the market departs substantially from the competitive norm. In the case of excess demand, rationing ensues. Services such as hemodialysis or major organ transplantation may not be available to all members of society.

Supplier-induced Demand

Figures 7–4 and 7–5 illustrate excess demand and supply, assuming constant initial supply, demand, price, and quantity conditions. An increase in the number of physicians in this market shifts the supply curve, resulting in a reduction in price and an increase in the quantity of care. Assuming that demand is inelastic with respect to price, physicians' incomes will decline, which will induce physicians to recommend additional units of service. This results in a shift in the demand curve. In this case, both price and quantity increase in response to the physician-induced demand. In contrast to the theoretical expectation that an increase in supply raises quantity and reduces price in a competitive market, find-

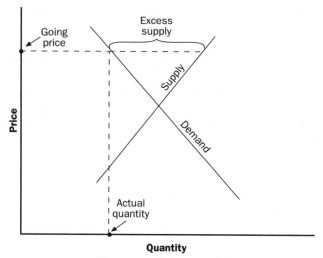

Figure 7–4   Excess supply.

ings suggest that an increase in the supply of physicians is accompanied by an increase in quantity and a constant or rising price.[9]

Such results are consistent with the demand-shift hypothesis. The health-care provider is hypothesized to shift demand to attain a target income. The target income is the amount of money earned through comparison with other physicians of the same specialty training and geographic location. Recent empirical studies of the impact of increases in the physician-population ratio on utilization indicated no decline in utilization associated with increases in physician supply. A modest positive relationship was found between utilization and the physician-population ratio. Estimated elasticities varied widely, ranging from 0.03 to 0.80.[9]

The inducement hypothesis questions the appropriateness of increased cost sharing by consumers as an approach to controlling utilization and moderating

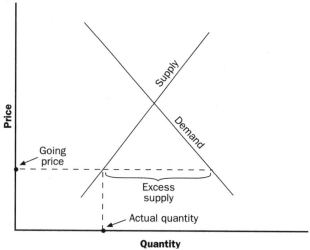

Figure 7–5   Excess demand.

growth in health-care expenditures. Additional cost sharing and the concomitant decrease in consumer-initiated demand not only reduce the earnings of physicians but also induce providers to increase demand, thereby reducing the impact of higher net prices on total health-care spending. Moreover, the inducement hypothesis suggests that controls placed on fees charged by physicians are unlikely to successfully constrain total spending on health services. Rather, price controls are likely to expand utilization and induce the substitution of more expensive services for less costly ones.[9]

Several important problems must be considered when undertaking empirical studies of the demand for health care. The first is the adequacy of using health-insurance information to obtain estimates of the price of health services. The second is the effect of provider influence on demand, for example, the extent to which supply creates its own demand. The third problem is the effect of health status on the demand for health care. Exclusion of a health status variable will bias the results in terms of the importance of the other independent variables. Empirical studies indicate that the demand for health services is inelastic with respect to price and income. The demand-for-health model recognizes that health services are purchased to obtain better health. Moreover, other items purchased, such as tobacco products, fatty foods, or alcoholic beverages, also have an impact on health status. One example of this model is that older persons, to retard the depreciation in health status caused by advancing age, increase their purchase of health services.[8,9]

The Effects of Changes in Price, Supply, and Demand for Health Care

The hospital sector is the most inflationary component of the health services industry. The average expense per hospital stay rose from slightly more than $127 in 1950 to $5359 in 1988. As is the case with other aspects of the health services industry, general inflation is responsible for the bulk of the increase in hospital expenditures. However, the increase in intensity, or acuity, per visit accounts for more of the increase in hospital expenditures than for physicians' or nursing-home services.[9]

The issue of the magnitude of economies of scale in the production of hospital services has been studied for many years. Recent evidence indicates only a slight tendency for average costs to decline as output increases. However, there is stronger evidence of scale economies for particular types of medical services. Case mix, for example, patient acuity and type of payer, is an important factor that must be taken into account when considering the effect of hospital size on average costs.[9]

State regulation of hospital costs has become increasingly widespread in the past 20 years. Rate regulation has been found to have a moderate impact on cost per admission, cost per patient day, and per capita expenditures. In addition, the growth in labor cost has slowed with prospective payment.[9]

During the 1980s, the federal government began to run up annual budget deficits in excess of $200 billion. As the amount of the national debt grew, a greater portion of the federal government budget each year was required to pay interest on the debt, which reduced the amount of dollars available for other discretionary spending. Since the beginning of the Medicare and Medicaid programs in 1966, total public spending on health care increased 40-fold and reached approximately $400 billion in 1994.[10]

At the beginning of the 1980s, several private- and public-sector initiatives sprang forth and acted both independently and interdependently to stimulate the beginning of economic competition among hospitals and physicians. The first of these initiatives occurred as a result of several events: American businesses were struck by double-digit inflation during the Carter administration, followed by a sharp economic recession during the Reagan administration. The volume of lower-priced imported goods rose substantially, as did competition from Japan and other countries. Many American businesses became aware of, and concerned about, the effects of steadily rising health-care premiums, which were increasing the costs of labor. Employers started to fear that, if left unchecked, rising health-care costs could thwart the ability to price their products competitively in a global market. Businesses sought to reduce costly inpatient hospital stays by beginning programs that mandated prehospital testing and screening and utilization review, required second opinions for surgery, and pressured insurance companies to cover the cost of less costly outpatient settings. Even before Medicare implemented diagnoses-related groups, these private-sector actions were causing a decline in hospital occupancy rates and the number of admissions.[5]

While prospective payment has succeeded in moderating the growth in current expenditures, there is little evidence that regulations designed to limit capital formation have succeeded. Even in situations where regulation of capital expenditures were successful in limiting growth in the number of beds, hospitals substituted investment in new services for beds. Both declining government support for capital regulation and industry are advanced as possible reasons for the ineffectiveness of controls on hospital capital formation.[9]

Cost Considerations in Provision of Care and Reimbursement for Physicians and Advanced Practice Nurses

PRICE OF SERVICES

All proposed health-care reform plans recognize the heightened demand for primary care services and providers. Greater availability of primary and preventive care has been tied to cost savings and improved quality. Nonphysician practitioners are cost effective with regard to the costs of their educational preparation and perhaps also with regard to their practice patterns and fees. How these professionals are paid and which of their services are covered have been contentious issues for more than two decades. This is evidenced by the patchwork of policies governing payment for their services, even within a single-payer system such as Medicare, and by substantial variation in payment rates among state Medicaid services.[11]

The extraordinary rise in health-care costs and the inability of nursing to show cost savings has been a barrier to obtaining direct payment. The portion of the gross national product comprised by health care grew from 5.3 percent in 1960 to 12.5 percent in 1990, increasing from $42 billion to almost $647 billion. Congress has shown its concern about the rise in the health-care budget by enacting new cost-containing Medicare payment systems for hospitals and physicians' services. Congress has exhibited restraint in the annual funding of other health programs, frequently only increasing funding to cover inflation. Reimbursement legislation for the services of APNs is almost always evaluated as a cost item. APNs are defined as nurse practitioners, clinical nurse specialists, certified nurse midwives, and certified registered nurse anesthetists (CRNAs). A summary of federal reimbursement for APNs is given in Table 7–1.[12]

The Congressional Budget Office believes that if the number of providers is increased, the costs for health care will increase because of the greater number of services provided. Congress is concerned about the rise in health-care costs and the increasing federal deficit. The large deficit is blamed for a sluggish economy, making members of Congress reluctant to increase spending on health care.[12]

Many Medicaid programs have considered the advantages of using nonphysician practitioners for primary- and maternal-care services and have established payment policies to encourage access to nonphysician practitioners. State Medicaid programs have significantly expanded service coverage and payment for nonphysicians in the following ways. First, state Medicaid policies, unlike those of Medicare, cannot limit coverage to rural settings. Nonphysician services are covered in all regions of a state. Second, more than half of the states that pay nurse practitioners and certified nurse midwives do so at the full physician's fee level. All states pay certified nurse midwives at a percentage rate that exceeds Medicare's level; two-thirds of the states pay nurse practitioners more than 85 percent of the physician's fee. Third, although Medicaid mandates require only pediatric and family nurse practitioner coverage, more than half of the states have allowed other types of nurse practitioners to participate as well.[11]

ACCESS ISSUES

Paying APNs directly allows them to provide care and to improve needed access to care. Many of the recent changes in federal health programs enacted by Congress were made to improve health-care access to underserved populations, such as nursing-home residents, low-income women and children, and people in rural areas. Direct reimbursement gives APNs recognition and visibility as pri-

TABLE 7–1

Federal Reimbursement for Nurses in Advanced Practice: Current Status Advanced Practice Nurses

Federal programs	Nurse practitioner	Certified nurse midwife	Certified registered nurse anesthetist	Clinical nurse specialist
Medicare, part B	Yes[a]	Yes	Yes	Yes[b]
Medicaid	Yes[c]	Yes	State discretion	State discretion
CHAMPUS[d]	Yes	Yes	Yes	Yes[e]
FEHB[f]	Yes	Yes	Yes	Yes

[a]Limited to nursing facilities and rural areas
[b]Limited to rural areas
[c]Limited to pediatric NPs and family NPs
[d]Civilian Health and Medical Program of the Uniformed Services
[e]Limited to certified psychiatric nurse specialists
[f]Federal Employee Health Benefit Program[12]

mary care providers. More than 35 million US citizens lack health insurance, and most of these people lack access to primary care.[13] To meet the needs of this uninsured population, additional primary care practitioners will be needed. Direct reimbursement of APNs eliminates one of the most significant barriers to greater utilization of these nurses.[12]

The Omnibus Budget Reconciliation Act (OBRA), enacted by Congress in 1990, allowed nurse practitioners and clinical nurse specialist services to be reimbursed when provided in a rural area. This law was enacted because Congress wanted to improve access to care for rural Medicare beneficiaries. Although the nurse practitioner and clinical nurse specialist must work in collaboration with a physician, they do not have to submit claims through their employer; they may submit claims directly. The payment level is at 85 percent of the fee schedule for outpatient services and at 75 percent for inpatient services.[12]

HEALTH-CARE PLANS AND HEALTH-INSURANCE POLICIES

The forces that evolved in the 1980s and early 1990s culminated in the development of health-care price competition because cost-conscious purchasers of health care sought to obtain greater value for each dollar spent. The evolution of managed health-care delivery has become a significant force with which APNs must be familiar.

Managed care involves the application of standard business practices to health-care delivery. Managed care purports to represent the best of the American free-enterprise system. New methods of providing finance and reimbursement for health-care services require hospitals and health-care providers to make tremendous transitions to entirely new business models.[14] Today, health-care providers are confronted with price competition and the need to rigorously control costs while at the same time facing increasing demands for data documenting the quality of clinical outcomes.[15]

For the first time in 1993, 51 percent of employees with employer-sponsored health insurance were enrolled in managed-care plans. In addition, many traditional insurance plans have managed-care features, insofar as they subject provider services to external utilization reviews, second opinions, and so forth. It was estimated that by the end of 1996, more than 120 million people will be enrolled in some form of managed-care organization (MCO), with some 75 million enrolled in preferred-provider organizations (PPOs) and 45 million in HMO plans. As payers, providers, and consumers of health care seek solutions to ever-increasing costs, managed care in the United States has experienced explosive growth. The purchasers of health care, including private and public payers, as well as patients, have become particularly interested in managed care as a flexible means for reducing health-care expenditures while preserving high-quality patient care. The most visible manifestation of the changing health-care market is the growth of managed care. Insurers are under intense pressure from employers to reduce premiums. Accomplishing this without reducing profits means decreasing costs, which in turn, requires insurers to limit expenditures, generally by controlling provider services. By the end of the decade, Blue Cross and Blue Shield plans expect to have between 80 to 90 percent of plan customers enrolled in managed-care plans.[14]

The manifestation of a more competitive health-care environment is taking the form of increasing enrollment in prepaid capitated health-care firms, such as HMOs, and the formation of larger integrated systems. Their growth will be aided by continuing regulatory and market-based adjustments designed to ensure that providers compete fairly, on the basis of price and quality. APNs can expect that more of the clinical and economic forces that shape their practices and determine their incomes will be driven by impersonal and unambiguous incentives that govern price-competitive industries: Providers and health professionals will be rewarded only to the extent that they keep their prices low and quality high.[8]

The evolution of prepaid capitated firms, or the managed-care industry, is a significant and positive development for APNs, whether they are employed by managed-care firms or decide to compete independently as solo providers or in group practice arrangements. From the economic perspective, the major difference between practicing as an employee of an HMO or practicing independently is that as an employee, the APN functions as an economic complement, whereas APNs in independent practice function largely as economic substitutes to an HMO or medical group practice.[8]

APNs are an economic complement so long as providing their services increases the productivity of the managed-care firm and the profits of the owners. The complementary role is not unlike that of hospital-employed registered nurses, whose nursing practice functions to increase the productivity of physicians by allowing them both to treat inpatients and to maintain an office-based practice. Because an HMO operates according to a prepaid capitated budget, it has an economic incentive to keep the total costs of providing health care as low as possible. In this way, any amount of unspent dollars can be retained as profit. Thus, HMOs have an economic interest to provide enrollees with more preventive care and health education, so that they can reduce future consumption of HMO resources by treating fewer enrollees for preventable acute and chronic illnesses. HMOs try to reduce admissions to costly hospitals, negotiate discounts on the purchase of pharmaceutical products and medical devices, and pursue other methods to reduce costs.[8]

Fagin[16] suggested that adequately educated APNs have proven competence and are capable of working without physicians' supervision. Many of the clinical services that APNs provide can closely substitute for those provided by physicians. Because APNs are less costly to an HMO in terms of salary and benefit requirements, they represent an economically attractive opportunity for an HMO to fill gatekeeping and other provider roles. As purchasers increasingly demand that HMOs lower the premiums charged per enrollee lest they induce their employees to enroll in a different and lower-cost HMO, price competition among HMOs is expected to intensify significantly. HMOs will face greater pressures to keep their costs low, which might further increase demand for APNs. Because managed-care firms will increasingly be motivated to keep their premiums competitively priced, it is anticipated that they will develop new roles for APNs and experiment with delivery models that will be tailored extensively around APNs. The purpose would be to find new ways to lower costs while simultaneously increasing enrollee satisfaction and attainment of desired clinical outcomes.[8]

For at least two economic reasons, APNs must anticipate that physicians and physician assistants (PAs) will resist the increasing employment of APNs. As more APNs become available, the total supply of health professionals will increase relative to the available number of managed-care positions. Consequently, this will place downward pressure on the salaries that managed-care firms are able to offer and still hire all the providers they want. As the supply of primary-care physicians increases, additional physicians will seek employment with managed-care firms and compete for available positions with APNs who have a comparative cost advantage.[8]

A second possible reason to expect physicians to resist the expansion of APNs in managed care is that many firms might adopt policies directing that APNs' caseloads comprise the "less difficult cases." But by having to care for "difficult cases," primary care physicians may be unable to obtain appropriate outcomes or levels of patient satisfaction to qualify for a year-end bonus. Hooker[17] reported that the Kaiser Permanente HMO System determined as far back as 1980 that 83 percent of the care provided by HMO physicians could be provided by an APN or PA. In primary care, that percentage is said to jump to 93 percent. In any health-care system, the highest cost is labor. If a health-care provider is able to provide the same services as physicians, with similar quality and outcomes, the only true barrier to this type of APN-PA utilization is physicians' attitudes.[17]

In the Hooker[17] study, research findings demonstrated that PAs and APNs could see as many or more patients per day as physicians at 50 percent less than physician's cost. From a workload standpoint, it appears that adult medicine physicians, PAs, and APNs at Kaiser Permanente Northwest see similar numbers of patients on hourly, daily, and annual bases. The types of patients seen by PAs and APNs in adult ambulatory settings are probably similar to those seen by physicians. From this standpoint, Hooker[17] concluded that "APNs and physician assistants were substitutes, rather than complements for, physician services" (p. 134).

Thus, APNs must understand that, although they present economic benefits to owners of HMOs, they represent an increasingly visible economic threat to primary-care and specialist physicians. For these reasons, it will be no surprise if organized medicine takes actions aimed at decreasing the supply of APNs. The main impediment to the attempts of APNs to obtain reimbursement has been organized medicine. The position that organized medicine has adopted is that APNs must practice under the supervision of a physician.[12] Mirr[18] noted that the lack of direct reimbursement for APN services decreases the overall effectiveness of these nursing professionals. Further, Timmons and Ridenour[19] reported that nurse practitioners have been billing patients for years under the title of physicians. This practice has promoted economic dependence of the APN on the physician.

COMPETITION

Advanced practice nurses need to understand who their competitors are, how many of them exist, where they are located, what services they offer, how much they charge, and how they are paid. This information will tell APNs a great deal about what other providers have found effective or ineffective, sparing practicing APNs from making time-consuming and costly mistakes. Knowing as much as possible about the competition will also make it possible for APNs to determine how they can fill gaps in service, how they can take advantage of market niches, and how they might provide care creatively and at a lower cost.[8] This type of knowledge can be obtained by contracting with health marketing research firms, by developing a strategic plan with consultation as necessary, and formulating an appropriate business plan based on the information gathered in this process.

Marketers take a large heterogeneous group of prospective buyers and divide them into smaller, more homogeneous groups who want approximately the same thing. This process is called **market segmentation;** each subgroup is called a **market segment.** Markets are segmented by variables such as age, sex, and income. Each segment is evaluated using a set of predetermined criteria. If two or more target markets are chosen, the organization is practicing a multisegment strategy. The process of gathering the information necessary to operate any business is called **market research.** Formal research techniques rely on systematic gathering of information from sources inside and outside the firm. Surveys, experimental designs, expert panels, and subscriptions to proprietary or syndicated research reports are typical of the formal research effort. Information that is routinely gathered, codified, analyzed, and stored is part of a marketing information system, which becomes a ready information source for decision makers.[20]

A marketing mix includes the following components:

- Product
- Branding
- Packaging
- Price
- Place
- Promotion
- Product positioning

Branding is important from the standpoint of professional identification: Clients must realize that health-care services are available from appropriately prepared and credentialed APNs. Packaging is a function of the image projected by the product, in this case, the APN. Clinical competence, affability, availability, and a professional demeanor help to prepare an appealing package when APNs market their services. Price is another important consideration with multiple objectives; nearly all objectives will have to be related to long-term profitability. The marketer must estimate demand at the price level and forecast the response of competitors. Marketers typically create channels of distribution to move the product from producer to user. Channel members must focus on the needs of the final consumer as well as their own needs. Promotion informs, persuades, or reminds customers about a product, such as advanced practice nursing services. Promotion management begins with an understanding of the target markets the firm has chosen to serve. This means one must know which media, such as newspapers, television, and so on, the market uses to get information and understand how it processes information and makes decisions. The organization or individual marketing services must develop a promotion strategy consisting of specific goals, plans to achieve them, an adequate budget to support this effort, and a method for evaluating results.[20]

A promotion plan includes some combination of promotion tools, referred to as the **promotion mix.** Like the marketing mix, it is a synergistic blend of elements. The four groupings of promotion tools are:

- Advertising
- Sales promotion
- Public relations and publicity
- Personal selling

Advertising is the use of impersonal messages sent through paid media, such as television, radio, newspapers, magazines, transit and highway billboards, telephone and business directories, and direct advertisements. Public relations activities are designed to foster goodwill, understanding, forgiveness, or acceptance. Publicity is not always favorable.[20] As the marketplace for healthcare providers contracts, a mixture of conciliatory and defensive posturing is seen in published interviews such as the following.

A newspaper interview with two APNs and a physician was titled "Nurse Practitioner Supervision at Issue: RNs Push for Collegial Practice."[21] The physician commented that nurses had the ability to "treat a sore throat" but lacked the

> medical education and judgment and hours and hours of supervised experience that will allow them to look at the entire differential of what [a] sore throat may be. (p. 3)

The physician's perception was that nurses and physicians should "be a team" and that patients should know whether they are seeing "a board-certified physician or a board-certified advanced practice nurse." Despite some positive comments from the nurse practitioners interviewed for this story, the physician was able to cast some doubt as to the capabilities of APNs. The economic threat that APNs represent to physicians leads to occasional difficulties with antitrust issues.

ANTITRUST ISSUES

The American Nurses' Association (ANA) and other advanced practice nursing organizations are watching the development of antitrust protection very carefully. ANA points out that regulations are necessary to prevent any of the following possible events:

- Use of practice arrangements that prohibit nurses from performing patient-care activities within the scopes of state nurse-practice acts
- Use of practice arrangements that limit the activities of nurses recognized as advanced practitioners
- Imposition of insurer limits on the availability and accessibility of liability coverage for nurses or the requirement for physician supervision as a prerequisite for coverage
- Use of insurance surcharges to increase malpractice premium coverage and other insurance-related impediments to physician-nurse collaboration
- Subjective or arbitrary insurance-reimbursement policies, such as denial of reimbursement for services performed within the scope of any licensed provider's practice if there is coverage for that service provided by the physician
- Denial of staff privileges at health-care facilities, including prescriptive authority for those authorized by state law to prescribe

Without federal protection and clearer guidelines, every time APNs are denied basic rights to practice, they would have to enter into lengthy litigation and demonstrate their legal right to compete. Case law exists that states that some specialty nurses and physicians do compete. See *Oltz v St Peter's Community Hos-*

pital, 861 F2d 1440, 1443 (9th Cir 1988) and *Bahn v NME Hospital*, 772 F2d 1467, 1471 (9th Cir 1975). Not only is this an issue of paramount importance to nurses, it is a priority issue of the Coalition for Quality Care and Competition, which represents more than 400,000 nonphysician providers. Issues important to this coalition include:

- Prohibition of any entity or plan from discriminating against a class of health-care professional
- Elimination of restrictions in current law that pose barriers for nonphysician providers from practicing in accord with state licensing acts
- Federal provisions guaranteeing nondiscriminatory access to qualified health providers being uniformly applied to all states, entities, and plans
- Replacement of the term *physician* with the term *qualified professional* in health-care regulatory language

Both of these positions go a long way in qualifying the needs of nonphysician providers in regulatory arenas. However, without federal protection and a mandate that states must adopt these provisions, the nonphysician provider will be in a situation of fighting for practice privileges and the right to provide care.[14]

If APNs in solo or group practice arrangements are to survive in a competitive market, they will need to be alert, seek ways to innovate and keep their costs as low as possible, and be willing to make frequent adjustments in the quality, pricing, and marketing of their services. It is recommended that APNs set their prices below the prevailing market price of services provided by physicians or their nearest competitors.[8]

Many policy makers and researchers agree that there are problems with physician oversupply and imbalance in specialty mix. Some have argued that these will be resolved as a more competitive health-care market develops, predicting that cost-conscious integrated systems will change the demand for physicians' services. As a result, physicians will experience lower incomes or potential unemployment, sending a signal to students and educators to change behavior. A systematic analysis has not been done assessing the impact of changes in the organizing and financing of health care on the physician labor market. Two types of changes are being seen in medical education:

1. The effect of increasing demand for generalists on changing specialty mix
2. The question of whether the market is creating incentives to train fewer physicians overall[22]

Although there have been changes in the marketplace, it is still too early to know whether these changes signal a departure from previous trends. Positions in generalist fields are becoming more attractive, but changes in incomes have been modest and the number of specialists continues to increase unabated. There is also little indication that job opportunities for physicians are contracting. However, given the length of training, the large pool of practicing physicians, and differing incentives existing in the educational and practice markets, it may be that the market forces are operant, but it is too soon to see widespread effects of a physician oversupply and imbalance in specialty mix.

To better understand the status of Medicaid payment for nonphysician services, the PPRC, working with the Intergovernmental Health Policy Project, conducted a survey of state Medicaid programs on payment policies. The survey was designed to determine whether state Medicaid payment policies enabled or restricted participation of physicians and nonphysicians in primary and maternal care. Survey results indicate that many states responded to federal Medicaid mandates by establishing nonrestrictive payment policies that enable certified nurse midwives and nurse practitioners to participate fully in the program. Not all states have been receptive to such policy expansions, as evidenced by policies that limit coverage or payment to certain nonphysician services or settings. Working within budget-neutral constraints in many cases, Medicaid programs continually balance two competing goals: improving access to care and containing the growth of Medicaid expenditures. Medicare and federal Medicaid mandates for nonphysician practitioner coverage are often the template for state payment policies.[11]

Key Terms in Finance and Reimbursement

FEE-FOR-SERVICE VERSUS CAPITATION

The traditional health-care billing system in which a health-care provider charges a patient separately for each service is the **fee-for-service system.** This type of system allows patients to have free choice in health-care providers and does not require providers to assume risk for the provision of care: For example, providers are more likely to be reimbursed proportionally for providing care in a fee-for-service system than in a managed-care system.

With the advanced practice nursing specialty of nurse anesthesia as an example, fee-for-service and traditional indemnity insurance plans will be described in the context of reimbursement for services provided by these APNs. In the early years of this century and through the 1950s, CRNAs were usually paid employees of either a surgeon or hospital. In rural areas, CRNAs often contracted with hospitals to provide services based on fee-for-service structures, that is, a set amount of compensation per case as opposed to straight salary for hours worked.[23]

Blue Cross and Blue Shield were among the first private payers to emerge during the 1930s. Early insurance plans paid only for physician or hospital charges, and they would not directly reimburse other health-care providers, such as CRNAs, psychologists, and physical therapists. To obtain payment for their services, these providers would submit charges to the hospital or physician. The hospital or physician would then obtain reimbursement for services as "incident to" their own and pass the money on to the nonreimbursed provider.[25]

Health-care costs escalated under the private payer systems of reimbursement. Reasons cited for this trend often were attributed to the failure of payers to reimburse lower-cost providers such as nonphysicians; preferential reimbursement of higher-cost care systems, such as hospitals, rather than ambulatory or outpatient services; and the insistence of physicians that harm would come to the physician-patient relationship if the fee-for-service structure were not maintained and strengthened.[23]

In an effort to control escalating medical costs, Medicare instituted a prospective payment system (PPS) in 1983. Initially, this legislation affected only Medicare, part A (hospital costs); however, it would soon have an effect on Medicare, part B (physician and nonphysician costs). Before 1983, Medicare reimbursed hospitals for CRNAs on a cost-based system, in which the hospital passed along the actual costs of providing the Medicare portion of CRNAs' services directly to Medicare.[23]

As a result of the Omnibus Budget Reconciliation Act of 1986, all CRNAs, regardless of their practice setting, were able to receive reimbursement from Medicare directly or to assign their billing rights to their employer. All CRNA services are subject to Medicare assignment (no balance billing). A subsequent law allowed rural hospitals with 500 or fewer surgical cases per year requiring anesthesia and one full-time CRNA to "pass through" the costs of anesthesia services. In 1992, final regulations were published that detailed procedural definitions of the 1986 legislation.[23]

Most health-insurance plans are undergoing rapid change, attempting to control spiraling health-care costs. APNs can expect reimbursement rates to decrease in the near future, affecting all types of APNs in various practice settings, whether self-employed or not. One thought is that fee-for-service reimbursement structures are a thing of the past, giving way to the more cost-efficient "managed-care" plans, where all providers, including physicians, are salaried. Despite this, organized medicine continues to cling to the notion that a fee-for-service system is the only means to maintain the integrity of the physician-patient relationship and fights vigorously to sustain the status quo.[23] As the penetration of managed care in major markets increases, terms associated with this care delivery system, such as **capitation,** need to be explained.

Capitation is prepayment for services on a per member per month basis. Providers are paid the same amount of money every month for a member regardless of whether that member receives services and regardless of how expensive these services are. To determine an appropriate capitation, it is important first to determine what will be covered in the scope of services, including all services that the provider will be expected to deliver. Certain services are difficult to define, such as diagnostic testing, prescriptions, surgical procedures (what if the same procedure is performed by the primary care provider and by a referral physician?), and so forth. Other services such as immunizations, office care, and so forth, are easier to define. Most performance-based compensation systems also hold the primary care provider accountable for nonprimary care services, either through risk programs, or through positive incentive programs. Providers need to be able to estimate costs for each capitated service.[24] Some other relevant concepts in managed care related to reimbursement are described in the next section of this chapter.

COPAYMENT, COINSURANCE, AND DEDUCTIBLES

A **copayment** is that portion of a claim or medical expense that a member must pay out of pocket. This is usually a fixed amount, such as $5 in many HMOs. **Coinsurance** describes aprovision in a member's coverage that limits the amount of coverage by the plan to a certain percentage, commonly 80 percent. Any additional costs are paid by the member out of pocket. It is a significant challenge for clinicians to provide services to clients with varying degrees of insurance coverage. A **deductible** is that portion of a subscriber's (or member's) health-care expenses that must be paid out of pocket before any insurance coverage applies, commonly $100 to $300. Deductibles are common in indemnity insurance plans and preferred provider organizations, but are uncommon in HMOs. Deductibles may apply to only the out-of-network portion of a point-of-service plan. Point-of-service plans provide a difference in benefits, for example, 100 percent coverage rather than 70 percent, depending on whether the member chooses to use the plan, including its providers, and is in compliance with the authorization system to go outside the plan for services.[24]

ADVERSE SELECTION

Adverse selection is a situation where an insurance carrier or benefit plan has a disproportionate enrollment of adverse risks, such as an impaired or older population, with a potential for higher health-care utilization than budgeted for an average population. Adverse selection occurs when premiums do not cover the cost of providing services.[25] Therefore, insurers may indicate that it is fiscally essential for them to avoid providing health-insurance coverage to higher-risk individuals.

COMMUNITY RATING

Community rating involves setting health-insurance premiums based on the average cost of paying for services for all covered people in a geographic area, regardless of their history or potential for using health services. Community rating is a method of calculating health-insurance premiums that sets the same price for the same health-benefit coverage for all individuals in a pool of insured and does not take into account such variables as the claims experience of the group, age, sex, or health status. Community rating helps to spread the cost of illness evenly over all health plan enrollees (the whole community), rather than charging the sick more for health insurance.[25]

EXPERIENCE RATING

Another method of determining the cost of health insurance to consumers is **experience rating.** With experience rating, health-insurance premiums are based on the average cost of actual or anticipated health care used by various groups and takes into account such variables as previous claims experience, age, sex, and health status. It is the most common method of establishing premiums for health insurance in private programs.[25] However, with increasing managed-care penetration in many markets and the move toward fully capitated systems, competition between insurance plans will likely intensify. Underbidding for contracts between competing managed-care plans may be part of that process, regardless of the methods used to derive premium costs.

Even when APNs are employed by large HMOs, it is important to be aware of issues such as fluctuations in the numbers of enrollees, because the current health-care marketplace is dynamic, and competing provider groups vigorously bid for contracts. APNs seeking to affiliate themselves with HMOs and PPOs need to consider what type of plan structure is employed. The plan may be a corporation, partnership, or corporation, for profit, or not for profit. The sponsorship of HMOs and PPOs provides a key to the underlying philosophy and initial purpose of the plan. The sponsorship could also reflect the receptivity of the plan to discussion regarding APN services. Typical sponsors include insurance companies, providers, investor ownership, consumer ownership, third-party administrators (PPOs), and entrepreneurial arrangements.[26]

Advanced practice nurses must ascertain the current arrangement between the managed-care organization and providers. To some degree, this is determined by the model of the HMO or PPO. The current arrangements will affect the approach that should be taken by the APNs in the negotiating process. The following information should be gathered:

- **Who are the existing providers for the plan and what hospitals are they associated with? What is the size of the network? How long have the providers been participating? How many new providers are added each year? How many providers have left the plan?**

- **Are the providers contracted with as a physician association, a joint venture, or as individual physicians or physician groups?** If the plan contracts with one large association of physicians, providers may have to "subcontract" with this organization before contracting with the plan. Even if contracting is possible directly with the plan, the physician association usually has more influence than in less-centralized organizations and may have to be included in discussions between APNs and the plan. If the plan contracts with groups or with individual physicians, the ability for new provider groups to contract directly with the plan is improved.

- **Does the plan contract with APNs such as nurse anesthetists, podiatrists, optometrists, chiropractors, and mental health professionals?** To the extent that a plan has already broadened its panel of providers beyond that of medical doctors, some of the groundbreaking work has already been achieved. Such plans already appreciate the quality of service and cost-containment ability of contracting with non-MD physicians. The doorway probably is open for nonphysician providers who can demonstrate the efficacy and cost effectiveness of their services.

- **What are the reimbursement arrangements with providers?** As much information as possible should be gathered on the current reimbursement and risk arrangement with existing providers. Such information will help determine the feasibility of various (discounted, capitation, fee schedule) arrangements which a group of APNs might consider, as well as the extent to which the plan typically shifts the risk to providers.[26]

- Entrepreneurial APNs need to be prepared to accept risk when contracting with managed-care entities. If clinical services performed by the APN cost less to provide than the contracted amount per member per month, profit is achieved. However, if the APN provides more services than the contracted amount, loss is incurred by the APN or APN group, not the managed-care organization.

GLOBAL BUDGETING

Global budgeting is an overall budget limit on health-care services, regardless of where the funds originate. Global budgets can take the form of a state or federal maximum limit on total health-care expenditures, but usually imply federal limits. In some contexts, global budgeting has come to mean setting a limit on spending within sectors, for example, specific allocations for physicians, APNs, or hospitals.[26]

Canada has used global budgeting for health care with varying results. One of the authors provided cardiac anesthesia services for British Columbia residents who were unable to undergo timely cardiac surgery in Canada. The Canadian government in that situation had to contract with the state of Washington to provide open heart surgery services. The National Health Service in Great Britain coexists with private indemnity insurance carriers. Certainly physicians and other health-care providers working for salaries under global budgets or in capitated systems have less financial incentive to provide services than under traditional fee-for-service care delivery.

Summary

Reimbursement for APNs has been discussed in the context of traditional economic theory. The economic system, particularly as it relates to health care, was described. Concepts such as market competition, disequilibrium, and supplier-induced demand were explicated. Cost considerations in the provision of services by, and reimbursement for, physicians and APNs were discussed in relation to the price of services, access issues, health-care plans, competition, and antitrust issues. Key terms in finance and reimbursement were defined.

Reimbursement is a challenging component of APN practice. APNs should be aware of market economics, use appropriate marketing strategies, and strive to provide high-quality, cost-effective services. As health-care providers assume more financial risk, fiscal rewards may be less predictable than in the past. However, APNs equipped with the necessary knowledge and skills can fill needed service niches in health care, practicing independently or collaboratively with physicians.

Suggested Exercises

1. A nurse practitioner who has been employed for 15 years is told that her position is being eliminated. She is told that her position is "too expensive" for the proposed hospital budget under a re-engineering plan. Consultants have told hospital administration to decrease fixed costs, such as payroll. The panel of patients seen by this nurse practitioner would be given the option of being seen by other health-care providers in the community. How might the nurse practitioner retain her practice while capturing the income stream generated by her services?

2. A nurse educator who is active in professional organization activities repeatedly cites the benefits of care provided by APNs. These benefits include safe and cost-effective care. At one forum, the educator is closely questioned regarding the availability data substantiating these benefits. How might the educator respond to these questions, based on the evolving health-care marketplace?

3. An nurse practitioner employed by an HMO contemplates relocating from an urban setting to a rural one, where she contemplates entering a joint practice arrangement with a physician who is anxious to collaborate with the nurse practitioner. However, both the physician and the nurse practitioner are unfamiliar with reimbursement mechanisms for services provided by nurse practitioners. What resources should these professionals consult to maximize reimbursement from their joint practice arrangement?

REFERENCES

1. Feldstein, P: The Politics of Health Legislation: An Economic Perspective. Health Administration Press Perspectives, Ann Arbor, Mich, 1988.
2. Buerhaus, P: Nursing, competition, and quality. Nurs Econ 10:21, 1992.
3. Fuchs, V: The Health Economy. Harvard University Press. Cambridge, Mass, 1986.
4. Enthoven, A: Managed competition: An agenda for action. Health Aff (Millwood) 7:25, 1988.
5. Feldstein, P: Health Care Economics, ed 4. Delmar Publishers, Albany, NY, 1993.
6. Cohen, J: Medicaid physician fees and use of physician and hospital services. Inquiry 30:281, 1993.
7. Lee, D, and Gillis, K: Physician responses to Medicare physician payment reform: Preliminary results on access to care. Inquiry 30:417, 1993.
8. Buerhaus, P: Economics and healthcare financing. In Hickey, J, Ouimette, R, and Venegoni, S (eds): Advanced Practice Nursing. Lippincott, Philadelphia, 1996.
9. Sorkin, A: Health Economics, ed 3. Macmillan, New York, 1992.
10. Center for Health Economics Research: The Nation's Health Care Bill: Who Bears the Burden? Center for Health Economics Research, Waltham, Mass, 1994.
11. Hoffman, C: Medicaid payment for nonphysician practitioners: An access issue. Health Aff (Millwood) 13:140, 1994.
12. Mittelstadt, P: Federal reimbursement of advanced practice nurses' services empowers the profession. Nurse Pract 18:46, 1993.
13. Lewin, I: To the Rescue: Toward Solving America's Health Care Crisis. Families USA Foundation, Washington, DC, 1993.
14. Faut-Callahan, M: Economics of anesthesia. Unpublished manuscript, 1995.
15. Bradford, B: Personal communication, April, 1996.
16. Fagin, C: The cost-effectiveness of nursing care. In Aiken, L, and Fagin, C (eds): Charting Nursing's Future: Agenda for the 1990s. JB Lippincott, Philadelphia, 1992.
17. Hooker, R: The Role of Physician Assistants and Nurse Practitioners in a Managed Care Organization. Association of Academic Health Centers, Kaiser Permanente Center for Health Research, Sacramento, 1993.
18. Mirr, M: Advanced clinical practice: A reconceptualized role. AACN 4:599, 1993.
19. Timmons, G, and Ridenour, N: Legal approaches to the restraint of trade of nurse practitioners: Disparate reimbursement patterns. Journal of the American Academy of Nurse Practitioners 6:55, 1994.
20. Fugate, D, and Freese, G: Nursing marketing. In Decker, P, and Sullivan, E (eds): Nursing Administration. Appleton & Lange, Norwalk, Conn, 1992.
21. Petrakos, C: Nurse practitioner supervision at issue: RNs push for collegial practice. The Chicago Tribune, Nursing News, p 3, 1996.
22. Schwartz, A: Will competition change physician workforce? Early signals from the market. Acad Med 71:15, 1996.
23. Simonson, D, and Garde, J: Reimbursement for clinical services. In Foster, S, and Jordan, L (eds): Professional Aspects of Nurse Anesthesia Practice. FA Davis, Philadelphia, 1994.
24. Kongstvedt, P: Compensation of primary care physicians in open panels. The Managed Health Care Handbook, ed 2. Aspen, Gaithersburg, Md, 1993.
25. Michels, K: Healthcare reform glossary of terms. Journal of the American Association of Nurse Anesthetists 62:19, 1994.
26. American Association of Nurse Anesthetists: Practice management in changing environments, Sections 4–1 and 4–2. The American Association of Nurse Anesthetists, Park Ridge, Ill, 1994.

Marketing the Role: Formulating, Articulating, and Negotiating Advanced Practice Nursing Positions

CHRISTINE E. BURKE, PhD, CNM
JEANNE PICHETTE BAIR, RN, MSN, CNM

Christine (Tina) E. Burke, PhD, CNM, has had a clinical practice in nurse midwifery since 1976, when she earned her master's degree in nursing from Yale University. Dr. Burke is an educator whose teaching credentials include positions at the University of Colorado, Georgetown University, George Mason University, and Yale University. Pentimento Praxis, Dr. Burke's consultation practice, was established in 1992 after completion of her doctorate in nursing from the University of Colorado. The scope of her consultations include creating caring communities, training teachers and community members in moral development and character education, caring for and preventing adolescent pregnancies, nurturing the perceptual palette, and providing parenting instruction. Dr. Burke lives in Denver, Colorado, with her daughter.

Jeanne Pichette Bair, RN, MSN, CNM, has had a full-scope midwifery practice since 1982, when she received her master's degree in nursing from the University of Pennsylvania. She has served on both the academic and the clinical faculty for 12 years, affiliated with the University of Pennsylvania, Columbia University, and the University of Colorado. Ms. Bair lives in Denver, Colorado, with her husband and their two daughters.

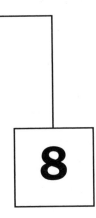

8

CHAPTER OUTLINE

THE TRADITIONAL MARKETING AP-
PROACH: THE 4 Ps
KNOWLEDGE OF PERSONAL VALUES,
PROFESSIONAL SKILLS, AND PRACTI-
CAL NECESSITIES
KNOWLEDGE OF PRACTICE REGULATIONS
KNOWLEDGE OF EXISTING SERVICES
KNOWLEDGE OF CLIENTS' HEALTH-CARE
NEEDS AND DESIRES
KNOWLEDGE OF THE TARGET POPULA-
TION'S UNDERSTANDING OF THE ROLE
AND SCOPE OF PRACTICE OF THE AD-
VANCED PRACTICE NURSE
KNOWLEDGE OF THE UTILIZATION AND
COST OF EFFECTIVENESS, AND SATIS-
FACTION WITH, ADVANCED PRACTICE
NURSING SERVICES
KNOWLEDGE OF SPECIFIC MARKETING
ELEMENTS
Substitution and complement functions

The product or service
The marketing plan
COMMUNICATION SKILLS
Networking
The job description
The cover letter
The résumé
The interview
EVALUATION OF JOB OPPORTUNITIES
The company
The position
The salary and benefits package
CLOSE OF THE DEAL
Contracts
Employment confirmation letter
Letter of acceptance
Noncompete agreement
MENTORS AND CAREER ADVANCEMENT
SUMMARY
SUGGESTED EXERCISES

CHAPTER OBJECTIVES

After completing this chapter, the reader will be able to:

1. Communicate the benefits that accrue to the target population or employer from utilization of the advanced practice nurse's (APN's) service offer through use of the four Ps.
2. Create a personal mission statement after reflection on personal values, beliefs, and quality-of-life issues that will influence your career pathways.
3. Interpret facts from major documents about cost, outcomes, and use of health services provided by APNs.
4. Create a marketing plan for an APN's service.
5. Create a succinct position statement for an APN's service that differentiates the service from alternatives and links it to target consumer needs and wants.

6. Demonstrate techniques and considerations in negotiating an advanced practice position from initial contact through the interview process to the contractual agreement.
7. Analyze existing network and use marketing techniques to further enhance and strengthen the resources.

Marketing, as a coordinated style of communicating information, is an essential skill for APNs. Success in the age of managed care and autonomous private practices and businesses demands an appreciation of market theories. APNs must understand a business plan as well as a nursing care plan to accomplish the goals of their independent practice. This chapter is *bifocal* in its presentation. The information shared is useful from either the *employer's* or *employee's perspective*. The skills necessary to gather and interpret marketing data, formulate marketing plans, and create essential written documents for the acquisition and development of APNs' services are presented through a marketing lens.

The Traditional Marketing Approach: The 4 Ps

The marketing process is guided by the four Ps:

- Product
- Price
- Place
- Promotion

These concepts help to assess the needs and the available resources to be used in the promotion of the APN service.

The first P, the **product,** is interpreted in an APN's business plan, not as material goods, but rather as human services. Unlike material products, these services lack tangibility, efficient storage capability for later use, and cannot be exactly replicated with each client, factors which pose some of the challenges of creating a marketing plan that accurately projects the future of an APN's service. The difference of human service is important because it is at the core of patient satisfaction. The development of an APN's service as a product includes the consideration of the **market segmentation,** or **target markets,** which describe who will be served; **product integrity,** or the balance of needs and resources; and the **competition,** or the other available health-care services in the community.

Price, the second P, is the identification of the right cost for the services. This price must be neither too high nor too low and also must meet the existing financial mandates of insurance companies, managed-care facilities, and federally funded Medicaid and Medicare plans. APNs' services can support their price for services from marketing research based on utilization and cost effectiveness. Proof that the services meet the needs of the patients and are financially efficient has been determined in recent research, which is discussed later in this chapter.

The third P is for **place,** or where these services are delivered. The demands of the consumers direct this marketing concern. The geographic location and physical convenience of the APN service play heavily into the clients' decision making among competitive health-care services. The more accessible and the more easily usable a service is, the greater the acquisition of health-care consumers. The simple matters of accessibility by public transporation, parking, and physically pleasant office spaces can ultimately sway potential clients from one service to another.

The final P is for **promotion,** or the ability to increase consumers' awareness of the APN's services offered and the communication of information that may attract consumers. The modes of promotion include advertisement, publicity, community presentations, and correspondence. In addition, the P for promotion also includes the manner in which the APN reflects the quality of the service in speech, dress, and the conduct of business. The best method of promotion is word of mouth by satisfied consumers. By its nature, this method of promotion is grounded in familiarity and trust, and a good word from a previous employer or consumer can do more for successful marketing than many costly advertising promotions.[1]

Employment is one of the obvious goals of advanced practice nursing education. This goal is met through one of three pathways:

1. Employment in an established health-care service that already employs APNs
2. Creation of new employment opportunities within a health-care system that has the potential for expansion to include nurse practitioners
3. Development of a private practice in the clinical or consultation arenas

In general terms, marketing is the activity that supports the buying and selling of products and services. The key to success in attaining employment involves matching the professional skills necessary for a job and the nurse practitioner. By analyzing the health-care needs of the target population and setting up a research-based plan to meet those needs, APNs are likely to create employment opportunities or, in marketing terms, to set up voluntary exchanges of goods and services.

A prerequisite to the successful marketing of an APN is knowledge. Each professional must spend time considering and developing self-knowledge and knowledge about the profession. Attention should be given to the following areas:

- Knowledge of personal values, professional skills, and practical necessities
- Knowledge of practice regulations
- Knowledge of existing services
- Knowledge of clients' health-care needs and desires
- Knowledge of the target population's understanding of the role and scope of practice of the APN
- Knowledge of the utilization and cost effectiveness of, and satisfaction with, advanced practice nursing services
- Knowledge of specific marketing elements

Knowledge of Personal Values, Professional Skills, and Practical Necessities

Developing a **personal mission statement,** or a statement of one's values, beliefs, and goals of practice, can assist in successfully communicating and selling one's view of health care. This statement will explain who you are. The personal mission statement typically includes one's values or guiding principles (e.g., trust, honesty, respect, responsibility, and caring) and one's professional skills and scope of services. Most importantly, it reveals the vision of the quality of life one needs (time for family, hobbies, political activity, and educational opportunities). This knowledge is usually acquired by introspection, by review of previous employment, and by consideration of personal needs, which are necessary for a reasonable life.

An example of guiding principles that have strongly affected the business community is Stephen Covey's *The Seven Habits of Highly Effective People*.[2] Mr. Covey developed a theory regarding the restoration of the character ethic. The habits are the intersection of knowledge, skill, and desire. *Knowledge* is the theoretical paradigm, or the what to do; *skill* is the how to do; and *desire* is the motivation. Covey divides these habits into three arenas:

1. The Private Victory

- Be proactive based on principles of personal vision.
- Begin with the end in mind guided by principles of leadership.
- Put first things first guided by principles of personal management.

2. The Public Victory

- Think win-win guided by principles of interpersonal leadership.
- Seek first to understand then to be understood guided by principles of empathic communication.
- Synergize guided by principles of cooperation.

3. The Renewal

- Sharpen the saw guided by principles of balanced self-renewal.

The importance of this work is its universal message about human effectiveness. The translation of these theories into nursing practice will help create a stronger, more professional vision.

Questions helpful in the introspective process are:

- What about your work do you enjoy the most?
- What other interests do you have?
- What skills do you do well?
- Which need improvement?
- What support do you need to attain a proficient level of practice?
- What made you leave jobs in the past?
- How will this affect your future employment?
- Do you prefer to work alone or on a team?
- What about your team members is necessary for good working relationships?
- How do you see your role in relation to the health-care system: What is your need for power or shared power?
- How do you handle stress?
- Will the job you are creating or applying for allow for some stress-reduction management, such as exercise?

- What are your family needs (child-care issues and emergency coverage, flexibility of hours to allow for family events)?
- How do you best communicate with others?

The time spent on a personal mission statement can save you from major career-related frustrations and problems. A considered mission statement can guide your job search with a clarity of purpose by defining both the professional and personal motivating factors. If salary and status hold greater value than free time and an active social life, focus the marketing efforts on demanding a financially fulfilling position. In all cases, be true to yourself.

Knowledge of Practice Regulations

The legal issues concerning advanced practice nursing are discussed in Chapter 7. Review this chapter and all related statutes and regulations. Place in a marketing portfolio the documents that will support an advanced nursing practice. Typically these documents include:

- State nurse-practice act
- State board of nursing regulations
- Prescriptive authority legislation
- Third-party reimbursement rules and regulations
- Practice protocols from similar APNs' services

Knowledge of Existing Services

Investigate the target market in which you wish to practice with an eye toward answering the following questions:

- What services already exist in the community?
- Who uses the services?
- What are the needs for these services based on the demographic data and the socioeconomic mix of the population (e.g., age, employment, unemployment, insured and uninsured)?
- Most importantly, what is not working with these services that an APN might be able to change (e.g., access to care, cost-effective care, patient education)?

Knowing the competition is the first step in creating a marketing strategy. Deciding how to position the service is the next. Positioning is a marketing strategy that works to separate the uniqueness of a product or service from the generic pack. It begins with knowing your service and the competition's service and then finding a niche that allows your service to stand out.[3]

Ask not what one has to offer, but what is needed by the consumer that an APN can meet. Knowing one's abilities and marketable skills is important, but it is more important to be in a position where someone will desire to use those services. This goal can be best accomplished by recommendations from people already highly respected by the target population or community. In a world full of well-qualified professionals, the APN or APN's service with strong recommendations will often rise above the competition and be hired.

Creating this market niche, the narrow market segment the APN can fulfill, can be accomplished by using a reverse marketing strategy. This consumer-driven process creates partners between the APN and the potential clients toward the common goal of health-care satisfaction. The positioning process, therefore, demands a needs assessment of the actual or perceived consumer needs. This is accomplished through the use of interviews, surveys, and questionnaires.[3]

Knowledge of Clients' Health-Care Needs and Desires

Knowledge of the needs and desires of the clients involves watching and reaching people. Mark McCormack, in *What They Don't Teach You at Harvard Business School*,[4] described seven fundamental steps to reading people:

- Listen aggressively to the what and how someone speaks.
- Observe aggressively and make note of all body language.
- Talk less and you will learn more, see more, and hear more.
- Take a second look at first impressions by reviewing what you first thought about a person or an idea.
- Take time to use what you have learned by reviewing what you know about your job and the clients, and then consider how you will present your services.
- Be discreet about what you have perceived about others and how they learn about your qualifications. Whenever possible, let others tell how great you are.
- Be detached enough to step back from a heated business deal and watch what is happening so that your reaction is not overreaction. Always try to act rather than react since this has more power.

Researching the health-care needs of a target population includes McCormack's ideas of reading people on the interpersonal level, and the more global tools for reading a community, such as surveys. These surveys should offer a broader perspective of the health-care needs from a mix of socioeconomic groups as well as from a variety of community members, consumers, health-care administrators, insurance agents, and peer professionals.

Knowledge of the Target Population's Understanding of the Role and Scope of Practice of the Advanced Practice Nurse

By survey, questionnaire, or personal contacts, determine the target market's level of understanding of an APN. Talk to prospective clients, employers, community leaders, insurance salespersons, hospital employees, and the medical community. Determine what, if any, previous experiences prospective employers have had with APNs.

Once the level of their appreciation of the APN has been determined, formulate a plan for educating or increasing the awareness of one's target population regarding the potential benefits of hiring an APN and their specific skills.

Knowledge of the Utilization and Cost Effectiveness of, and Satisfaction with, Advanced Practice Nursing Services

Review and collect current literature that supports the role of the APN. Resource assessment and use are at the core of every economic strategy plan. A marketing plan should respect not only the fiscal and structural resources of the health-care system but also the human resources necessary for health-care provision. Encourage prospective employers or consumers to read the literature on utilization and suggest that they take the time to evaluate what costly physicians' services they might substitute with APNs' services. Research has shown that nonphysician health-care professionals provide high-quality primary care and increased consumer access to care.

On the most basic level, APNs earn smaller salaries and, therefore, solely in terms of salary and benefits, cost less than physicians. More importantly APNs are more likely to prescribe improved nutrition, exercise, stress management techniques, and health promotion, modalities which are less likely to directly affect the clinic, hospital, or institutional budget. In addition, APNs are less likely to send each patient home with a prescription, potentially saving health-care dollars.

Research in primary care has described the level of productivity and cost associated with patient delegation of nonphysician health providers (NHPs), nurse practitioners, and physician assistants, and physician providers. These studies reveal that four NHPs can replace two to three physicians. The addition of an NHP to an office or clinic setting increased the total office visits by 40 to 50 percent. The substitution of one NHP for one physician resulted in an average savings of more than $34,000 dollars per year.[5] Similarly, Greenfield et al.[6] found that in an NHP system in a health-care setting in which protocols were used, a 20 percent reduction on visit costs was realized. A meta-analysis of studies on nurse practitioners and CNMs provides our profession with excellent support for the use of professionals in these advanced practice nursing roles.[7] A 1986 study reported by the Office of Technology Assessment (OTA)[8] concluded that nurse practitioners and CNMs provided a quality of care equivalent to the care given by physicians. This study also concluded that in the areas of communication and preventive care, the nurses were much more adept than physicians. A second study conducted in 1987 by Crosby, Ventura, and Feldman[9] reported findings similar to the OTA study. This study concluded that:

- Patients are satisfied with their care from nurse practitioners.
- The interpersonal skills of APNs are better than those of physicians.
- The technical quality of APNs is equivalent to physicians' care.
- APNs' patient outcomes are equivalent or superior to physicians' patient outcomes.

- APNs facilitate continuity of patient care and improved access to care in rural and other settings and provide care to underserved populations.

In November 1995, The Health Research Group of Ralph Nader's Public Citizen released a unique consumer guide to certified nurse midwifery practices in the United States. The report concluded that CNMs will play an increasing role in American obstetric care because of the quality of care, cost-effectiveness, and overall patient satisfaction described by CNM clients.[10] The Nader group found that 87 percent of CNMs serve low-risk clients, that 92 percent provide obstetric and gynecological care, that cesarean section rates for CNM clients were half that of the overall US rate, and that CNMs use less technology and more patient education in prenatal visits. The endorsement of the use of CNMs by this prestigious research group can assist all CNMs to support their place in a health-care system. These research findings can be incorporated in the marketing plan. Gathering research studies such as this for the marketing portfolio will act as a strong base of support, especially in systems that appreciate statistical proof of health-care outcomes.

Knowledge of Specific Marketing Elements

SUBSTITUTION AND COMPLEMENT FUNCTIONS

In this changing health-care climate, many physicians are concerned about their power, their income, and even their jobs. The rules are changing too quickly and too dramatically, causing discomfort for many providers, physician and non-physician alike. APNs have frequently found employment in areas less desirable for physicians. These areas are typically rural areas or underserved inner-city clinics, which were not financially lucrative and were therefore less desirable to physicians.

In these areas, there is little argument about how nurse practitioners can be used both as substitution for, and in complement with, physician providers. For clarity, it helps to define these terms in the context of this chapter. **Complement** is defined as[11]:

- Something that completes, makes up a whole, or brings to perfection.
- The quantity or number needed to make up a whole. Either of two parts that complete the whole or mutually complete each other.

Substitute is defined as one that takes the place of another, a replacement.[11]

In an underserved area any competent health-care provider can reasonably argue for positions providing care that otherwise would be unavailable. This could mean working with a physician or physicians to "mutually complete" a health-care partnership. It also could be as a substitute for a physician, "taking the place of" a physician in an area without one.

The arguments for positions in more competitive areas often are more difficult to make and may be less well received. In these areas, it is wise to focus on how APNs are different rather than how they are the same. If APNs are "the same as" physicians, it is often more difficult to break into the health-care system where physicians are abundant. Practitioners may be more marketable if they "mutually complete" a health-care partnership than attempt to replace one. In marketing roles in these settings, it is important to stress that APNs provide similar services but with an emphasis on health and prevention.

In the ever-changing health-care environment, APNs can no longer afford to be just clinicians. Marketing has become crucial to survival. **Marketing** is defined as the act or process of selling or purchasing in a market, an aggregate of functions involved in moving goods from producer to consumer.[11] Some factors to consider in the marketing process include:

- What is the product or service?
- How is it different from others?
- How is it better?
- Are APNs more consumer oriented, more cost effective, and so forth?

THE PRODUCT OR SERVICE

The product or service generally *is* the APN, but the individuation depends on the particular area of practice. APNs are professionals with specialized knowledge or skills that are applied within a broad range of patient populations in a variety of practice settings.[12]

- Certified nurse midwives are individuals educated in the two disciplines of nursing and midwifery, who possess evidence of certification according to the requirements of American College of Nurse-Midwives.[13] Nurse midwifery practice is the independent management of care of essentially normal newborns and women occurring within a health-care system that provides for medical consultation, collaboration, or referral.
- Certified registered nurse anesthetists are registered nurses who have completed a nurse anesthesia program accredited by the Council on the Accreditation of Nurse Anesthesia Education Programs[14] and have been certified by the Council on Certification of Nurse Anesthetists.
- Clinical nurse specialists (CNSs) serve as role models in delivery of high-quality nursing care to patients.[15] The CNS's client is the nurse, and the focus is on nursing staff education, system analysis, and providing direct and indirect nursing care.[16]
- Nurse practitioners (NPs) provide a full range of primary health-care services with a holistic patient and family focus. The NP's client is the patient, and the focus is on providing direct patient care.[17]

THE MARKETING PLAN

After all the information has been collected from introspection, research data, personal communications, and target population surveys, the APN can create a **marketing plan,** or outline of strategies for promotion of services. Marketing plans contain five major elements:

1. The statement of the purpose and the main objectives
2. The product description or what the APN's service has to offer
3. The big picture: Where will the APN and APN's service be in 5 years?
4. The immediate action plan or steps for getting to the big picture

A. Describe your market: _____
   Age: _____
   Family size: _____
   Annual family income: _____
   Location: _____
   Health-care decision patterns: _____
   Reason to seek CNM care: _____
   Other: _____
   (Geographically describe your service area)
   (Describe your client base economically)
   How large is your market? _____
   Women of childbearing age or birth rate: _____
   Growing _____ Steady _____ Decreasing _____
   If growing, annual growth rate _____
B. Describe the service you will provide: _____
C. Describe your pricing/billing practices: _____
D. Describe the place you will provide services: _____
E. Describe referral sources: _____
F. Describe your competition: _____

G. Describe plans for practice promotion and continued marketing: _____

   _____

H. Describe any barriers to practice that might exist: _____

   _____

I. Describe any consumer or professional networking that will be done: _____

   _____

Figure 8–1 Developing a marketing plan. (Adapted from Collins-Fulea, C,[18] p. 25.)

5. The marketing tools and strategies to be used. These include interviews, networking, and advertisement.

   Fig. 8–1 is an example of a marketing plan adapted for CNM practice.[18]

   A marketing plan should not be considered concrete, but rather, ever changing. It should be reviewed routinely and revised as needed to reflect changes in professional development or the needs of the target market. The possibility of health-care and welfare reform in our country, for example, could change access to care. APNs must be ready to adapt to that change.

Communication Skills

NETWORKING

"Mid-level providers" are ideally positioned for the radical changes sweeping the health-care field, but they will surely experience much struggle in the process. One way to cope with the inevitable struggle is through networking.

Networking is not new! It has been done on both an informal and a formal basis since the beginning of mankind. A **network** is simply a group of individuals with similar interests and/or problems who join together to provide support and to exchange information. With the advent of computer technology, contacts are no longer limited by geography or phone bills. Networks easily span incredible distances, allowing even the most rural practitioners easy access to a peer group.

Informal Network

An informal network has traditionally been part of the male-dominated business world, especially in the upper levels of certain disciplines. The network comprises acquaintances, colleagues, and friends from school, church, family, sports, and business. When a man needed a favor, he contacted someone in his network. Men grow up knowing how to network, partially because of the emphasis on team sports during boys' formative years. They learn quickly and well that they need one another in order to win the game, to get ahead.[19]

Formal Network

Professional organizations are a good example of a formal network. These organizations, through their membership, are able to quickly disseminate information and take action. When federal legislation is proposed that might have a negative impact on the public's health, the American Nurses' Association (ANA) is able to contact its network of state associations requesting that they enlist the support of their membership to oppose the bill. Networking can be an immeasurable benefit to success and happiness in an advanced practice role. Through networking, one can:

- Build support systems
- Share resources and avoid reinventing the wheel
- Identify similar practice issues, such as restraint of trade; credentialing difficulties; and physician opposition, direct or subtle[20]

The best place to learn about job opportunities is through one's network of friends and acquaintances. Networking, as related to job searches, is the process of enlisting other people to help one find employment. Most job openings are filled by word of mouth.[21] One never knows who can help!

- Build a base of contacts with alumni groups, professional organizations, PTA, and children's sports leagues
- Expand this contact base
- Get and use referrals
- Follow up on all leads

All leads are worth pursuing. When contacting someone from the network, let that person know that you are looking for a job and would welcome advice, suggestions, or ideas. It is probably better not to ask directly for a job. This can put people off and decrease the probability of assistance. The most important thing that one can get from people are names of other people. Word of mouth is the most effective way to find a job. Other methods include:

- Newspaper advertisements: Only 10 to 15 percent of job openings are advertised in newspapers.
- Large-scale mailing of résumé: The success rate for receiving a call for an interview is only 2 percent.
- Temporary work: It can be a foot in the door and an opportunity for permanent work.
- Executive recruiters (headhunters)
- Employment agencies
- Recruiting databases
- Going online with your résumé
- Browsing through job listings

The APN can get indirect knowledge of changes in job markets by reading the business pages and local business journals for hints to the "hidden job market." These include promotion announcements, transfers, retirements, company expansions, company relocations, announcements, awards, mergers, and take-overs.[22]

THE JOB DESCRIPTION

The purpose of the job description is to clarify the scope of practice and expectations of a professional position. See Fig. 8–2 for an example of a job description. The job analysis mentioned previously helps create the framework of skills, educational requirements, licensure, reporting relationships, working conditions, and specific functions and responsibilities needed to fulfill a job description.

The job description is a guide for the prospective employee regarding these issues of practice. The components of the job description include:

- The job identification, which includes the official title, the salary, and the department of operations, if applicable.
- The job summary, which gives an overview of the scope of the job. The who, what, when, where, and why questions regarding the position should be succinctly answered in this summary.
- The functions and principal responsibilities, which should list the position functions and responsibilities precisely. These include such functions as physical assessment, laboratory results reviews, patient education, documentation, student teaching, clinic maintenance, community outreach, staff development, and research.
- The list of skills required, which should describe attributes such as good judgment, good interpersonal skills, and ethical practice.
- The working conditions, which should describe physical or time and space issues, including hours of patient care in clinic, on-call requirements, office space, clinic or hospital locations, and potential occupational hazards.
- The education and experience, which should state the minimum preparation necessary to practice and often includes a statement of preferred education and experience for the position.
- The reporting relationship, which is the key to the power structure in one's job. This section should accurately describe who reports to whom and if anyone is reporting to the APN.

POSITION TITLE: Certified Nurse-Midwife (CNM)

DEPARTMENT: OB/GYN   **GRADE:** 15a

JOB SUMMARY: Provides comprehensive, primary health care to a select population of essentially healthy women. Participates in the care of women with medical complications in collaboration with Obstetricians-Gynecologists.

Principal Functions and Responsibilities:
1. Performs accurate history and physical examinations on essentially healthy women.
2. Provides primary care in an ambulatory setting to women, including ordering and evaluating of diagnostic tests and management of minor complications.
3. Provides inpatient obstetrical care for essentially healthy women, including labor management, delivery of infant, repair of lacerations/episiotomies and management of minor complications. Initiates emergency care as needed.
4. Provides individualized client teaching and counselling utilizing the nurse-midwifery philosophy.
5. Identifies deviations from normal and consults, co-manages, or refers as appropriate.
6. Completes necessary documentation.
7. Participates in research and continuing-education activities.
8. Instructs and supervises nurse-midwifery students as assigned.
9. Performs other duties as assigned.

Skill and Ability Requirements:
1. Considerable degree of independent judgment, to monitor and respond to changes of a client's condition.
2. Interpersonal skills to work effectively with clients and other members of the health care team.

Work Conditions:
Normal client-care environment with some exposure to biological hazards and infectious diseases.

Education and Experience Requirements:
Graduation from an accredited school of Nurse-Midwifery
Certification by ACNM or ACC
State Licensure

Reporting Relationships:
1. Reports to the Director, Nurse-Midwifery Services
2. Indirectly supervises personnel involved with the care of assigned clients.

APPROVED BY: _____   **DATE:** _____

Figure 8–2   The job description. (From Collins-Fulea, C,[18] p. 114, with permission.)

The job description will act as the template for the cover letters, résumés and the interviewing process.

THE COVER LETTER

The cover letter accompanies a résumé as a request for consideration for a job. It is the first impression one will make on a potential employer. The letter should be addressed to the appropriate person, clearly written, with no spelling or grammatical errors. It needs to describe the specific job one is interested in, the time frame of one's availability, and contact information (i.e., a phone number, fax number, e-mail and street address); and it should be written in a professional business style. The proper business format for the cover letter is as follows:

- The applicant's name and address
- The date
- The name and address of the person to whom one is sending the résumé
- The salutation (i.e., "Dear Dr. . . .")
- The opening statement, which gives the reason one is writing and indicates the job in which the APN is interested
- A brief paragraph stating why one is interested in the specific clinic or health-care facility
- A closing paragraph, which includes a request for an interview and offers references if desired
- The complimentary closing (i.e., "Sincerely" or another acceptable closing, with a signature and a typed name beneath the signature.

If the résumé is enclosed, be sure to write "enclosure" at the bottom left side of the letter. *Remember, keep copies of all of correspondence.*

The cover letter is typically only one typewritten page (Fig. 8–3). This brevity requires the writer to consider what is most essential to entice the

---

C. Brenda Penburke, CNM, PhD
4 Yale Street
New Haven, Conn. 40511
Telephone: 203-455-1267

November 12, 1995

Dr. Lilly Sen
Walrus Woman's Center
4563 Utopia Way
Astoria, Oregon 46042

Dear Dr. Sen:

I am a certified nurse-midwife, presently employed at Planned Parenthood of New Haven, Connecticut. I am considering a move to Astoria and am very interested in the position of Advanced Practice Nurse in your family planning clinic.

I have twenty years' experience in all aspects of nurse-midwifery but most particularly in the areas of well-woman gynecology and family planning.

I have enclosed my résumé for your review. Please feel free to contact me if you require additional information or references. I am looking forward to hearing from you.

Sincerely,

C. Brenda Penburke, CNM, PhD

Figure 8–3   An example of a cover letter.

prospective employer to read the résumé and to communicate that information in a well-written and clearly presented manner. The cover letter should be written individually for each potential position. It should be printed on a good quality bond paper and proofread carefully for any errors in grammar, spelling, and format.

THE RÉSUMÉ

Résumés vary in length and style, but all function to give a detailed outline of one's professional credentials, education, and experience. A résumé should be tailored to meet the needs and requirements of a specific job. Federal government positions generally require very short résumés (one to three pages), while their applications are very detailed. Academic résumés, or curriculum vitae, are typically fairly lengthy. The educational demands of an academic position are supported by previously given lectures, courses, and publications. Therefore, it is essential to list more fully all of these data.

There are two basic types of résumés:

1. The chronological résumé
2. The outcome or functional résumé

The chronological résumé provides a brief description of one's job history. This type is best used by those persons with a stable job history, with no more than 1 month between jobs. The outcome résumé does not describe the job history, but rather focuses on areas of proficiency and expertise. This type is best used when an APN has changed fields or is reentering the job market.[23]

As a part of the networking process, sharing résumés with others within the nursing profession may give some perspectives on how to support a job candidacy. In the creating your résumé, consider the essential components of the job being sought and present previous employment or education in this light. Be sure that the résumé accurately describes your skills and does not mislead a potential employer. Have a colleague read the résumé and the job description for the position being sought. This peer pal can comment on its accuracy and presentation.

The general components of a résumé include:

- Name
- Address, phone, fax, e-mail address
- Educational background and degrees earned
- Professional employment, other previous employment, if applicable
- Community service
- Research interests
- Grants written
- Publications
- Speaking engagements
- Honors and awards
- Consulting activities
- Professional memberships
- Military history

Keep demographic data (i.e., age, children, marital status, dates completed school) out of a résumé to avoid being screened out by any of these noncontributing factors.

Résumé writing is fundamentally an organized written communication of one's skills, education, and experience. To more effectively stress your previous experience, use action words to generate images of a "doer," or a person who takes the initiative to get a job done. Some of these action words are *administered, assumed responsibility, supervised, designed, handled, managed, prepared,* and *taught.*

Consider reviewing specific health-career résumé texts or using a professional résumé-writing service to increase the potential power of the document. Writing good résumés is like any other skill that develops with good modeling and persistent practice. An excellent resource is *Résumés for Health and Medical Careers.*[23]

THE INTERVIEW

The interview is the active phase of the exchange of information between an APN and a potential employer. The applicant and the interviewer create a purposeful relationship to exchange information about the persons involved in, and expectations of, a specific job. During this process, both parties have an opportunity to gather information to support the "correct fit" of the applicant to the position.

Simple cues such as one's attire, manner of speech, body language, demeanor, and timeliness create the first impression. If one is well groomed, comfortable, dressed appropriately in business attire, prepared to answer questions to support the skills and educational requirements for the job, and has arrived on time, the applicant will appear in a good light.

Prepare for the interview by finding out as much as possible about the position, the organization, the location, and the actual job requirements. Develop a list of questions to help clarify areas of concern. Review the personal mission statement and ask questions related to issues that make job satisfaction high (i.e., salaries and benefits, educational support, vacation and holiday time, local professional networks, and personal relationship needs). Consider your strengths and weaknesses and how you can see yourself growing in the position. Ask what mutual benefits might be gained in this relationship. Be prepared to answer questions about educational background, human relationship skills, communication style, teaching skills, and leadership roles.

Do not be afraid to ask for some of the same information from a potential employer. Remember, the goal of the interview is to match people to positions and to other people. What one gives and what one gets are the basis for marketing as a voluntary exchange of goods and services.

Planning for the interview is the key to success. Consider these eight keys to getting a job offer as suggested by Dorothy Leeds in *Marketing Yourself*[24]:

- Be prepared.
- Be ready to turn negatives into positives.
- Ask questions to keep control.
- Listen actively to content and intent of questions asked.

- Don't answer any questions not fully understood.
- Ask for the job.
- Follow up.

Practice enough to be relaxed and comfortable to allow your best self to shine through.[25]

After each interview, make a dated summary of the scope of questions, the perceived responses to the answers, and all promised follow-up. Finally, write a thank-you note that includes any follow-up information and a clear statement of your desire for the job.

Evaluation of Job Opportunities

When assessing a job offer, it is important to look at three factors:

1. The company
2. The position
3. The salary and benefits package

THE COMPANY

Many resources are available for research on companies that may be of interest. Local libraries have business directories that will provide detailed information about specific businesses. Included in these directories are the name of the business, names and titles of key personnel, complete address, phone number, number of employees, kind of business, type of location, and number of years in business.

THE POSITION

It is helpful to get a written job description for any position negotiated. If the job description is available before interviewing, it can be a useful guide for questions and clarification of the position. If a job description is not available, request that one be written before accepting the position. Minimally, get a definition of what duties will be expected, who will supervise the position, and where the job will be performed. Find out what orientation or on-the-job training will be provided.

THE SALARY AND BENEFITS PACKAGE

The salary offered or requested should meet or exceed the salary for similar positions in the area. It should be a salary with which one feels comfortable. *Beware of salaries that are much higher or much lower than the norm for that area.* If the salary is high, this may indicate a job that is undesirable for some reason and therefore hard to fill. If the salary is unusually low, this may indicate the lack of financial stability in the company or perhaps an undervaluing of the position by the company. A good benefits package is worth 20 to 40 percent of the salary. While successful negotiation is crucial to survival and growth in the profession, not many of APNs possess these important skills.

Before beginning contract negotiations, it is important to have a clear goal. Negotiate from strength. Know the product. Know the negotiators, be familiar with the company, and reaffirm the personal mission statement previously devised.

Salary

Before beginning negotiations, know what salaries are typical for similar positions in the community. If a salary range is discussed, such as $55,000 to $60,0000, simply state that $60,000 would be acceptable. It is probably best not to quote a specific figure unless the limits of the salary range for the job are known. The employer might be willing to offer more than is requested. A counteroffer can always be made if the salary quoted is unacceptably low.

Benefits

Items to negotiate include:
- Full family medical and dental insurance
  - Indemnity plan or managed care
  - Acceptable panel of providers
  - Point-of-service clause
  - Pregnancy coverage
  - Prescription plan
  - Vision plan
  - Orthodontics
  - Preexisting conditions clause
- Vacation days
- Paid holidays
- Sick days
- Retirement benefits
  - Time required for vesting
  - Safety of investments in the pension plan
- Life insurance
- Long-term disability plan
- Optional short-term disability
- Optional long-term care insurance
- Dependent-care reimbursement account
- Health-care reimbursement account
- Tax-deferred annuities
- Malpractice insurance
- Opportunities for advancement and career development
- Corporate cellular phone rates
- E-mail access
- Tuition waivers

- Continuing education: travel and registration fee
- Professional dues
- Subscriptions to professional journals
- Payment of consulting physician
- Provision of office space, supplies, personnel, and computers
- Payment of answering service and/or pagers

Close of the Deal

CONTRACTS

Defining the parameters of the job through formal contracts, letters of agreement, memoranda, or even verbal agreements is a necessity. Employees without written contracts can legally be considered "at-will" employees. **At-will employees** are those who may be fired without cause at any time. Likewise, an at-will employee can quit any time.[18] A **contract** is defined as[11]:

- An agreement between two or more parties, especially one that is written and enforceable by law
- The writing or document containing such an agreement

An **employment agreement,** such as in Fig. 8–4, is a type of contract describing an agreement between an employer and an employee that specifies duties and compensation, as well as the rights and responsibilities of each party.

If not offered a contract by the prospective employer, another approach is to supply one. This may seem like a formidable task, but there are many sources of assistance. There are computer software programs, such as Family Lawyer by Quicken.[26] Basic contract forms can be purchased at many office-supply stores. These resources provide a basic framework with which to begin. Most employment contracts are fairly straightforward. In negotiating phased-in compensation or a partial buy-in of a practice, have an attorney review the contract to ensure adequate protection. Contracts typically have similar areas of content. A basic employment contract should include date of agreement, name and address of the employee and employer, specific duties of the agreement, salary and fringe benefits, termination of employment agreement, and signatures of both the employer and employee.

EMPLOYMENT CONFIRMATION LETTER

Get the offer in writing for your own protection. If a verbal agreement is offered, request that the employer "clarify the job" in a written memorandum. If no written offer is made, it is advisable to send a letter to confirm the understanding. The letter should include a clause stating that the job will be defined by the letter unless the employer responds in writing.

LETTER OF ACCEPTANCE

A **letter of acceptance** is used by prospective employees to confirm the employee's understanding of the terms and conditions of the employer's offer of employment and to formally accept the offer.

EMPLOYMENT AGREEMENT

This Employment Agreement ("Agreement"), effective as of _____ (date), by and between _____ (name) of _____ (address), "the Employer," and _____ (name) of _____ (address), "the Employee."

1. EMPLOYMENT. Employee agrees to provide to Employer the services described in attached job description.

2. PAYMENT. The Employer agrees to provide Employee with an annual salary of $ _____.

3. MALPRACTICE. The Employer agrees to provide institutional malpractice insurance coverage for any duties performed within the scope of the Employee's job description. The Employee is not covered by this policy for any activities not specified in the job description.

4. VACATION/SICK DAYS. After completing the probationary period of not more than 90 days, each Employee accrues 0.8 sick days/month and 1.5 vacation days/month. Sick days may be accumulated up to 60 days. Vacation days must be used by the Employee's anniversary date each year.

5. CONTINUING EDUCATION. The Employer agrees to provide 7 days and $ _____ annually for continuing education, to be effective after completion of one year of employment.

6. COMMUNICATIONS. The Employer agrees to provide pagers and answering service to the Employee at no cost. Employee is entitled to corporate cellular phone rates (Employee provides cellular phone). Employee will be reimbursed for work-related calls by submitting an annotated monthly voucher.

This Agreement may be terminated for any reason by either party with a 14-day notice during the probationary period. After achieving Permanent Employee status, either party must give at least 30 days' notice prior to termination.

This Agreement is rendered null and void by falsification of information provided during the application process.

_____
Signature of Employee

_____
Signature of Employer

_____
Date

Figure 8–4 An example of an employee agreement.

NONCOMPETE AGREEMENT

A **noncompete agreement** is made by an employee (the noncompeting party) not to leave the current employer (the protected party) and become a competitor in the same market.[17] See Fig. 8–5 for an example of a noncompete agreement. Frequently, these agreements specify an amount of time (e.g, 3 years) and a geographic area (e.g., within a 5-mile radius of the office of the protected party). In addition, these agreements may include a clause that prevents the noncompet-

---

NONCOMPETE AGREEMENT

This Agreement is effective as of _____ (date), by and between _____ (name and address), "the Employer," and _____ (name and address), "the Employee".

For a period of _____ (specify amount of time) after leaving the employment of _____, the Employee, will not directly or indirectly engage in _____ (area of practice) within a _____ (specify a distance or specific geographical area) of _____ (address of employer).

In addition, the Employee agrees not to directly solicit transfer of care of any clients of Employer for a period of _____ (specify amount of time).

_____
Employer (Protected party)

_____
Employee (Non-Competing Party)

_____
Date

Figure 8–5   An example of a noncompete agreement.

ing party from soliciting business (e.g, contacting patients to inform them of the new practice location). It is important to understand the terms of these agreements. Failure to do so may severely impair one's ability to relocate if the job does not work out.

Mentors and Career Advancement

The final concept for discussion is that of mentors and career advancement. **Mentoring** is a relationship between a novice and an expert in any given profession in which advice is shared toward a mutual goal of career advancement. This relationship has as its most important functions[27]:

- Preparation for the leadership role
- Promotion of career success and advancement
- Enhancement of self-esteem and self-confidence
- Increased job satisfaction
- Strengthening of the profession

Building a mentor relationship on a strong foundation of similar values, goals, and abilities is necessary for successful career advancement. The personal mission statement, which was discussed earlier, can help again in this relationship. Knowing oneself and knowing the character of the mentor become the cornerstones for a successful match.

The characteristics of good mentors consist of a set of behaviors that include guiding, supporting, and teaching as well as good communication skills, good judgment, appropriate use of power, well-honed people skills, an ordered personal life, and a good sense of humor.[28]

The novice professional who attracts a good mentor has been shown to possess six major character traits:

1. Good performance
2. Right social background
3. Striking appearance in a suit (either gender)
4. Social affiliation with the mentor
5. Flair for demonstrating the extraordinary
6. High visibility

The best age difference between mentor and protégé is said to be a half generation, or 8 to 15 years. A greater age difference may create a parent-child relationship. Prospective protégés in their late 20s and early 30s generally look for a match with mentors in their 40s.[29]

A single role model, or mentor, does not always meet the needs of every novice professional. An alternative to the traditional mentor-model is proposed by Haseltine et al.[30] These authors have urged young professionals to actively participate in the creation of their professional identity by choosing advisors and considering multiple role models. The process of career goal attainment can be furthered, not just with a single mentor, but a group of professionals who work at different levels of career advancement. The *patron system* is a continuum of benefactors whose roles are to guide, support, and advocate for the novice. It is composed of *peer pals*, *guides*, and *sponsors*.[30] The peer pals are people with whom who you share information and strategies and, most importantly, who act as sounding boards for your new ideas. Guides offer invaluable information about the organizational structure and are able to offer suggestions for avoiding the wrong people or pathways as well as for pointing out the right people and shortcuts toward a goal. The role of a guide may be a coworker but also it may be an administrative-support person, such as a secretary or research assistant. The sponsor is a less powerful replacement for the mentor. Often these three alternatives—peer pals, guides, and sponsors—are more attainable to the novice professional and may be available immediately. The perfect mentor relationship may be discovered during this networking process. This patron system functions on a more horizontal plane than the vertical, hierarchical mentor system. The advantage of this horizontal link is the wider range of contacts for information and career advancement. Remember that career advancement and support should be built on mutual trust and a fair exchange of information.

SUMMARY

The use of these marketing strategies allows APNs to present both themselves and their role in the most effective manner. It also clarifies the major points of reference regarding the job for the employer as well as for the prospective employee, allowing each to make a decision regarding employment based on a foundation of well-defined facts.

Suggested Exercises

1. A colleague of another discipline claims that APNs are not particularly cost effective and that no evidence exists about how clients perceive the quality of care provided by these professionals. Relate the findings from major studies of the cost and quality of advanced practice nursing and outline indicators that have been consistently evaluated to determine quality of advanced practice nursing care.

2. A physician colleague challenges you that one of the sources of resistance to APNs is that they compete with physicians' practices. Give examples of how nurses in advanced practice can substitute or compensate to provide medical care in underserved areas of health care. Recall that underserved can have several interpretations, such as insufficient numbers of providers, inadequate insurance system, poor geographic access, and so on.

3. **Résumé and cover letter:** Specify a hypothetical professional job opportunity for which you would like to apply. In response, write a cover letter and enclose your professional résumé.
   Professional practice statement (PPS): Develop your individual PPS (i.e., job description) for the hypothetical job sought. This assignment builds on the work of the cover letter and résumé. The PPS must include clinical, administrative, research, and education components. Although it will not be necessary to create supporting policy statements or clinical privilege lists, these considerations should help to frame the writing of the PPS.

4. Role-play an interview, including discussion of salary and benefits.

5. What analogies can be made to the characteristics and functions of a mentor? What concerns or cautions are frequently made regarding gender? Evaluate the logic of these assumptions, identify unstated assumptions, and propose solutions or conclusions.

6. Consider your present employment. Create a list of possible peer pals, guides, and sponsors. What made you choose these people? How could you introduce the idea of their cooperation in the patron system?

REFERENCES

1. McNeil, NO, and Mackey, TA: Unpublished material, 1995.
2. Covey, SR: The Seven Habits of Highly Effective People. Simon and Schuster, New York, 1989.
3. Gallagher, SM: Promoting the nurse practitioner by using a marketing approach. Nurse Pract 21:36, 1996.
4. McCormack, M: What They Don't Teach You at Harvard Business School. Bantam Books, New York, 1984.
5. Schweitzer, S: The relative costs of physicians and new health practitioners. In Staffing Primary Care in 1990: Physician Replacement and Cost Savings. Springer, New York, 1991.
6. Greenfield, S, et al.: Efficiency and cost of primary care of nurses and physician assistants. N Engl J Med 298:305, 1978.
7. Brown, SA, and Grimes, DE: Nurse Practitioners and Certified Nurse-Midwives: A Meta-Analysis of Studies on Nurses in Primary Care Roles. American Nurses Publishing, Washington, DC, 1993.
8. US Congress, Office of Technology Assessment: Nurse Practitioners, Physicians As-

sistants and Certified Nurse-Midwives: A Policy Analysis. US Government Printing Office, Washington, DC, 1986.

9. Crosby, F, Ventura, MR, and Feldman, MJ: Future research recommendations for establishing nurse practitioner effectiveness. Nurse Pract 12:75, 1987.

10. Gabay, M, and Wolfe, SM: Encouraging the Use of Nurse-Midwives: A Report for Policy Makers. Public Citizens Publication, Washington DC, 1995.

11. Morris, W (ed): The American Heritage Dictionary of the English Language. Houghton Mifflin, Boston, 1981.

12. American Association of Colleges of Nursing: Position Statement: Certification and Regulation of Advanced Practice Nurses. Washington, DC, 1994.

13. American College of Nurse-Midwives: Essential Documents: Definition of a Certified Nurse-Midwife. Washington, DC, 1978.

14. Council on Accreditation of Nurse Anesthesia Education Programs: Standards for Accreditation of Nurse Anesthesia Education Programs. Park Ridge, Ill, 1994.

15. Moloney, MM: Professionalization of Nursing: Current Issues and Trends, ed 2. JB Lippincott, Philadelphia, 1992.

16. Boyd, NJ: The merit and significance of clinical nurse specialists. J Nur Adm 21:35, 1991.

17. Mallison, M: Nurses as house staff. Am J Nurs 93:7, 1993.

18. Collins-Fulea, C (ed): An Administrative Manual for Nurse-Midwifery Services. Kendall-Hunt Publishing, Dubuque, Iowa, 1996.

19. Puetz, BE: Networking for Nurses. Aspen Publishers, Rockville, Md, 1983.

20. Petras, K: The Only Job Hunting Guide You'll Ever Need. Poseidon Press, New York, 1989.

21. Kent, GE: How to Get Hired Today! VGM Career Horizons, Lincolnwood, Ill, 1991.

22. Casey, R: How to Find a Job: Your 30 Day Action Plan. Thomas Nelson Publishers, Nashville, 1993.

23. Editors of VGM Horizens: Résumés for Health and Medical Careers. NTC Publishing Group, Lincolnwood, Ill, 1996.

24. Leeds, D: Marketing Yourself. HarperCollins, New York, 1991.

25. Fisher, R, and Ury, W: Getting to Yes: Negotiating Agreement without Giving In. Houghton Mifflin, Boston ,1981.

26. Parsons Technology: Quicken: Family Lawyer. Intuit, Hiawatha, Iowa, 1995.

27. Vance, C: Is There a Mentor in Your Future? Imprint 36(5):41, 1989.

28. Alleman, E et al: Enriching mentor relationships. Personal Guide Journal 62:329, 1984.

29. Hunt, DM, and Michail, C: Mentorship: A career training and development tool. Academic Management Review 8:475, 1983.

30. Haseltine, DP, Rowe, MP, and Shapiro, EC: Moving up: Role models, mentors and the patron system. Sloan Management Review 19:51, 1978.

CHAPTER 9

Collaborative Practice: How We Get from Coordination to the Integration of Skills and Knowledge

Collaborative Practice: How We Get from Coordination to the Integration of Skills and Knowledge

SARA TORRES, PhD, RN, FAAN
LINDA M. DOMINGUEZ, PhD, RN

Sara Torres, PhD, RN, FAAN, received her doctorate in psychiatric mental health and research from the University of Texas at Austin in 1986, her master of science in psychiatric mental health from Adelphi University in 1975, her bachelor of science in nursing from the State University of New York at Stony Brook in 1972, and her associate's degree in arts and science from the State University of New York at Farmingdale in 1971. She is associate professor and chair of the Department of Psychiatric, Community Health, and Adult Primary Care at the School of Nursing, University of Maryland at Baltimore. Dr. Torres's major academic and research interests focus on the Hispanic community and include work in family violence in the Hispanic community (particularly wife abuse), the delivery of cross-cultural health care, and the mental health of Hispanic women (anxiety and depression). She is a nationally recognized expert and frequently sought consultant in this area. Dr. Torres has given presentations on these topics at state, national, and international conferences and has published numerous articles in the area of family violence, culture, and Hispanic women.

Linda M. Dominguez, PhD, RN, received her doctorate in nursing from the University of Arizona in Tucson in 1996. Dr. Dominguez obtained both her master of science in adult health in 1987 and her bachelor of science in 1972 from Arizona State University in Tempe. During her doctoral studies, the university presented her with the Centennial Achievement Doctoral Student Award for outstanding personal growth, integrity, and contributions to community. Dr. Dominguez has presented her qualitative research on women with the human immunodeficiency virus / acquired immunodeficiency syndrome (HIV / AIDS) and women of Mexican heritage with HIV / AIDS at state and national conferences. Currently, Dr. Dominguez works in quality management in managed care.

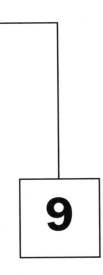

9

CHAPTER OUTLINE

WHERE WE HAVE BEEN AND WHERE WE
WANT TO ADVANCE

COLLABORATIVE PRACTICE: WHERE WE
CAN BE

Definition of collaborative practice

*Characteristics of collaborative relation-
ships*

Benefits of collaborative practice

Collaborative models

Intradisciplinary models

Interdisciplinary models

COLLABORATIVE PRACTICE: WHAT IT
SHOULD BE

*Crucial components of collaborative prac-
tice*

*Considerations involving gender and eth-
nic groups*

*Social forces mandating collaboration in
the health-care arena*

REMOVING THE BARRIERS: HOW WE GET
THERE

Education

Intradisciplinary support

*Support from the administrative environ-
ment*

Enhancement of political savvy

SUGGESTED EXERCISES

CHAPTER OBJECTIVES

After completing this chapter, the reader will be able to:

1. Explain the rationale and benefits of collaborative practice.
2. Compare and contrast the different models of collaborative practice.
3. Analyze the essential components of collaboration as used by individuals of different gender and ethnic groups.
4. Analyze barriers to collaborative practice.
5. Formulate strategies for the removal of barriers to collaborative practice.
6. Analyze interdisciplinary and social factors that support collaborative practice.

Where We Have Been and Where We Want to Advance

I f Santayana was correct that "those who cannot remember the past are condemned to repeat it,"[1] then a brief sketch of the stereotypical mid-twentieth-century nurse is a fitting introduction to this chapter on collaborative practice. Nursing was a "women's career," with all suggestions of subservience and sexism that the phrase implies.[2] Most nurses were "trained" in hospitals to be task oriented. They were discouraged from questioning and were expected to submit to hospital routines. Nurses were taught to show deference to physicians and were not free to think or act in the best interests of the patient. Consequently, patient advocacy became a subordinate function of the nurse, who had assumed a subordinate position within the hospital hierarchy.[3,4] Hospital privileges of patient care and decision-making functions were domains reserved exclusively to the physician. Collaboration between nurses and physicians was not considered.

Cultural, social, and economic forces, too numerous to recite, have transformed the nursing archetype. Nowhere is this change more striking and more exciting than in the role of the advanced practice nurse (APN) in collaborative practice. This chapter presents various definitions and models of collaborative practice among APNs and other health-care professionals. In our examining these models, crucial elements of collaborative practice and related operational dimensions that may either enhance or impair collaboration are elucidated. Elements of collaborative practice are further analyzed as to their applicability to male and female health-care providers belonging to different ethnic groups. In addition, recent developments, such as the Pew Commission's recommendations concerning nursing's autonomy, are addressed.[5–7] Finally, strategies directed toward minimizing or eliminating barriers to collaborative practice are proposed.

Collaborative Practice: Where We Can Be

Notwithstanding the advances in medicine, nursing, and related fields, it is becoming increasingly difficult for a single health-care provider to meet the complex needs of patients. The delivery of health care requires the expertise and combined abilities of individuals with diverse skills and knowledge who collaborate to deliver high-quality care.

DEFINITION OF COLLABORATIVE PRACTICE

Various perspectives and definitions found in the literature depict collaboration as a joint and cooperative enterprise undertaken by health-care providers to integrate team members' perspectives and expertise. Examples of definitions of collaborative practice are presented in Table 9–1. On analysis of these definitions, general characteristics of collaborative practice begin to emerge. Examples of these include collaboration as a complex evolutionary process, as the sharing and integration of team members' skills and expertise, as a collegial relationship of equal authority, as a willingness to work as a team member, and as a process within a horizontal structure.[8–12]

TABLE 9–1
Definitions of Collaborative Practice

Arcangelo,[8] 1994
Collaborative practice is one that "allows all members of the healthcare team to share their expertise in the provision of primary care" (p. 3).

Arslanian-Engoren,[9] 1995
Collaboration is "a complex evolutionary process of establishing oneself, at the advanced practice level, in a collegial relationship" (p. 73).

Evans and Carlson,[10] 1992
"Collaborative practice is therefore a joint effort that involves team-oriented persons who work as colleagues within a horizontal rather than a vertical hierarchy" (p. 1671).

Lamb and Napodano, [11] 1984
Collaboration is "the integration of the perspectives and skills of each team member, and a process of complex problem solving. Collaboration implies the generation and evaluation of new problems and plans which result directly from the integration of individual contributions rather than simply the coordination of individual ideas" (p. 26).

Norsen, Opladen, and Quinn,[12] 1995
Collaborative practice means "working together in a joint effort toward a mission of excellent patient care" (p. 44).

Horizontal frameworks differ from vertical or hierarchical structures in that participants have equal authority and share decision-making responsibilities equally.[12] Communication within horizontal structures is generally characterized as open and free flowing. In contrast, vertical structures usually have chains of authority that are hierarchical. The leader of this hierarchy generally has more privileges or decision-making authority than other members of the chain. An example of a vertical structure is the traditional physician and nurse hierarchy characteristic of many hospital settings. In this traditional structure, the physician is regarded as the leader, and the nurse is consequently relegated to a lesser position. In contrast, the aim of collaborative practice is to equalize the power and authority among all members of the group regardless of any members' backgound. However, although equality is promoted in collaboration, the person with the most expertise in a particular area is recognized as having the most influence.[13] Influence is dynamic and is reconfigured as needs dictate.

CHARACTERISTICS OF COLLABORATIVE RELATIONSHIPS

The structure of collaborative relationships and multidisciplinary relationships may have many configurations (Table 9–2). In **intradisciplinary** collaborative practice, the members belong to the same discipline, although their backgrounds may be different. Intradisciplinary collaborative practice also denotes the relationship between the APN and the client.

An **interdisciplinary** collaborative relationship is one in which individuals of different disciplines explicitly form a collaborative team. Just as in intradisciplinary collaborative practice, collaborative practice between the APN and physician or of an APN within an interdisciplinary team is two or more professionals working in proximity to each other. Genuine collaborative practice demands that an APN and physician or other health-care team members work together as colleagues, demonstrating high levels of interpersonal skills.[12,14,15]

TABLE 9–2
**Examples of Intradisciplinary, Interdisciplinary, and
Multidisciplinary Relationships**

Intradisciplinary collaboration	APN and head nurse
	APN and RN
	APN and APN
	APN and patient and/or family
Interdisciplinary collaboration	APN and physician
	APN and social worker
	APN and pharmacist
	APN and dietitian
	APN and physician, social worker, pharmacist, and dietitian
Multidisciplinary team (no collaboration)	APN, physician, social worker, pharmacist, and dietitian

For the purpose of this chapter, a **multidisciplinary** team is one in which individuals of different disciplines come together within a vertical structure to coordinate patient care. For instance, the APN may consult a social worker and a dietitian for the purpose of developing a plan of care, or a physician may consult an APN for information on preventive interventions. However, in these examples, there is a hierarchical or vertical structure in which only one health-care provider (the physician or APN) has sole responsibility for seeking others' advice, making decisions, coordinating care, or developing patient interventions.

In collaborative practice, both the APN and physician or other members of an interdisciplinary team may provide primary health care to patients, share joint responsibility for patient interventions, have equal decision-making authority, and integrate their skills and knowledge for the provision of care within the scopes of their respective practices.[10,11,16] The ability to provide care within one's scope of practice exemplifies autonomy in collaborative practice.

The scope of each practitioner's responsibility can be defined by the relevant discipline's standards of practice, state practice acts, and institutional standards. In collaborative practice, a team member's area of expertise defines which member is authorized to carry out the integrated plan of care.[8] Therefore, potential autonomy exists within each practitioner's boundaries of skill, competence, and scope of practice. The collaborative team bestows trust on and empowers its members to act on the plan of care.[11,17]

Historically, collaborative relationships between the nurse and physician have been difficult to establish, in part because of the oppressive relationship that nursing has endured with physicians.[9,18] Collaboration requires personal and professional maturity and security, because APN and physician interdisciplinary team members will have to learn new attitudes and behaviors.[18] The desire to work together as colleagues stems from the recognition that each member in the collaborative enterprise has unique yet complementary skills that will lead to quality of care in practice.

BENEFITS OF COLLABORATIVE PRACTICE

Quality of care, increased access to care, decrease in time to obtain care, and decrease in costs are major benefits of collaborative practice.[8,12,19] A synergistic effect is expected to emerge from collaborative practice. The combined and maximized efforts of an interdisciplinary group of health-care providers who work together and share their expertise result in a more beneficial patient outcome than that achieved by an individual or independent health-care practitioner.[8,18] APNs and other health-care providers who collaborate to provide appropriate patient-centered interventions can readily consult with each other to develop a plan of care. Time is saved for both health-care providers and patients. For example, time and resources are spared when patients are assessed by a team at a single facility. By not having to send the patient to another facility to consult with another health-care provider, the practitioner spares the patient from having to navigate to another facility to obtain another health consultation. Further, health-care costs are decreased when the patient's care is well coordinated and is based on recommendations from those who have collaborated and integrated each other's expert advice.

Increase in personal satisfaction is another benefit of collaborative practice. APNs and health-care providers who engage in collaborative practice find it rewarding to work in a horizontal structure in which egalitarian relationships prevail. The environment in collaborative practice is a positive one in which collegial relationships exist, complementary expertise is acknowledged, autonomous practice is the rule, and communication is open. Mutual confidence, trust, and respect further enhance the collaborative enterprise. Practitioners experience the excitement of being creative, productive, and effective in practice.[20] A sense of professionalism, achievement, and work satisfaction arises from professional growth gained by working with other colleagues and sharing knowledge.[14,21] APNs and health-care providers in collaborative practices take pride in their work and strive to maintain their group's high standards of care, outcomes which in turn lead to a sense of achievement that may contribute positively to patient care and to the development of patient interventions.[9,19]

Finally, because collaborative practice is patient centered, it can, or should, be a flexible and dynamic enterprise.[12] Because the needs of the patient determine the goals of care and the nature of the interventions to be provided, the responses from patients who have received such care have been enthusiastic.[20]

COLLABORATIVE MODELS

Various types of intradisciplinary and interdisciplinary collaborative models have been described in the literature and are presented in Table 9–3. The arrangements of the models differ in interesting ways, but the common purpose of these models is the provision of high-quality patient care.

INTRADISCIPLINARY MODELS

The **integrative practice model** described by Kopser, Horn, and Carpenter[22] required the clinical nurse specialist (CNS), the clinical nurse manager, and staff development specialist to work in a collaborative enterprise within a major university hospital. This model is a patient-centered model that integrated patient goals with the nurses' mission to provide high-quality interventions. In this model, the primary roles of these three practitioners differed, but their secondary role responsibilities overlapped. For instance, the primary role functions of the CNS, clinical nurse manager, and staff development specialist were clini-

TABLE 9–3

Examples of Collaborative Practice Models

Type of Model/ Practitioners Involved	Author(s)/Year	Purpose	Characteristics of Model	Results of Testing Outcomes
Intradisciplinary (integrative practice model): CNS, clinical nurse manager, staff development specialist	Kopser, Horn, and Carpenter,[22] 1994	Provide quality interventions	Patient-centered ■ Practitioner's primary roles differ; however, secondary role responsibilities overlapped. ■ Collaborative components included trust and respect, shared goals, open communication, knowledge of roles, leadership qualities, and maturity.	Increase in scores related to quality of care, professional growth, and number of primary nurses
Intradisciplinary (collaborative management nursing practice model): CNS, nurse manager	Caruso and Payne,[23] 1990	Provide optimal patient care, personal/professional satisfaction, and lower cost of care	■ Patient and institutional staff-centered ■ Horizontal structure ■ Egalitarian ■ Integration of role responsibilities	No outcomes measured
Intradisciplinary: CNSs, head nurses	Clang and Gagen,[24] 1992		■ Acute-care setting ■ Collaborative components: comparable education, horizontal structure, similar philosophy related to nursing and patients, roles and functions clearly delineated, active collaboration, mutual respect	No outcomes measured
Intradisciplinary: CRNA, occupational health nurse	Huffman,[25] 1983	Share patient's medical history with CRNA in hospital emergencies. CRNAs provide in-services	■ Collaboration for the provision of information for anesthesia management	No outcomes measured

Table continued on following page

TABLE 9–3

Examples of Collaborative Practice Models (Continued)

Type of Model/ Practitioners Involved	Author(s)/Year	Purpose	Characteristics of Model	Results of Testing Outcomes
Interdisciplinary (joint accountability model): CNS, physician, head nurse	Walton, Jakobowski, and Barnsteiner,[26] 1993	Is based on patient and institutional needs	<ul><li>Hierarchical model</li><li>Role and function determined by head nurse and physician</li><li>CNS's position jointly funded by nursing and medicine</li></ul>	No outcomes measured
Interdisciplinary: CNS, physician	Arslanian-Engoren,[9] 1995	Provide a phenomenologic study to describe the lived experience of collaboration	<ul><li>Mutual trust and respect</li><li>Collegial relationships</li><li>Defined roles</li><li>Lead to a positive experience</li></ul>	No outcomes measured
Interdisciplinary (collaborative management): CNM, physicians	Avery and Del Guidice,[27] 1993	Provide best possible care for all mothers and babies	<ul><li>Supportive environment</li><li>Agreement to collaborate</li><li>Competency</li><li>Communication</li><li>Practice within scope of practice</li></ul>	No outcomes measured
Interdisciplinary: Nurse, physicians, nursing staff	Gleeson, et al,[21] 1990	Meet the needs of patients and maintain continuity and quality of care	<ul><li>APN collaborates to manage more acute and/or more serious health problems than those treated on an outpatient basis.</li><li>APN works with new technology used in acute-care settings.</li><li>APN provides comprehensive day-to-day care simultaneously for many patients.</li></ul>	No outcomes measured

Table continued on following page

TABLE 9–3

Examples of Collaborative Practice Models (Continued)

Type of Model/ Practitioners Involved	Author(s)/Year	Purpose	Characteristics of Model	Results of Testing Outcomes
			▪ APN has daily interaction with unit staff members.	
			▪ APN assumes the role of hospital staff educator and nursing consultant.	
			▪ Model is patient-population centered as well as staff nurse centered.	
			▪ APN reports to director of nursing and informally responsible to medical staff.	
			▪ APN acts as a liaison between patients and their families, physicians, and allied health services.	
Interdisciplinary: APN, physician, team members	Norsen, Opladen, and Quinn,[12] 1995	Provide excellent patient care	▪ A joint endeavor	No outcomes measured
			▪ Patient-centered goals	
			▪ Cooperation, assertiveness, responsibility, communication, autonomy, coordination	
			▪ Articulation of scope of practice, roles, and responsibilities	

cal practice, clinical management, and education. Their secondary responsibilities, such as clinical leadership, nursing research, and education responsibilities, were interrelated. Primary role responsibilities determined the manner in which secondary functions were assigned. Significant in the implementation of the integrative practice model was that outcomes were measured using a computer-based system to monitor quality. Increased scores were obtained in the areas of nurses' professional growth, number of primary nurses, and quality of care delivered, which indicated the advantages of the integrative practice model.[22]

The aims in the intradisciplinary **collaborative management nursing practice model** described by Caruso and Payne[23] were to achieve optimal patient care, personal and professional satisfaction, and lowered health-care costs. This model, which used adaptation and crisis theory as its framework, was used on a high-risk antenatal unit. A salient characteristic of this model was the equitable and horizontal authority structure between the CNS and nurse manager. Role responsibilities were integrated to obtain the shared goals of comprehensive high-quality patient care and of the advancement and promotion of professional nursing practice. Standards of care were mutually agreed on, as were unit-based goals, policies, and procedures. Strategies to retain staff and develop a satisfying work environment were jointly developed. Although this model demonstrated that collaborative management, the strategies instituted to promote a satisfying work environment, and autonomy had resulted in the institution's financial soundness by decreasing nursing staff turnover rate and increasing efficiency of nurses, empirical measurements used to support such findings were not described.

Clang and Gagen[24] described collaborative practice between a diabetes CNS and a head nurse on a 21-bed unit. After working together for 3 years, the CNS and head nurse analyzed the elements of their joint efforts that created a positive relationship and improved quality of care in their unit. These included having comparable education; working within a horizontal structure; having a similar philosophy related to nursing and patients; having roles and functions clearly delineated; engaging in collaborative activities; and visibly demonstrating mutual respect to staff, patients and their families, and physicians. There were no qualitative nor objective measurements, however, to support these authors' claims of improved relationships and increased quality of care from collaborative practice.

Huffman's[25] intradisciplinary model of collaboration was an older one that described the relevance of certified registered nurse anesthetists (CRNAs) working together with occupational health nurses for the purpose of sharing information. Inquiry into the elements of collaboration were not the focus of this model. However, collaborative components such as cooperation and sharing information were identified as important components of this intradisciplinary model.

INTERDISCIPLINARY MODELS

In Walton, Jakobowski, and Barnsteiner's collaborative practice model,[26] an example of a joint appointment versus a collaborative practice arrangement was presented. In this model, implemented in a pediatric teaching hospital, the CNS was jointly accountable to two supervisors, a chief physician, and a director of nursing practice and research. The CNS's responsibilities were agreed on by each supervisor, and the CNS's position was jointly funded by both nursing and medicine. Responsibility for the evaluation of the CNS was shared by medicine and nursing. The CNS functioned within the traditional domains of practice, education, consultation, and research and had formal authority in both the medical and nursing departments. For example, the CNS's input was used by physicians to develop an appropriate plan of care for patients. Further, the CNS had the influence to affect nursing practice so that the plans of care could be implemented. The formal structure of this collaborative practice model was hierarchical. Although the authors enumerated various family, professional, and institutional benefits of this model, specific outcome measurements were not described.

Arslanian-Engoren's phenomenologic study[9] examined the lived experience of four CNSs who collaborated with physicians in practice. The following recurrent themes were identified by the author as essential for successful collaboration:

- Experience of mutual trust and respect
- Establishment of collegial relationships
- Need to define one's practice role
- Maintenance of a nursing perspective
- A positive experience
- An advanced education
- Clinical preparation
- Professional maturity

Avery and Del Guidice[27] described collaborative management as an integral part of nurse midwifery patient management. Although these authors' article recognized that certified nurse midwives (CNMs) collaborated with various health-care providers, the focus was on the relationship between CNMs and physicians. The intent of the article was to provide guidelines for the establishment and optimal maintenance of such an enterprise. The guidelines presumably promoted a collaborative climate that included such elements as:

- An environment supportive of collaborative practice
- The patient choosing collaborative management over exclusive medical management when both are appropriate options
- The CNM and physician agreeing to comanage patients
- Explicit and clearly written criteria and guidelines for defining high-risk patients and situations
- The CNM and physician sharing of an accurate and clearly articulated patient database
- A clearly outlined plan of care that is mutually agreed on and documented on the medical record
- Competence in practice
- Agreement that the CNM must function within the safe boundaries of practice and make referrals if a patient is beyond this practitioner's level of competence

This model recognized the frequent conflict between the CNM and physician when attempting to engage in collaborative management. The guidelines offered are an attempt to decrease discord and to stimulate positive interactions within a collaborative enterprise.

The model of collaborative care described by Gleeson et al.[21] was implemented in a multispecialty children's hospital. In this model, the pediatric nurse practitioner had multiple responsibilities and was accountable to patients, their families, hospital staff, and community. Aside from doing physical assessments and having history-taking responsibilities, the APN functioned as a liaison between the patient and the family as well as the patient and various health services both in the hospital and/or clinic and in the community. Other professional responsibilities included being a role model and serving as a resource for other nurses, publishing articles, organizing community self-help groups, and participating in speaking engagements in the community. Although various benefits were generally identified as a result of utilization of this model, empirical outcome measurements were not presented.

Norsen, Opladen, and Quinn[12] described collaborative practice components between APN and physician dyads at the University of Rochester Strong Memorial Hospital. Collaborative practice at this institution was implemented in 1979. At that time, the goal of collaborative practice was to provide direct-care services to a growing population of patients who had undergone cardiac surgery. With time, the basis for establishing collaborative practice was broadened to meet the increasingly complex needs of patients, hospital, insurers, and government regulators. The overall aim of nurses and physicians engaged in collaborative practice was to work jointly toward the provision of high-quality care. Key attributes of collaborative practice identified by these authors included:

- Cooperativeness
- Assertiveness
- Responsibility
- Communication
- Autonomy
- Coordination

Operationalizing this model required the establishment of an interdisciplinary team whose composition was based on the mission and goals of the team, a system that promoted and maintained the collaborative undertaking, and collaborators' knowledge of the factors that contribute to successful collaboration. This model further recognized that the APN must undertake direct and indirect care activities, have a tolerance for role flexibility, be able to work under ambiguous situations, and embrace change in a dynamic environment.

It is significant to note that with the exception of the research by Arslanian-Engoren,[9] the descriptions of these models were anecdotal. Further, as indicated in Table 9–3, only limited empirical outcome measurements to verify actual benefits of these models were noted. It is obvious that additional research on collaborative practice is warranted.

Collaborative Practice: What It Should Be

Literature that deals with collaborative practice generally identifies autonomy, competence, collegiality, interaction and communication skills, and trust as crucial ingredients for successful collaboration.[9,10,12,18,28] Because of the importance of these elements, they are further described in this section in relation to individuals of different gender and ethnic groups. For instance, it is important to consider whether these components of collaborative practice are valued, appreciated, and accepted by specific gender and ethnic groups. This section presents a brief description of salient differences among major gender and ethnic groups to illustrate that what is valued by some, or even most people, may not be equally valued by others. Finally, other prevalent social forces mandating collaboration in the health-care arena are considered.

CRUCIAL COMPONENTS OF COLLABORATIVE PRACTICE

Successful collaborative practice is more than working in physical proximity to others. It requires the willingness of collaborators to work together with attitudes that facilitate and express a value for autonomy, competence, collegiality, interaction and communication skills, and trust in the collaborative enterprise.[18,28] If individual partners embrace such attitudes, ongoing success will be facilitated in those behavioral and/or institutional changes needed to foster a collaborative climate. Further, favorable attitudes need to be actively and consistently promoted by and among the collaborators to maintain continued success.

Autonomy

In any collaborative practice, it is important that APNs, physicians, and other team members have the autonomy to practice within their scopes of practice. In part, autonomy is obtained and articulated through certification within one's scope of practice, state practice acts, and institutional standards. It is imperative that hospital structures be examined in relation to providing a supportive climate where collaborators have control over their professional activities and quality of the environment.[10] In practice, it is equally important that autonomy be imparted or legitimized by members in the intradisciplinary and interdisciplinary collaborative teams. Members of a collaborative enterprise foster each other's autonomy by demonstrating confidence, respect, and trust, which enables the team members to function independently within their scopes of practice.[9,12,18] Moreover, an egalitarian climate is essential for autonomy. Sherman[17] described a strategy implemented in a prosperous large corporation that empowered its employees to create a new process. In this strategy, there were no supervisors, there were no plans on how to begin the process, and there also were no hierarchy, titles, and job descriptions. The employees were left to integrate each other's input to complete their mission. Initially, the team was thrown into chaos because they were functioning with limited guidance. However, by tackling small tasks one at a time, this team succeeded in building their skills and, ultimately, in accomplishing their assignment.

Competence

Competence in practice is fundamental to the establishment of trust and respect among collaborating practitioners.[13] Further, competence is more than a demonstration of adequate clinical skills. In general, to be competent in an advanced clinical role, one must have acquired an education that facilitates the development of the professional maturity, self-confidence, and motivation necessary to effectively combine direct- and indirect-care responsibilities in a dynamic health-care environment.[12] For example, APNs need to be flexible in roles that require them to provide care, educate patients and staff, conduct research, and be a consultant for others. Advanced graduate education enables APNs to view situations from many perspectives, analyze situations, and engage in critical thinking. One of the challenges being faced by APNs is criticism from physicians, federal and state regulatory agencies, and the public related to the nature and amount of education APNs receive. Large discrepancies exist between APNs and physicians regarding training and educational requirements. To be considered equal in the collaborative process, APNs may need to standardize educational requirements. In November 1994, the American Association of Colleges of Nursing advocated that all advanced practice nursing certification must meet recognized national standards, a graduate degree in nursing and uniform standards to certify nurses in advanced practice.[29]

When forming a new collaborative practice, individuals are often unaware of the competence and expertise of the other potential partners. Strategies need to be developed so that collaborators may come to know and, it is hoped, appreciate the skills and talents of others. Alpert et al.[18] described strategies that were purposefully implemented to increase group cohesiveness and knowledge about each other's responsibilities. Nurses and physicians spent a day together to become familiar with each other as individuals and practitioners and to learn more about each other's responsibilities and decision-making abilities. Turns were taken in reporting on patients during rounds. Strategies to enhance socialization were also implemented. These activities further assisted in learning more about an individual's integrity and credibility.

Collegiality

Collegiality in collaborative practice pertains to the cooperation, equality, and sharing of responsibilities by all involved. Collaborators must be willing to cooperate and jointly participate in collaborative relations.[10] In the collaborative process, it takes a mature and secure individual to acknowledge and respect another team member's opinions. In addition, each collaborator must be willing to analyze and sometimes acknowledge a better, albeit different, way of doing things and to be flexible enough to adapt and accept change.[12,22]

Intertwined in the notion of shared responsibilities is the element of equality. Team members in successful partnerships generally work within a horizontal structure. For example, in collaborative practice, an APN and physician have joint responsibility for the provision of high-quality care as well as for decision making. However, the ultimate decision may rest with the team member who has the most expertise in the area of concern.[9,10] The responsibility for coordinating interventions to promote efficient provision of patient care can also be shared. Sharing this responsibility reduces duplication of effort and ensures that the most qualified person completes the task at hand. Because responsibility of organizing components of the plan of care usually falls to one individual, the job of coordinating plans of care may be rotated among the different members.

Strategies for team building must be incorporated within ongoing practices. This is necessary especially when certain individuals entering collaborative practice have not been trained to function as part of a team. Burchell, Thomas, and Smith[28] identified several strategies for team building:

- Joint examination of the practice infrastructure
- Purpose
- Physical setting
- Interpersonal dynamics
- Exercises to examine dominant group behaviors

Interaction and Communication Skills

The demonstration of effective communication skills is crucial to the success of any collaborative endeavor. All members need to exchange information and ideas directly and share in discussion to integrate information and make decisions.[12] Assertive behavior is a desirable attribute for practitioners; by being assertive, practitioners ensure that their differing viewpoints are discussed before a consensus is obtained on the best possible intervention for a patient.[12,22] Advocacy for a patient or issue should be focused, rational, and factually accurate. The practitioner must be sufficiently assertive to be able to speak up, ask questions, or go out on a limb to negotiate a plan of care that will benefit the patient.

From the foregoing, it is clear that collaboration is an interactive process. Mere technical competence and/or a sufficient knowledge base is insufficient for successful collaborative practice. The collaborative climate is improved when practitioners demonstrate psychological intelligence, or what Daniel Goleman called "emotional intelligence (EQ)."[30] EQ consists of emotional skills useful for effective communication and interaction with others. Having emotional intelligence enables collaborators to know when to laugh at another's jokes, when to have confidence or trust in another's abilities, and when to know another is emotionally overloaded—skills necessary for successful collaboration. Goleman[30] described five domains of emotional intelligence:

1. Knowing one's emotions
2. Managing emotions
3. Recognizing emotions in others
4. Handling relationships
5. Motivating oneself

Self-awareness is fundamental to EQ and allows practitioners to know their emotions as well as providing ongoing insight into their inner states. Both strong feelings and a lack of such feelings can impede their reasoning and decision-making abilities. Collaborators who have the ability to monitor and understand their own emotions are better able to analyze situations, including their own emotional reactions, and to use intuitive abilities to read and grasp the meaning of others' behavior patterns. Such self-awareness enables them to keep emotions in balance and allows for responses to be gauged appropriately to the circumstance. The ability to gain control over one's emotions or the art of soothing oneself in the wake of emotional upheaval is an essential life skill.[30] Team members who are able to manage their emotions are better able to get on with the work at hand without being deterred by personal emotional upheaval.

The ability to recognize others' emotions and to have empathy is a basic component of EQ and a useful skill in collaborating with others. Having empathy assists one to recognize social signals, such as another's tone of voice, gestures, and facial expressions, all of which provide valuable information about another person's feelings or wants. Because collaboration is an interactive process, practitioners who can recognize others' emotions have an edge in shaping encounters, in influencing others, in prospering in relationships, and in making others feel comfortable.[30]

Lastly, individuals who have a high degree of EQ are identified as being self-motivators. Those who are self-motivators possess such characteristics as high levels of hope, resourcefulness, self-assurance, flexibility, and the good sense to break down large tasks into smaller, more manageable ones. The ability to motivate oneself is a beneficial characteristic for practitioners engaged in collaborative practice and can be especially useful in jointly addressing conflicts.

Trust

Trust is viewed as a building block and as a common element in the collaborative enterprise.[9,12] Mutual trust and respect for each other as human beings and for each other's clinical competence and decision-making abilities evolve over time. Trust and respect develop as individuals work in collaboration and come to know and appreciate each other's skills.[9] Working in a climate of trust and respect fosters feelings of satisfaction and serves as a unifying force in the collaborative endeavor.[12,27] As indicated by Norsen, Opladen, and Quinn[12]:

> Without the element of trust, cooperation cannot exist, assertiveness becomes threatening, responsibility is avoided, communication is hampered, autonomy is suppressed, and coordination is haphazard. (p. 45)

CONSIDERATIONS INVOLVING GENDER AND ETHNIC GROUPS

Do not assume that what is right for one group of individuals is also right for another. This caveat is appropriate to situations involving gender and ethnic differences. The preceding sections presented many of the components of collaborative practice that were identified as fostering and as crucial to collaboration. We now examine this information in the context of collaborators who belong to different gender and ethnic groups. Such a perspective reveals the applicability of these collaborative components to different gender and ethnic groups, as well as difficulties in different clinical settings. To avoid stereotyping individuals, it is important to remember that gender and ethnic group generalizations do not hold for everyone of the particular gender or ethnic group. Although there are many common values and experiences, just as many variations exist among individuals of a particular group.[31]

Differences in developmental experiences and socialization have led to consequent differences in the way men and women view their world. An example of this is supported in the research on moral development by Gilligan.[32] In this study, women more so than men made moral decisions based on the context of the situation, relationships, and connectedness and within the context of care, that is, of doing no harm. Gilligan's ethic of care differed from Kohlberg's ethic of justice,[33] which had generally been perceived as typical moral decision making. According to Kohlberg, moral decision making is rigidly guided by rules and the principle of universality; that is, moral judgments made in one scenario will be made the same way in similar scenarios regardless of time, place, or persons involved.

Similar to gender considerations, one needs to examine how the components of collaborative practice would pair with values of other ethnic groups. For example, white middle-class Americans want to master their environment. In contrast, Asian Americans, Native Americans, African Americans, and Hispanic Americans prefer to live in harmony with their environment.[31] Another example pertains to "people relations." White middle-class Americans strive for independence, whereas Asian Americans, Native Americans, African Americans, and Hispanic Americans prefer collateral relationships.[31] It is important not only to inquire into the value dimensions of different ethnic groups but also to analyze how collaborative components would match with a particular ethnic group's values. For example, assertiveness in communication is generally valued in collaborative practice. However, the appropriateness and ease of communicating assertively may be different for men and women of different ethnic orientations. How easy would it be for an Asian, a Hispanic, or a woman to engage in assertiveness? Is assertiveness an attribute of all ethnic groups?

More research is needed that examines the extent of appropriateness and applicability of the components of collaborative practice to individuals of different gender and cultural groups. Research and theory development are crucial pathways to expanding the knowledge base of nursing.[34] Collaborative practice theories also need to be examined for their utility and appropriateness with individuals of different gender and ethnic groups. Acknowledging and studying gender and ethnic group differences can only advance knowledge. As Spradley[35] so eloquently indicated, "Cultural diversity is one of the great gifts bestowed on the human species" (p. viii).

SOCIAL FORCES MANDATING COLLABORATION IN THE HEALTH-CARE ARENA

Social forces are influencing the transformation of our health-care system by specifying collaborative endeavors that should be undertaken to upgrade the system and to make it operate more in synchrony with the public's health-care needs. Consumers, insurers, lawmakers, and policy analysts have come together in recent years to criticize the inefficiencies and inconsistencies of the current health-care system, from the education of health-care professionals to the delivery of costly and discriminating care.[6,36,37] The Pew Health Professions Commission, an influential public-policy analysis group, has recently described its vision for the future US health-care system. The Pew Commission envisions health care as moving more toward primary care, with an emphasis on prevention and population-based practice. The commission strongly urges the effective use of available resources and affirmation of the rights of health-care consumers by decreasing costs while improving access and quality.

While some of the Pew Commission's recommendations, such as standardizing entry-to-practice requirements and removing practice barriers, have been welcomed by the nursing profession, other suggested strategies have created much concern. Certain collaborative mandates of the commission are viewed as an impingement on the autonomy nursing has long fought to achieve. Specific recommendations that threaten nursing's autonomy include:

- Establishment of multiple levels of nursing education programs reflective of needed contributions to the dynamic patient-care system
- Development of interdisciplinary collaboration in teaching, practice, and research for continued care of chronic patients
- Continuation of nursing graduate-level clinical training programs for nurses in areas where health-care services can reduce cost and improve access and quality
- Establishment of interdisciplinary state boards for each discipline

To date, the ANA has expressed both interest in and concern over the foregoing health workforce regulation mandates. The ANA realizes possible infringements that the Pew Commission's recommendations may have on the practice of nursing and its autonomy and on the quality and safety of patient care.[5] Specific areas of concern include:

- Removal of unnecessary restriction on the scope of practice without the abolishment of all distinctions between health-care professions, including their occupations, skills, knowledge, and abilities
- Assessment of intraprofessional competencies in disciplines that contain different specialty areas of practice
- Establishment of interdisciplinary oversight boards to regulate, approve, amend, or reject board decisions
- Consolidation of the structure and function of interdisciplinary health professions boards, such as the consolidation of medicine and nursing care boards

The ANA continues to analyze the possible impact of the commission's strategies and maintains an active dialogue with the commission on these issues.

Removing the Barriers: How We Get There

Advanced practice nurses know where they want to be relative to collaborative practice. Some of the roadblocks that they must overcome include limited recognition of their skills and competencies, impediments to autonomy in practice, struggles gaining authority to prescribe medication, and issues of irregular reimbursement. This section addresses these roadblocks and encourages particular psychosocial-political strategies to assist APNs to attain their goals.

EDUCATION

Knowledge is power, both for attaining and maintaining autonomy and for providing a basis for clinical competence. To date, no minimum entry-level educational standard for advanced practice nursing exists, and the education of APNs varies greatly.[27] At this time, only the CNS and NP groups require graduate (master's or doctorate) degrees for advanced practice. Despite much debate, graduate education is not a mandate. Although it is anticipated that CRNAs will be required to have a master's degree for certification by 1998, the degree will not necessarily have to be in nursing.[38] Furthermore, continuing education requirements for APNs are generally well below those of physicians.[38] The inconsistencies in entry-level education, types of education, and limited continuing education requirements may be detrimental to the acceptance and advancement of the expanded practice role in nursing.

As a group, APNs claim to be knowledgeable and competent practitioners who are worthy of legal autonomy, authority, and egalitarian relationships in collaborative practice.[27,39] These claims must be supported by providing consumers of health care, insurers, lawmakers, and physicians with necessary and reliable evidence. In addition, historical knowledge related to nursing's development needs to be retained and periodically examined. Nursing must not forget its past to keep from losing its autonomy.

INTRADISCIPLINARY SUPPORT

Support for the widespread acceptance of advanced practice in nursing must be generated from within the ranks of the nursing profession. Faculty and professional organizations in nursing have much work to do to support advance practice nursing.[29] APN faculty has a general responsibility to educate health-care consumers and community groups to expound on the value and competencies of advance practice in nursing. Moreover, nursing curricula need to be continuously examined for their appropriateness in meeting the needs of patients in an evolving health-care system. Entry and certification standards for APNs, as well as the content and amount of continuing education requirements, must be monitored to promote the ongoing acceptance of advanced practice nursing.[39] Finally, research in nursing needs to be maintained and promoted in nursing curricula.

Nursing must be cognizant of the strides made in gaining its autonomy to guard against losing independence in the future. Nursing's history should be presented in academic settings and include discussions of feminist perspectives that illuminate the social woes that continue to intrude into the practice of nursing. Traditional socialization of nursing influenced by immutable, suppressive social perspectives generally and specifically affects the advanced practice of the profession. Only when the general nursing population learns of its oppression can nurses begin to recognize and acknowledge their own worth, abilities, and accomplishments.

Support for advanced practice nursing has to continue to be provided by APNs' specific professional organizations. For example, the International Confederation of Midwives (ICBM) assists in the development of the National Midwifery Association by providing information and equipment.[40] The public advancement of CNMs is further promoted by ICBM's collaborative efforts with international organizations such as the United Nations, World Health Organization, and United Nations International Children's Emergency Fund (commonly known as UNICEF).

The ANA continues to support various advanced practice organizations. Approximately one-quarter of the budget and staff of the Department of Practice in the ANA are assigned to deal with the major issues of concern pertinent to advance practice organizations.[38] The bulk of ANA issues and ANA activities related to supporting APNs center on:

- Reimbursement
- Prescriptive authority
- Legal recognition
- Monitoring of federal use of definitions related to collaboration that really mean supervision
- Assistance in developing a core definition of advanced practice nursing and standards

Reimbursement and prescriptive authority of APNs continue to be indiscriminately constrained nationwide. In response, the ANA provides legal recognition, legislation, and lobbying and works with regulatory agencies to address APNs' concerns. The ANA employs eight lobbyists in Washington. Moreover, the ANA keeps the various APN organizations informed of legislation pertinent to them and provides consultation regarding appropriate responses to various legislation. The ANA also works with APN organizations in their efforts to develop core definitions of advanced practice, articulate advance practice nursing's scope of practice, and standardize statements for advanced practice. These core definitions and standards are being developed with the understanding that individual specialty areas may use or tailor them to their particular needs.

SUPPORT FROM THE ADMINISTRATIVE ENVIRONMENT

Advanced practice nurses have the knowledge and skills to diagnose and treat uncomplicated illness, provide health education, link patients with community resources, counsel, and provide health promotion and disease prevention strategies.[8,16] Yet barriers to practice, such as limited prescriptive authority, restricted reimbursement, and regulation of practice continue to be found in certain states, prompting APNs to continuously justify themselves and their actions.[39,41] Much of the reluctance in the acceptance of APNs stems from the lack of public awareness regarding the abilities and competencies of APNs[42] and from certain medical professionals who have limited regard for any group of professionals who may be perceived as encroaching upon their territory.[39]

Administrative support may be gained by more clearly articulating the scope of practice and by demonstrating the cost-effective benefits of collaborative practice involving APNs.[12,19] Analysis of hospital structures may be necessary to remove barriers that prohibit APNs from receiving competing credentials and thereby being able to practice autonomously in such settings, receive full reimbursement, and have authority to prescribe medications. Moreover, supportive hospital administrations that practice collaboration in management set the standards for others in practice to follow.[10]

ENHANCEMENT OF POLITICAL SAVVY

Securing support from federal and state governing entities, as well as from the public, demands that APNs become astute about, and active in, the political process. APNs must begin to speak the right language. Learning the nature of politics is learning the realities of the process that are based on the power of money and the ability to attain votes. Pearson[43] proposed three strategies that would enable APNs to become powerful players in the political arena. Suggested strategies include:

- Learning the nature of politics
- Collaborating with other advanced practice nursing organizations to identify common goals to be attained
- Learning evasive political techniques to attain incremental legislative gains

To become "players" in the political arena, APNs are urged to organize and fund lobbyists who will represent them as a unified entity. Advanced practice nursing organizations must also collaborate with each other to determine and address common legislative issues. Lastly, an effective approach to legislative gains entails patience and the use of "smoke screens" to get a piece of legislation to pass under another bill.

Speaking the right language entails that APNs be explicit and use concrete language that laypeople can understand to describe what they are trained to do. APNs must not be shy about advertising their ability to diagnose, treat, and prescribe in a manner that is safe, cost effective, and equal or superior to physicians. Buppert[39] advocated that nurses present hard facts and figures to support their value in the provision of high-quality care. Research data presented for this purpose must be impeccable in design and conducted by impartial investigators to withstand the opposition's criticisms. APNs must actively work to gain the confidence and support of the public, including health-care consumers, insurance company decision makers, businesses, media, and politicians.[43]

Advanced practice nurses, individually and collectively in professional organizations, can join forces and publicize the positive effects that APNs have on patient outcomes and communities to enhance their acceptance.[39,44] Nurses need to publicize their valuable skills and services using common modes of communication, such as the media and magazines geared to the layperson.

Suggested Exercises

1. What are the current relationships and perspectives about APNs and physicians, APNs and other nurses, and APNs and the public?
2. Discuss the multiple psychosocial-economic factors that may enhance or constrain collaborative practice between APNs and physicians or between APNs and multidisciplinary groups of health-care providers.
3. What are the psychological pros and cons to interdisciplinary education among health-care providers?
4. Does collaborative practice guarantee that APNs will be moral agents for clients?
5. What are the benefits and contraindications to having public input on nursing board decisions?
6. What are the pros and cons to having physicians on nursing boards?

REFERENCES

1. Bartlett, J: Familiar Quotations: A Collection of Passages, Phrases and Proverbs Traced to Their Sources in Ancient and Modern Literature. Little, Brown, Boston, 1982.
2. Meleis, AI: Theoretical Nursing: Development and Progress. JB Lippincott, Philadelphia, 1991.
3. Davis, AJ, and Aroskar, MA: Ethical Dilemmas and Nursing Practice, ed 2. Appleton-Century-Crofts, Norwalk, Conn, 1983.
4. Yarling, R, and McElmurry, B: The moral foundation of nursing. ANS 8:63, 1986.
5. American Nurses Association: Report on Revamping the Licensure System: A Look at the Pew Workforce Regulation Recommendations. ANA, Washington, DC, November 1995.
6. Langfitt, TW: Foreword to Health Professions Education for the Future: Schools in Service to the Nation. Report of the Pew Health Professions Commission. University of California at San Francisco, 1993.
7. Task Force Report: Reforming Health Care Workforce Regulation: Policy Considerations for the 21st Century. UCSF Center for the Health Professions, San Francisco, 1995.
8. Arcangelo, VP: The myth of independent practice. Nursing Forum 29:3, 1994.
9. Arslanian-Engoren, CM: Lived experiences of CNSs who collaborate with physicians: A phenomenological study. Clinical Nurse Specialist 9:68, 1995.
10. Evans, SA, and Carlson, R: Nurse-physician collaboration: Solving the nursing shortage crisis. J Am Coll Cardiol 20:1669, 1992.
11. Lamb, GS, and Napodano, RJ: Physician-nurse practitioner interaction patterns in primary care practices. Am J Public Health 74:26, 1984.
12. Norsen, L, Opladen, J, and Quinn, J: Practice model: Collaborative practice. Critical Care Nursing Clinics of North America 7:43, 1995.
13. Sparacino, PSA: Opportunities for the advanced practice nurse: Encroachment or collaboration? Clinical Nurse Specialist 8:122, 1994.
14. Bradford, R: Obstacles to collaborative practice. Nursing Management 20:72I, 1989.
15. Kane, RA: Interprofessional Teamwork (Manpower Monograph No. 8). Syracuse University, Syracuse, NY, 1975.
16. Mundinger, MO: Advanced-practice nursing: Good medicine for physicians? N Engl J Med 330:211, 1994.
17. Sherman, S: Secrets of HP's "muddled" team. Fortune 133:116, 1996.
18. Alpert, HB: 7 Gryzmish: Toward an understanding of collaboration. Nurs Clinics North Am 27:47, 1992.
19. Sebas, MB: Developing a collaborative practice agreement for the primary care setting. Nurse Pract 19:49, 1994.
20. Stein, LI, Watts, DT, and Howell, T: Sounding board: The doctor-nurse game revisited. N Engl J Med 332:546, 1990.
21. Gleeson, RM: Advanced practice nursing: A model of collaborative care. The American Journal of Maternal Child Nursing 15:9, 1990.
22. Kopser, KG, Horn, PB, and Carpenter, AD: Successful collaboration within an integrative practice model. Clinical Nurse Specialist 8:330, 1994.
23. Caruso, LA, and Payne, DF: Collaborative management: A nursing model. J Nurs Adm 20:28, 1990.
24. Clang, ED, and Gagen, JA: Head nurse and CNS: Teaming up. Nursing Management 23:104, 1992.
25. Huffman, LM: The nurse anesthetist and the occupational health nurse: Professionals with much to contribute to each other. Occupational Health Nursing 31:23, 1983.
26. Walton, MK, Jakobowski, DS, and Barnsteiner, JH: A collaborative practice model for the clinical nurse specialist. J Nurs Adm 32:55, 1993.
27. Avery, MD, and Del Guidice, GT: High-tech skills in low-tech hands: Issues of advanced practice and collaborative management. J Nurse Midwifery 38:2S, 1993.
28. Burchell, RC, Thomas, DA, and Smith, LS: Some considerations for implementing collaborative practice. Am J Med 74:9, 1983.
29. Booth, RZ: Leadership challenges for nurse practitioner faculty. Nurse Pract 20:52, 1995.
30. Goleman, D: Emotional Intelligence: Why It Can Matter More Than IQ. Bantam Books, New York, 1995.
31. Sue, DW, and Due, D: Counseling the Culturally Different: Theory and Practice. John Wiley & Sons, New York, 1990.
32. Gilligan, C: In a Different Voice: Psychological Theory and Women's Development. Harvard University Press, Cambridge, Mass, 1982.
33. Kohlberg, L: Moral stages and moralization. In Likona, T (ed): Moral Development and Behavior. Holt, Rinehart & Winston, New York, 1976.
34. Walker, LO, and Avant, KC: Strategies for Theory Construction in Nursing, ed 2. Appleton & Lange, Norwalk, Conn, 1988.
35. Spradley, JP: Participant Observation. Harcourt Brace Jovanovich, Orlando, Fla, 1980.
36. Dower, C: Regulatory Issues for the Health Care Workforce: The Federal Role in Health Care Workforce Regulation, No. 4:2. The Pew Health Professions Commission and the Center for the Health Professions, San Francisco, Winter 1994–1995.
37. Dower, C, and Finocchio, L: Health Care Workforce Regulation: Making the Necessary Changes for a Transforming Health Care System, No. 4:1. The Pew Health Professions Commission and the Center for the

Health Professions, San Francisco, Winter 1994–1995.

38. O'Neal, D: Personal communication, April, 1996.

39. Buppert, CK: Justifying nurse practitioner existence: Hard facts to hard figures. Nurse Pract 20:43, 1995.

40. Raisler, J: The international confederation of midwives: Past history, present activities, and future challenges. J Nurse Midwifery, 39:326, 1994.

41. Mahoney, DF: Employer resistance to state authorized prescriptive authority for NPs. Nurse Pract 20:58, 1995.

42. Kassirer, JP: What role for nurse practitioners in primary care? N Engl J Med 330:204, 1994.

43. Pearson, LJ: Annual update of how each state stands on legislative issues affecting advanced nursing practice. Nurse Pract 20:13, 1995.

44. Brooten, D, and Naylor, MD: Nurses' effect on changing patient outcomes. Image J Nurs Sch 27:95, 1995

CHAPTER 10

Clinical Research in the Advanced Practice Role

CHAPTER

Clinical Research in the Advanced Practice Role

JULIE REED ERICKSON, PhD, RN, FAAN
CHRISTINE SHEEHY, PhD, RN

Julie Reed Erickson, PhD, RN, FAAN, is assistant professor of nursing at the University of Arizona College on Nursing. According to the Carnegie-Mellon Association criteria, the University of Arizona is a research I university. After completing her master's degree, Dr. Erickson practiced for 5 years as a pulmonary clinical nurse specialist in pediatrics. After completing her doctorate, Dr. Erickson received federal grant funding to study the implementation and outcomes of community-based interventions for AIDS risk reduction among adult intravenous drug users, treatment of homeless adult drug users, and substance abuse prevention among high-risk minority youth. She teaches undergraduate research and graduate statistics courses at the University of Arizona.

Christine Sheehy, PhD, RN, has a doctoral degree in public policy from Virginia Commonwealth University. Between 1989 and 1990, she taught in the master's and doctoral programs and was project director for the master's-level geriatric–nurse practitioner option at the University of Arizona College of Nursing. After a 2-year period as director of health services research for the Maricopa Health System, she returned to the academic setting at Arizona State University in Tempe. Dr. Sheehy's substantive expertise is in the area of health-policy analysis, quality-of-care and health-outcome measurement, and chronic illness and aging. She has also worked as a temporary consultant for the World Health Organization in the Western Pacific Region.

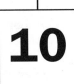

10

CHAPTER OBJECTIVES

After completing this chapter, the reader will be able to:

1. Analyze the influence of the "research-practice gap" on advanced practice nurses (APNs) as *consumers* of research and the implications for clinical care.
2. Compare and contrast the research experiences and characteristics of the four APN groups, including their respective strengths and limitations.
3. Delineate strategies for one's own APN role to enhance utilization of research findings in clinical practice and relate these to other topics in this text, such as critical thinking, change and leadership theories, and excellence in practice.
4. Synthesize information about research priorities for APNs and the relevance to advanced practice nurses as *researchers*.

According to Diers,[1] *decision making* is what most characterizes advanced practice, and underlying decision making are *clinical judgment, scholarly inquiry,* and *leadership.* Clinical judgment includes systematic data gathering, ordering of phenomena, and discriminating analysis of observations. Scholarly inquiry involves performing logical analysis of findings, raising interpretation beyond the facts to higher levels of conceptualization, and reinforcing clinical judgment and vice versa. Both clinical judgment and scholarly inquiry use the scientific method and should reflect the rigor of the research process. The *work* of advanced nurses is *practice,* and the *product* is *patient care;* therefore, leadership in the advanced practice role supports the scientific processes by[1]:

- Interpreting the context of practice
- Demonstrating influences on care
- Leading changes in practice

Nurse clinicians use research methods every day to evaluate patient outcomes and responses to treatments and procedures and to solve problems and answer questions about delivery of care.[2,3] Knowledge of research enables one to read critically, to evaluate published research, and to function as a change agent in planning, implementing, and sustaining innovation in practice (Fig. 10–1).

The scientific orientation of clinical nursing practice was formed by Florence Nightingale, who instructed nurses to use objective, sound observations, not just as information or interesting facts, but to save lives and to increase the comfort and safety of those for whom they cared.[5,6] As far back as the 1890s, this mandate heralded the need to methodically relate interventions to desired improvement in outcomes. Her use of the scientific approach to practice led Nightingale to claim the profession as a "science of nursing."[7]

The scientific process is inherent in the clinical decision making of advanced practice nursing and in the achievement of high-quality patient care. Research must be an integral part of the advanced practice role:

- To support APNs in becoming more *influential in determining health-care policy*
- To provide a *common language* that encourages sharing of information
- To enhance the *bridging of medical and nursing* perspectives in provision of health care

Nursing will become increasingly influential in health-care policy formulation to the extent that nurses can demonstrate competence in their knowledge and actions.[8] To justify advanced practice roles in a rapidly changing and competitive health-care market, APNs must address accountability by measuring and evaluating outcome of their care. Research provides a critical component of what legitimizes nursing as a health-care profession.[9] According to Hawkins and Thibodeau[8]:

> Research is the means by which outcomes can be validated, the value of nursing management demonstrated, and the practice quantified as unique and, in some cases, superior to that of other health care professionals. (p. 112)

Research also provides essential information to policy makers about health-care options.[10]

"Advanced-practice nurses also engage in a variety of activities consistent with the goals of the profession. These activities include. . . participation in research and utilization of scientific findings to improve patient outcomes" (American Nurses Association {ANA}, *Nursing: A Social Policy Statement*, 1994 Revision, p. 17).[13]

"As a leader or change agent, the nurse-midwife demonstrates: . . . The ability to evaluate, apply and collaborate in research. . . " (American College of Nurse Midwives {AANM}, *Core Competencies for Basic Nurse-Midwifery Practice*, 1993, p. 5).[14]

One of the primary roles of the Clinical Nurse Specialist is research, and implementing it can be done by the conduct of research or its utilization (Stetler, Bautista, Vernale-Hannon & Foster, *Nursing Clinics of North America*, 1995).[15]

"Nurse practitioners are committed to seeking and sharing knowledge that will promote quality health care and improve clinical outcomes by conducting research and applying the research findings of others" (American Academy of Nurse Practitioners {AANP}, *Scope of Practice for Nurse Practitioners*, 1993, p 1).[16]

"The nurse practitioner uses research findings as a basis for practice and improves health care through participation in research" (American Nurses Association {ANA}, *Standards of Practice for the Primary Health Care Nurse Practitioner*, 1987, p 8).[17]

"The purpose of research at the master's level is to prepare a practitioner for the utilization of new knowledge to provide high-quality health care, initiate change, and improve nursing practice...course work should provide graduates with the knowledge and skills to:. . . access current and relevant data. . . analyze the outcomes of nursing interventions. . . utilize information systems. . . initiate a line of inquiry into comprehensive data bases in order to utilize available research in the practice of nursing" (American Association of Colleges of Nursing {AACN}, *The Essentials of Master's Education for Advanced Practice Nursing*, 1996, pp. 6–7).[18]

Figure 10–1 Defining the role of research in advanced practice.

Research provides a common language for communicating with other health professionals about the contributions of nursing to patient care[2] and disseminates information about nursing's effectiveness that is crucial to survival of the APN role.[11] In addition, because APNs work with interdisciplinary colleagues whose training required research,[1] using scientific methods provides a standardized vocabulary for exchanging findings and interpreting clinical information. Finally, because the advanced practice role typically bridges nursing and medical functions, APNs are ideally situated to share research findings, evaluate care plans, and contribute to the scientific basis of care.[12]

The research function of APNs can be operationalized as both a *consumer* of research findings, and as a *researcher*. Both orientations, consumer and researcher, are consistent with expectations enumerated in policy statements and standards of practice directed at the four APN groups of clinical nurse specialist (CNS), nurse practitioner (NP), certified nurse midwife (CNM), and certified registered nurse anesthetist (CRNA).[13–18]

Research methods are the proper subject for research courses in advanced practice training. The purpose of this chapter is not to undertake an exhaustive and likely duplicative description of methods, but rather to provide insights into selected dimensions of operationalizing research in the APN role. Among the four groups of APNs, many research concerns and issues are shared. However, differences arising from the historical development of each role and the context in which care occurs may be a strength or limitation for research in one group or another. Elucidation of the development and care associated with a role can alert the APN to pitfalls and emphasize areas of potential research optimization. The chapter also addresses practical ways that the research component of APN roles can be actualized and broad areas of research priority.

Advanced Practice Nurses as Consumers of Research

Research utilization implies that the consumer[5,19,20]

- Reads the literature
- Makes critical judgments on the purpose, methods, results, and conclusions of a research study
- Evaluates the clinical applicability of the research
- Uses relevant findings in clinical practice
- Evaluates the effects of the new treatment on clients
- Disseminates the findings to others providing care to patients

THE RESEARCH-PRACTICE GAP

The literature has repeatedly confirmed that research findings with important implications for care are not widely used in clinical settings, despite clear evidence that use of the findings would improve patient care.[2,21,22] That is to say, a *research-practice gap* exists. Although the fundamental reason for doing nursing research is to develop a body of knowledge relative to practice,[23] research has little value unless it is applied.[4] Titler and Goode[23] suggested that

> the conduct of research is essentially unfinished unless the findings are synthesized and applied in practice to improve patient outcomes. (p. xv)

Many authors attest that a key responsibility of APNs is to help close the research gap by implementing research findings in practice settings.[10,24–28] Several barriers have been identified as contributing to the research-practice gap:

- The belief that research holds an *"ivory tower" mystique*
- A preference for research *investigation as superior to utilization* of research findings
- Inadequate *personal and administrative empowerment*
- Unavailability of *clinically relevant studies* in the research literature
- *Computer illiteracy*
- *Insufficient skill and/or experience in interpreting studies*

The Ivory Tower Mystique

Perhaps because of the perceived complexity of research methods, a *mystique* has evolved about research and researchers. Hawkins and Thibodeau[14] viewed the major barrier to inclusion of research in advanced practice as the belief that research is separate and magical. However, nurses collect data every day, make hypotheses on the desired outcomes of care, evaluate their clinical judgments for each patient encounter, write up their findings, and discuss their observations with others in clinical conferences. Ferrell, Grant, and Rhiner[2] believed that involvement in research means abandoning research as an ivory tower–academic activity and viewing research as clinical problem solving using scientific methods. Research cannot be limited to the few nurses who are doctorally prepared or to nurses in research positions in clinical settings.[2,29]

Investigation as Superior to Utilization

Graduate education often understates the importance of research utilization because "the emphasis in educational settings has for many years been conduct of research"[10] (p. 457). Although efforts have been made to increase the research utilization training of nurses, research application remains minimal,[30] and investigations are infrequently replicated in clinical settings.[16] APNs frequently articulate the conduct of research to be the gold standard of the research role.[10]

APNs need to understand and be skilled in study design, sampling, reliability, and statistics.[1] However, the emphasis on learning and practicing these skills should be balanced by an equally endorsed orientation toward the use of such skills to interpret and apply findings reported in the research literature. Replication studies, in addition to original research for honor's and master's degree theses, would reinforce the importance and value of research utilization.[30] Knowledge of research is necessary to read critically and to evaluate published research and to function as change agents capable of planning, introducing, and sustaining innovation in a practice setting.[4]

The publication of clear and intelligible reports would help APNs to better use research findings. Many of the published reports suffer from[10,30]:

- Use of research jargon
- Emphasis on measurement instead of measures
- Focus on statistical methods rather than their meaning
- Presentation of statistical analyses that are not easily understood
- Failure to explore fully the clinical implications of the findings

Research communications need to be carefully examined by nurse researchers and research journals.[21]

Inadequate Personal and Administrative Empowerment

There is some evidence that APNs have a poor self-image; that is, they do not see themselves as capable of shaping their own practice.[14] As an extension, APNs and nurses in general have expressed concern that they do not have enough power or authority to change patient-care practices even if research supports such initiatives.[21,30] Inadequate time due to heavy workload and competing priorities has been identified as discouraging research efforts in clinical settings.[10,19,21,30] Other barriers to research among APNs include[10,19,21,30,31]:

- Inadequate facilities and organizational infrastructure for research
- Lack of administrative incentives

- Resistance and lack of cooperation in the work setting by administrators, other health-care professionals, and nursing staff
- Practice changes recommended from the findings that may be too costly to implement
- Previous negative experiences with research
- Isolation from knowledgeable colleagues

Hawkins and Thibodeau[14] suggested that greater clinician-researcher interaction is critical to overcoming the self-image barrier. As described later in this chapter, many collaborative arrangements can be instituted to increase this interface and to foster mentoring relationships. To counter the authority barrier, Funk et al.[21] advocated for increased nurse control over practice through decentralization and shared governance. Administrators can help create time for research activities by incorporating these activities into staff job responsibilities, allowing time for literature reviews, exploration of new ideas, and pilot projects on new practices.[21] Administrative backing in the form of supporting attendance at conferences and continuing education opportunities, funding to support studies, providing access to library and consultative services, photocopying, and funding of pilot projects is also greatly needed.[10,19,21,30–32] Additional strategies include instituting research journal clubs, forming research committees, promoting research presentations, subscribing to journals that emphasize research implementation in practice such as *Applied Nursing Research* and *Clinical Nursing Research*,[30] and developing formal mechanisms for incorporating research findings.[21]

All nurses must contribute to making research utilization a reality. According to Titler and Goode[23]:

> Advanced practice nurses must embrace the pivotol leadership role they play in the synthesis and implementation of research findings. Staff nurses are essential in making the practice changes a reality at the bedside. . . . Nursing administrators at all levels of the organization must create practice environments that support and reward use of research. . . . Nurse educators must teach students the "hows" and "whys" of research utilization. (p. xv)

Unavailability of Clinically Relevant Studies

The lack of clinically relevant studies inhibits research utilization.[19,30,33] Hawkins and Thibodeau[14] found that the nursing journal with the largest number of readers publishes few, if any, research studies. Often, years lapse between the start of a clinical study and the publication of results in nursing research journals.[31] Until recently, the paucity of clinically relevant and well-designed studies was due to the historical development of several APN roles.

NURSE PRACTITIONERS There were three fairly distinct phases in development of the NP role[34]:

1. The "precursor period" during which the expanded role was initially conceived
2. The subsequent phase of progressive role definition, legitimation, and competencies
3. Role consolidation and maturation

Because some momentum for the NP role came from concern about shortage of physicians and the problem of access, underlying early research was the[35]

unstated assumption that primary care services as defined and provided by physicians were adequate in every respect except quantity. (p. 71)

The emphasis on "access" led researchers to study patient outcomes in terms of the extent to which access was achieved (e.g., number of visits), comparing NPs to physicians (MDs), and considering medical care to be standard and/or uniform.[35] Diers and Molde[35] stated:

The overwhelming majority of research on nurse practitioners has not dealt with a conceptual understanding of the *practice*; rather, the independent variable has been conceived of as the *practitioner*. (p. 74)

Further, because NPs were often seen as a subset of medical practice, the dependent variable, or patient outcome, was also cast or defined in traditional medical terms, and when other measures were included, they typically were patient satisfaction and acceptance.[35]

Most original studies

- Evaluated the roles of NPs in relation to physicians
- Assessed client acceptance
- Were descriptive in design
- Were conducted by investigators with limited research expertise
- Used retrospective analysis that suffered from incomplete data retrieval[32]

According to Stanford,[32] one notable exception was the study by Lewis and Resnik,[36] which employed randomized assignment of patients to control and experimental groups, follow-up, and multiple outcomes, including satisfaction with care, patients' knowledge about their illnesses, and system variables about the number of missed appointments and the utilization of hospital services.

After these early efforts, studies of NPs were done mostly by physicians, sociologists, and program evaluators (i.e., non-nurses); used primarily questionnaires for data collection; did not use longitudinal designs; and lacked rigor in pretesting of instruments for reliability and validity and appropriate statistical analyses.[32,34,35,37] Not all studies suffered from these weaknesses, however. A well-known exception was the Burlington randomized trial, which employed randomized controlled design, psychometrically tested instruments, and specification of patient outcomes.[32,38]

Recent studies[32]

- Have greater sophistication in methods
- Have more NPs involved in the investigations
- Address analysis of nursing components of practice pursued, including process and outcomes and factors that influence NP performance (e.g., scope of the extended role, patient assignment, economic issues)

The fact that many clients of NPs are chronically ill poses a substantial challenge to research. Selecting measures and relating interventions to outcomes of care are more difficult when studying persons who have multiple and complex health-care needs.[35] Conversely, the fact that NPs frequently work in primary-care settings is clearly an advantage. The practice population and setting usually include a wide range of health-maintenance and illness problems that afflict persons from infancy to old age, support ongoing relationships between patients and nurses that are needed for prospective and longitudinal studies of interventions and outcomes, and support collaborative research between nurses and other health-care providers.[39]

CLINICAL NURSE SPECIALISTS Similar to NPs, the literature before 1990 offers more information about the "role" of the CNS than about the "effectiveness" of these practitioners in patient care.[40] Most published reports described what a CNS "does" but say little about what this advanced practice role "achieves."[41]

Perhaps CNSs have an advantage in length of experience and clarity of expectations about research because the entry-level requirement for practice has always been the master's degree. However, the tasks of documenting CNS practice and delineating the effects of interventions on patient outcomes are hampered by the complexity of the role and wide variation in its implementation.[42] Thus, it is difficult to identify which of the activities are most effective in achieving outcomes.[42] In several studies where CNSs collaborated with other disciplines on patient outcomes, distinguishing the effects of individual team providers on outcomes is difficult.[42]

CERTIFIED NURSE MIDWIVES Of all the advanced practice groups, CNMs appear to have had the greatest leverage in documenting and reporting their contributions. Many clinically relevant and well-designed studies are available. Among the explanations for this success are:

- The availability of *data on effectiveness*
- *Establishment of linkages* between data on effectiveness and health-policy issues and / or concerns
- Well-defined and sensitive *outcomes measures*

Data on Effectiveness From inception of the role, CNMs were encouraged to keep statistics, and since 1972, this requirement has been formally acknowledged.[43] The statistics were primarily intended for self-evaluation of clinical programs but were drawn on as data from which effectiveness studies were reported.[43] "Effectiveness" usually meant program effectiveness, linked to the reason the nurse midwife was brought into a situation, which usually was to improve access to health care for childbearing women and babies who were not receiving adequate services.[43] Much data on infant and maternal mortality, as well as improvements in access for women in rural areas, were collected from studies done by the Metropolitan Life Insurance Company for the Frontier Nursing Services between 1925 and the mid-1950s.[43]

In the mid-1950s, midwifery made a "deliberate" and "successful" attempt to provide services in hospitals, because most women were delivering in that setting.[43] Effectiveness had been documented in rural and underserved populations. Once CNMs were practicing in hospitals, effectiveness included comparison of care given by CNMs and physicians using medical criteria, such as amount of analgesia given, duration of stages of labor, type of delivery, and complications. These effectiveness studies helped to justify CNMs' role not only to the public, but also to other professionals.[43]

By the 1960s and 1970s, effectiveness meant reduction of mortality rates, evidence of medical efficacy, quality of life, and cost effectiveness. In the early 1970s, CNMs expanded into the private sector, and studies focused on patient acceptance and physician receptivity in addition to the effectiveness questions.[43] The effectiveness evaluations were largely conducted so CNMs would be accepted by the professional community and have access to childbearing women. Diers and Burst[43] stated:

> Thus the effort was to prove being "as good as" physician care, to prove being "safe," to prove being "acceptable," and to prove being "cost-effective." (p. 72)

According to Diers and Molde,[35] the practice of CNMs was more developed through accreditation mechanisms, professional association positions, and legal parameters than through other nursing expanded roles. Therefore, greater standardization exists, and it has been possible to study much about nurse midwifery practice.

> For example, investigators have clearly examined both the effect of nurse-midwifery practice on medical or obstetrical outcome (morbidity, mortality, complications) and the effect of the nursing component in nurse midwifery on compliance (with postpartum recommendations, prenatal visits, or diet advice). (p. 79)

Establishment of Linkages Nurse midwifery has been very successful in influencing health policy about changes in care, reimbursement, and other policy agendas.[43] This influence is explained partly by the quantity and quality of the effectiveness data.[43,44] The data sets were more complete than usual record keeping because much of the data collected was required for public-health statistical reports, had procedures for verifying reliability, and was collected repeatedly longitudinally.[43] The primary reason for collecting and analyzing the data in the studies was to support a clinical position, not to build a body of knowledge; hence findings are closely tied to policy issues rather than to a theory base.[43] Although many studies were based on retrospective analysis, the integrity of that data is likely more robust than data collected in other areas of advanced practice nursing. Further, CNM findings are relevant to practice problems,[16] variables were easy to understand, outcomes were self-explanatory, and implications are obvious, connecting data to issues policy makers worry about.[43] The nurse midwifery literature has, to a great extent, avoided obstacles to policy creation, including isolated research findings, disjointed investigations, and infrequent replication resulting in several strong studies that provide support for the role.[16]

Outcome Measures Nurse midwives have had fewer problems in defining patient outcomes because of the obvious validity of the dependent variables (e.g., neonatal mortality), and the dependent variables (e.g., infant birthweight) are fairly sensitive to different practice interventions (e.g., nutritional counseling).[35,43] According to Diers and Molde[35]:

> Because the normal obstetrical situation is relatively less complicated methodologically (though not necessarily clinically) than internal medicine, considerable progress has been made in devising measures of the effect of nurse midwives and in describing the independent variable. (p. 79)

Numerous studies reported in the 1980s and early 1990s provide support for the positive outcomes of nurse midwives.[45,46] Anderson and Murphy[47] described the outcome planned home births ($N = 11,788$), over a 5-year period, including hospital transfers, practice protocols, risk screening, and emergency preparedness. Beal[48] evaluated the nature of nurse midwifery care and the relationship of clinical practice to outcomes in order to identify differences in intrapartum management between CNMs and physicians. Variables included patterns of administration of intravenous fluid, amniotomy, electronic fetal monitoring, pain medication, pitocin augmentation, lengths of the three stages of labor, total hospitalization time from labor until delivery, mode of delivery, incidence of episiotomy and laceration, and Apgar scores.[48] Yeates and Roberts[49] studied the relationship between nutritional intervention by CNMs and the outcome of birthweights. Corbett and Burst[50] investigated the relationship between CNM interventions of bearing-down technique in second stage of labor and energy expenditure, mean duration of the second stage, and Apgar scores. Although the last two studies had small samples,[49,50] the second did employ random assignment to control and intervention groups.

CERTIFIED REGISTERED NURSE ANESTHETISTS Research on CRNAs is scant. According to Waugaman[51]:

> There has been little incentive to conduct outcome studies in anesthesia since the Centers for Disease Control & Prevention (CDC) has asserted that the incidence of adverse outcomes, morbidity and mortality is too low to justify a nationally conducted study. (p. 51)

The majority of CRNAs and anesthesiologists practice in an interdisciplinary care team, yet little research exists on this practice model.[51,52] The medical direction ratios (that is, the number of nurse anesthetists per physician) for delivery of anesthesia care in the anesthesia care team model have not been substantiated in outcome research.[51]

COMPUTER ILLITERACY

Most nurses, including APNs, probably do not make use of the information highway to help locate clinically relevant studies. The Internet, a global network, can connect colleagues with similar interests by electronic mail and by the World Wide Web (WWW). In searching for research areas, the WWW is most useful. An address preceded by HTTP is a Web page. The Internet also makes possible participation in discussion groups about numerous topics. Two examples are Internet Relay Chat and USENET.

Many hospitals have computer terminals linked to the Internet that can access national data bases.[30] The article by Biddle et al.[53] compares manual index data search sources to their computer counterparts. However, a search of the literature can be done without access to a medical library. A dial-access system, which incorporates a computer, a modem, a telephone line, and a software package, allows one to search the Medline and Catline databases.[53]

For home use, one can choose among many Internet service providers. Prodigy and Compuserve are major national providers that typically charge a flat rate for a fixed amount of user time, plus additional charges for the number of minutes exceeding the flat-amount allocation. Often, local providers provide similar services but at lower rates. Even if one has no regular access to computing services at home or in the workplace and limited or no access to good medical libraries, many public libraries provide Internet access and will set up an electronic mail account. The *Online Journal of Knowledge Synthesis for Nursing,* which is published by Sigma Theta Tau, is also an excellent source of information.[23] Several additional resources are listed in Table 10–1. Beginning competence in computer applications is a must for APNs.

Insufficient Skill and/or Experience in Interpreting Studies

The inability of clinicians to understand research reports limits research utilization.[19,33] APNs often lack adequate knowledge and an explicit set of criteria for judging the applicability of research findings to practice. APNs may recognize the term "research utilization," but few are formally educated in use of a specific model for utilization.[10] Models for research utilization are helpful in incorporat-

TABLE 10–1
Online Sources of Information

ONLINE DATABASES OR SOURCES OF DATA
1. Clinical Performance Measure Database: available through the Agency for Health Care Policy and Research. The database is in Access 1.0, and the documentation (which is voluminous) is in WordPerfect 6.0 and up. This database comprises data from JCAHO, HEDIS, HCFA, and Rand.   Go into http://www.ahcpr.gov:808/, click on Conquest 1.0, and download. Then on your local drive, just go and click on the executable files; they are self-extracting.
2. Healthcare Cost and Utilization Project (HCUP-3): National Inpatient Sample Release (NIS) 2, 1993, data available May 1996. The 1993 NIS data include: (a) 6.5 million inpatient stays in 900 hospitals from 17 states; (b) clinical and resource use variables usually found on discharge abstracts; (c) weights to produce national estimates; (d) hospital identifiers to link with American Hospital Association's Survey of Hospitals. This 6-CD set can be purchased for $160 from National Technical Information Service (703-487-4650) or on the Internet at hcupNIS@cghsir.ahcpr.gov.

ONLINE SOURCES OF GRANT FUNDING
1. Mental health grants: http://www.nimh.nih.gov/   E-mail to: LISTSERV@LIST.NIH.GOV. Leave the "subject" blank; in the body of the message, type: only subscribe NIHGDE-L, your first name, and your last name.

ONLINE INFORMATION AND NETWORKING
1. <NURSENET@UTORONTO.BITNET>: a global forum for nursing issues.
2. Nurse Forum in the American Nurses Association's (ANA's) online service with CompuServ and includes access to the Internet, the WWW, and electronic mail. For customer information, contact 800-274-4ANA
3. In Netscape, go to File and type www.achoo.com and then press "enter." Under Business of Healthcare, there is a nursing site (in blue).
4. http://www.reutershealth.com/: a site of news for health.

ing research findings into practice[21] and in increasing knowledge about application of those findings.

Three major models for research utilization in clinical settings were developed and tested in nursing. The models are quite similar in many respects but are distinguished by their intended goals. The first project for nursing research utilization began in 1975 by the Western Interstate Commission for Higher Education (WICHE) Regional Program for Nursing Research Development.[27] Five components were described as necessary for nurses to achieve the goal of change in practice[27,54]:

1. Access to research findings
2. Ability to critically evaluate studies
3. Competence in change theory and strategies
4. Approaches to managing risk taking
5. A plan for implementation and criteria by which to evaluate the effects

One outgrowth of the WICHE model was the formation of information systems, including a list of nurse researchers by areas of interest and/or expertise, a compendium of nursing instruments, a compilation of funding sources, and a list of research priorities derived from a Delphi survey.[27,55]

Developed in the late 1970s, the Conduct and Utilization of Research in Nursing (CURN) model delineated six phases to achieve the goal of putting research knowledge into nursing practice.[5,15,56] The six phases are:

1. Creating an atmosphere for change by identifying specific patient-care problems
2. Evaluating current scientific knowledge of the clinical problem, institutional policies, and potential costs
3. Determining the fit of the nursing practice innovation
4. Carrying out clinical trials
5. Deciding to accept, reject, or change the innovation
6. Disseminating the innovation to other nursing practice units

The collaboration of nurse clinicians and nurse researchers was critical in all six phases of the CURN model.

The Stetler/Marram[57] Model for research utilization has been tested and refined into six phases. The six phases are:

1. Literature review of a clinical problem
2. Critiquing the research
3. Evaluating its clinical applicability
4. Determining the potential use of the research findings
5. Translating the findings into practice
6. Evaluating the expected outcomes

Stetler's approach to the goals of enhancing knowledge and increasing use of research findings reflects a model of critical thinking that has been applied many times and in different settings.[10,58] In particular, the 1995 article by Stetler et al.[10] demonstrates the functioning of a research utilization interest group, contains a worksheet to apply the model and strategies, and suggests strategies and/or tips to help ensure success of such a forum.

Collaboration

Collaboration must be encouraged between academic and clinical institutions for mutual support in establishing research programs and programs for research utilization.[18,31,59] Blending of research resources is critical to providing a scientific basis for advanced nursing practice and providing answers to clinical questions that arise every day.[59]

Dufault[31] examined a model of collaboration using a consortium of nurse researchers, staff nurses, clinical managers, clinicians, and nurse administrators to enhance research utilization and development. Sprague-McRae[18] advocated either a collaborative intradisciplinary or a collaborative interdisciplinary team to validate clinical practice and to support NPs as primary investigators in the research process. More research by clinical practitioners, either alone or in collaboration with academic researchers, will likely overcome the barrier of finding relevant literature on clinical problems. The American Nurses' Association Cabinet on Nursing Research[60] endorses the partnership of clinicians and researchers in research utilization.

There are many barriers to the utilization of nursing research to affect change in clinical practice and improve clinical outcomes. These barriers include the ivory tower mystique about research, the perception that the conduct of research is superior to the application of research findings, inadequate personal empowerment, lack of administrative support, lack of clinically relevant studies for some APN groups, and insufficient skill among APNs to access, critique, and interpret studies. On the positive side, many strategies for overcoming the barriers exist. Ultimately, overcoming barriers to effective research utilization is accomplished by developing intellectual curiosity, by thinking reflectively about one's actions, by promoting and valuing innovation,[4] and by creating an environment that supports questioning, evaluating current practice, and seeking and testing of research-based solutions.[30]

Advanced Practice Nurses as Researchers

Scientific inquiry (i.e., research) and the continuing discovery of new knowledge are crucial to a profession,[2,61] and have as the goal the generation of knowledge for science-based clinical practice.[15] As mentioned earlier in this chapter, research contributes to the validation of nursing outcomes, the explanation and quantification of the unique nature of advanced nursing practice, and the documentation of the superiority of nursing care when higher quality exists.[14] Krywanio[3] stated that the NP is critical to identifying issues that are important in clinical research as well as in providing firsthand insight into the research process. This unique perspective and insight into care processes and care outcomes are held by all APNs across a variety of clinical settings.

Hawkins and Thibodeau[14] suggested that not every APN has the array of research skills needed to carry out a clinical research study. Diers[1] stated that a major advantage for an APN is to complete a research thesis that can be integrated into clinical practice and can serve as a model for future clinical investigations. However, a difference of opinion exists on the need for a research thesis in a graduate program. The American Association of Colleges of Nursing[13] concluded that in a professional master's degree program, a research thesis is not an appropriate requirement.

Advanced practice nurses can assume many roles in the conduct of research. Hawkins and Thibodeau[14] suggested the roles of subject, research assistant, consultant, content expert, nursing expert, collaborator, or principal investigator.

COLLABORATION

Collaboration is advantageous to the conduct of clinical nursing research.[62,63] The collaborative approach pools complementary talents, research skills, and clinical experiences from among its members,[64] and may be interdisciplinary or intradisciplinary. For example, in one interdisciplinary interpretation, a NP might consult with a clinical nurse researcher on the design of the study protocol, sources of funding, and implementation.[3] Sprague-McRae[18] suggested that intradisciplinary research collaboration occurs between nurse researchers–nurse clinicians, nurse researchers–nurse researchers, or nurse clinicians–nurse clinicians. Havelock and Havelock[65] recognized intradisciplinary collaboration as building on the strengths of practice-based and academic-based models of clinical research. Dufault[31] used a model of reciprocity between nurse clinicians and nurse scientists. In Dufault's model, clinicians learn research methods and gain an appreciation of research, while scientists learn about clinically relevant problems and the challenges of conducting clinical investigations.

The interdisciplinary research team can involve nurse clinicians, nurse researchers, physicians, finance officers, psychologists, sociologists, anthropologists, attorneys, nutritionists, statisticians, and other health-care professionals. The chosen mix of disciplines depends on the clinical problem being investigated, the setting of the study, the desired talent pool of team members, and the goals of collaboration. Sprague-McRae[18] suggested that interdisciplinary research collaboration increases the visibility of nurse clinicians as uniquely skilled and contributing members of the health-care team, promotes positive working relationships among health disciplines, and distributes the workload of a clinical investigation. Consulting with experts (either formally or informally) and piloting of studies are always advisable.

IDENTIFICATION OF RESEARCHABLE TOPICS IN CLINICAL PRACTICE

Whatever collaborative arrangement APNs choose, another important decision concerns identifying what should be investigated. Research ideas arise from one's own interests, observation of a recurring problem or unexplained phenomenon, suggestions of colleagues, and published results that recommend areas of further study.[53] The study topic should be of great interest to the researcher, because the implementation of a study is long and involved and because it is necessary to sustain motivation to carry out the project.[53]

General Areas of Research Priority

Although the term **outcome** has recently been popularized, the need to study the impact of nursing interventions on client response has been espoused for years.[6,66–70] Gurka[67] and Peglow et al.[68] insisted that to document effectiveness, clinical research must focus on both the *process* and *outcome* of the activities of APNs. Health-care *costs*, cost effectiveness, and financing[14,68,71]; health-care *delivery; interdisciplinary* dynamics and the *interface of nurses with other disciplines*[14,32]; and *quality* of care[68] are other aspects that must be woven into study designs. Lengacher et al.[72] reported an acute need for outcome research on the *design and use of nursing practice models*. It is reasonably well accepted that "risk adjustment" is important to measurement of outcomes. However, the research method by which that is accomplished and the variables contributing to risk adjustment formulas are still being debated and therefore are not fully established. Examples of variables that may be included are measures of severity (e.g., diagnosis, comorbidity, complications) and additional case-mix modifiers, such as age, the contribution of depression, and other patient characteristics that influence outcomes, such as functional level and cognitive status.[44,73,74] Case mix differs in measurement depending on the setting in which patients are seen. For example, diagnoses-related groups apply to hospital settings, whereas ambulatory-care groups are under development for outpatient settings. A comprehensive discussion of risk adjustment is not possible within the context of this chapter, but its rapid growth in development suggests that the reader may wish to pursue independent reading more fully. Resources on this subject and sources of measurement are included in the bibliography of this chapter.

Crummer and Carter[75] suggested studying the *critical pathway model* for its ability to define current practice and to meet the goals of nursing case management. Lusk and Kerr[76] saw increased *hazards facing employees in the work site* as important to study. Prichard et al.[66] encourage exploration of the *influence of technology*, because nursing practices may be eliminated or altered as technological advances occur. Examination of the *evaluative component* of the Stetler-Marram research utilization model, implementation of research findings in an *interdisciplinary* manner, and *research utilization competencies* are also needed.[10] *Qualitative studies* about styles of practice are also increasingly important.[32]

It should also be noted that research questions can be examined using *existing data*. For example, birth-certificate data provided by the Natality, Marriage and Divorce Statistics Branch of the CDC contains information on mother's age, parity, starting date of prenatal care, birth weight, and 1-minute Apgar score, which can be used as was the case in the midwifery study.[45] Nurse midwives have used existing data for many years, in studies of CNM effectiveness.[43,44] Molde and Diers[44] suggested that patient-care charts provide data and that encounter forms are another good source. NP research would be improved if existing data were systematically tabulated in each setting.

Sources of data could be greatly increased and comparability and benchmarking across APN patient groups improved by the routine collection of assessment data using standardized assessment instruments. Valid and reliable instruments assessing coping, functional status, quality of life, stress, and other variables of interest to APNs are available in the literature. An APN planning a research study should carefully consider using established instruments to avoid the exacting, tedious process of instrument development and, more importantly, to allow comparisons with published findings. APNs should also look to existing taxonomies for standardized nursing language, performance measures, decision making, and classification of nursing interventions.[77–80]

Selected Research Priorities Specific to Advanced Practice Nurse Groups

With regard to NPs, Stanford[32] suggested the following areas as warranting continued investigation:

- Development of theoretical models to help link research, theory, and practice
- Improvement in methods, including sampling and defining comparison groups and target populations
- Implementation of longitudinal studies
- Refinement and extension of findings that can be generalized
- Determination of more appropriate instrumentation

Diers and Molde[35] recommended that if NP care is defined to encompass dimensions of nursing in addition to medical criteria, many more dependent measures can be identified for patients, such as outcomes for persons with chronic illnesses, measures of counseling and patient knowledge, standards of care, and appropriate units of study for cost analysis. Gerace[39] expanded on the preceding theme of selecting outcome measures for study. Gerace stated that because much of the practice of NPs is based on meaningful interactions with patients, *qualitative* rather than quantitative research may be more appropriate. Clinical practice domains might include nutritional assessment and counseling, the patient's perspective of chronic illness and associated self-care needs, family systems, patient education, the NP role in team interaction and telephone encounters[39], and the influence of differences in practice patterns.[32]

Outcome studies should be designed to *improve* rather than merely evaluate styles of practice, including the helping relationship, and with a policy framework in mind.[44] Molde and Diers[44] caution:

> Explaining the outcomes, however, requires a systematic search of the characteristics of the care, the provider, the context, the relationship of patient to clinician, and the resources broadly conceived in the setting. (p. 364)

For CNSs, Rizzuto[42] urged formal documentation of the *process of consultation* and further investigation of patient outcomes and the type and frequency of outcomes achieved. Hamric[71] suggested that studies are needed on cost effectiveness of CNSs and their role in improving patient outcomes.

Areas for research by CRNAs appear to be wide open and fertile. Waugaman[51] advised outcome research to provide necessary evidence for state and federal governments to make decisions about health-care reform. Elements of such research might include:

- Provider data
- Paradigms of cost equality and efficiency relative to case management techniques application in a variety of institutional settings
- Participation of CRNAs in continuous quality improvement programs that can be maintained individually and in a national data bank

Cromwell[81] added two important avenues to pursue. First, in the "team model" of physician anesthesiologist–CRNA practice, there is substantial regional variation in the number of CRNAs supervised (i.e., the ratio of physicians to CRNAs), and little is known about the impact. As a result, significant opportunities exist to demonstrate possible improvements and differences in cost and outcomes. Second, anesthesia is an ideal laboratory for studying substitution effects.

According to Cromwell:

> Anesthesia, therefore, provides an excellent example of what can go wrong with the workforce mix when you pay for inputs (i.e., types of providers) rather than outputs (i.e., the services delivered). (p. 220)

Despite all their accomplishments, CNMs still have many interesting research topics to pursue and challenges to overcome. Ament[16] reported that CNMs still face barriers to practice in many areas of the country, including difficulty with reimbursement from state and private sources, denial of hospital privileges, uncertain access to malpractice insurance, and lack of uniform prescriptive authority. Hence, much more documentation of outcomes and dissemination of findings to policy makers are needed. Positive outcomes of midwifery provide support for increased use of midwives and suggest the need for systematic studies of the cost savings associated with midwifery care.[45,46]

Mead[82] suggested study of the fit between the theory of research and the practicalities of everyday midwifery. Lehrman[83] examined a theoretical framework for nurse midwifery. Declerca[45] stated that further research into the content of midwifery care is recommended.

Summary

Every professional nurse must contribute to the flow of information from one organization to another, from academia to practice, and from written journals to bedside care givers.[23] For nursing, it is critically important that clinical research influence health policy.[16]

The scope and standards of practice for APNs mandate utilization of research in clinical practice as well as a role in generating research to build the scientific base of nursing. The demands for time and skills to meet these research expectations are enormous. However, the APN should confront the challenge using models of research utilization and research collaboration already in the professional literature. APNs are in the unique position to expand nursing practice, to prove the value of advanced practice, and to build knowledge for future generations of nurses.

Suggested Exercises

1. Carefully consider your own experience in research utilization.
   a. Write down the barriers that were present as you attempted to put research into practice.
   b. Write down the supports that were present on a personal and administrative level as you attempted to put research into your practice.

c. Characterize how consistent or inconsistent your experience with barriers and supports is with the literature reported in this chapter.

d. Given your past experience and the information in this chapter, describe barriers, strategies for overcoming barriers, and support mechanisms that you would anticipate in your next attempt at research utilization.

e. Review each of the research utilization models described in this chapter. Discuss the usefulness, value, and viability of each model in your current work environment. Select the model that could prove successful in putting research into your current clinical practice. Write down five steps in implementing the research utilization model in your work environment.

2. Carefully consider your own experience in conducting research.

a. Write down what roles you assumed in the conduct of research. Describe your experiences in each role. Determine your desire to repeat the roles in other research studies and your desire to take on new roles.

b. Review your research skills. Document your current strengths and weaknesses. Comment on what new skills you need, what skills could be provided by a collaborator, and what skills you have no desire to develop.

c. Review the research collaboration models presented in this chapter. Discuss the usefulness, value, and viability of the models given your research expertise and your current work environment. Select a model that may prove to be successful in carrying out new research or replicating previous studies.

d. Think carefully about your current clinical practice. Write down four research questions, four research hypotheses, and/or four nursing outcomes that could be studied in your practice. Write down five steps that you could take in further exploring a question, hypothesis, and/or outcome. Think through how you would find the time, resources, and other supports within and outside of your current work environment to carry out research.

REFERENCES

1. Diers, D: Preparation of practitioners, clinical specialists, and clinicians. J Prof Nurs 1: 41, 1985.
2. Ferrell, B, Grant, M, and Rhiner, M: Bridging the gap between research and practice. Oncol Nurs Forum 17:447, 1990.
3. Krywanio, M: Integrating research into private practice through consultation. Nurse Pract 19:47, 1994.
4. Sleep, J: Research and the practice of midwifery. J Adv Nurs 17:1465, 1992.
5. McGuire, D, Walczak, J, and Krumm, S: Development of a nursing reseach utilization program in a clinical oncology setting: Organization, implementation, and evaluation. Oncol Nurs Forum 21:704, 1994.
6. Nightingale, F: Notes on Nursing: What It Is and What It Is Not (commemorative 1992 edition). JB Lippincott, Philadelphia, 1859.
7. Nightingale, F: Notes on Nursing: What It Is and What It Is Not. Dover Publications, New York, 1969.
8. Hawkins, J, and Thibodeau, J: The role of research in advanced practice. In Hawkins, J, and Thibodeau, J: The Advanced Practitioner: Current Practice Issues. Tiresias Press, New York, 1993.

9. Huber, G: Clinical nurse specialist and staff nurse colleagues in integrating nursing research with clinical practice. Clinical Nurse Specialist 8:118, 1994.

10. Ament, LA: Strategies for dissemination of policy research. J Nurse Midwifery 39:329, 1994.

11. Papenhausen, J, and Beecroft, P: Communicating clinical nurse specialist effectiveness. Clinical Nurse Specialist 4:1, 1990.

12. Sprague-McRae, J: Nurse practitioners and collaborative interdisciplinary research roles in an HMO. Pediatric Nurs 14:503, 1988.

13. American Nurses' Association: Nursing: A social policy statement. American Nurses' Association, Kansas City, Mo, 1994.

14. American College of Nurse-Midwives: Core Competencies for Basic Nurse-Midwifery Practice. American College of Nurse-Midwives, Washington, DC, 1993.

15. Stetler, CB, et al: Enhancing research utilization by clinical nurse specialists. Nurs Clin North Am 30:457, 1995.

16. American Academy of Nurse Practitioners: Scope of Practice for Nurse Practitioners. American Academy of Nurse Practitioners, Austin, Tex, 1993.

17. American Nurses' Association: Standards of Practice for the Primary Health Care Nurse Practitioner. American Nurses' Association, Kansas City, Mo, 1987.

18. American Association of Colleges of Nursing: The Essentials of Master's Education for Advanced Practice Nursing. American Association of Colleges of Nursing, Washington, DC, 1996.

19. Pettengill, M, Gillies, D, and Clark, C: Factors encouraging and discouraging the use of nursing research findings. Image J Nurs Sch 26:143, 1994.

20. American Nurses' Association: Guidelines for the Investigative Function of Nurses. American Nurses' Association, Kansas City, Mo, 1981.

21. Funk, S, et al.: Barriers to using research findings in practice: The clinician's perspective. Appl Nurs Res 4:90, 1991.

22. Heater, B, Becker, A, and Olson, R: Nursing interventions and patient outcomes: A meta-analysis of studies. Nurs Res 37:303, 1988.

23. Titler, MG, and Goode, CJ (Guest eds): Preface. Nurs Clin North Am 30:xv, 1995.

24. Briones, T, and Bruya, M: The professional imperative: Research utilization in the search for scientifically based nursing practice. Focus on Critical Care 17:78, 1990.

25. Edwards-Beckett, J: Nursing research utilization techniques. J Nurs Adm 20:25, 1990.

26. Kirchhoff, K: A diffusion survey of coronary precautions. Nurs Res 31:196, 1982.

27. Phillips, L: A Clinician's Guide to the Critique and Utilization of Nursing Research. Appleton-Century-Crofts, Norwalk, Conn, 1986.

28. Rogers, E: Diffusion of Innovations. The Free Press, New York, 1983.

29. Martin, M, and Forchuk, C: Linking research and practice. International Nurs Rev 41:184, 1994.

30. Funk, SG, Tornquist, EM, and Champagne, MT: Barriers and facilitators of research utilization. Nurs Clin North Am 30:395, 1995.

31. Dufault, M: A collaborative model for research development and utilization: Process, structure, and outcomes. Journal of Nursing Staff Development 11:139, 1995.

32. Stanford, D: Nurse practitioner research: Issues in practice and theory. Nurse Pract 12:64, 1987.

33. Miller, J, and Messenger, S: Obstacles to applying nursing research findings. Am J Nurs 78:632, 1978.

34. Edmunds, MW: Evaluation of nurse practitioner effectiveness: An overview of the literature. Evaluation and the Health Professions 1:68, 1978.

35. Diers, D, and Molde, S: Some conceptual and methodological issues in nurse practitioner research. Res Nurs Health 2:73, 1979.

36. Lewis, CE, and Resnik, BA: Nurse clinics and progressive ambulatory patient care. N Engl J Med 277:1236, 1967.

37. Shamansky, SL: Nurse practitioners and primary care research: Promises and pitfalls. In Werley, H, and Fitzpatrick, J (eds): Annual Review of Nursing Research. Springer, New York, 1985.

38. Spitzer, WO, et al: The Burlington randomized trial of the nurse practitioner. N Engl J Med 290:251, 1974.

39. Gerace, TM: Primary care nursing: A model for research. In Norton, PG, et al (eds): Primary Care Research: Traditional and Innovative Approaches. Sage Publications, Newbury Park, Calif, 1991.

40. Lipetzky, P: Cost analysis and the clinical nurse specialist. Nursing Management 21:25, 1990.

41. Beyerman, K: Making a difference: The gerontological CNS. Journal of Gerontological Nursing 15:36, 1993.

42. Rizzuto, C: Issues in clinical nursing research: Documenting clinical nurse specialist role functions and outcomes. West J Nurs Res 17:448, 1995.

43. Diers, D, and Burst, HV: Effectiveness of policy related research: Nurse-midwifery as case example. Image J Nurs Sch 15:68, 1983.

44. Molde, S, and Diers, D: Nurse practitioner research: Selected literature review and research agenda. Nurs Res 34:362, 1985.

45. Declerc, ER: The transformation of American midwifery: 1975 to 1988. Am J Public Health 82:680, 1992.

46. Rooks, J, et al: Outcomes of care in birth centers. N Engl J Med 321:1804, 1989.

47. Anderson, RE, and Murphy, PA: Outcomes of 11,788 planned home births attended by certified nurse-midwives: A retrospective descriptive study. J Nurse Midwifery 40:483, 1995.

48. Beal, MW: Nurse-midwifery intrapartum management. J Nurse Midwifery 29:13, 1984.

49. Yeates, DA, and Roberts, JE: A comparison of two bearing-down techniques during the second stage of labor. J Nurse Midwifery 29:3, 1984.

50. Corbett, MA, and Burst, HV: Nutritional intervention in pregnancy. J Nurse Midwifery 28:23, 1983.

51. Waugaman, WR: Outcome research: The gold standard for professional practice. Nurse Anesthesia 4:51, 1993.

52. American Society of Anesthesiologists: Statement to the Committee on Finance, US Senate (Position on FY 93 Budget Proposals). Park Ridge, Ill, February 18, 1992.

53. Biddle, W, et al: An introduction to research: A primer for the nurse anesthetist. Journal of the American Association of Nurse Anesthetists 59:421, 1991.

54. Kruegar, J, Nelson, A, and Wolanin, MO: Nursing research: Development, collaboration, and utilization. Germantown, Md, Aspen Systems, 1978.

55. Lindeman, CA, and Krueger, JC: Increasing the quality, quantity, and use of nursing research. Nurs Outlook 25:450, 1977.

56. Horsley, J, Crane, J, and Bingle, J: Research utilization as an organizational process. J Nurs Adm 8:4, 1978.

57. Stetler, C: Refinement of the Stetler/Marram Model of application of research findings to practice. Nurs Outlook 42:15, 1994.

58. Hanson, JL, and Ashley, B: Advanced practice nurses' application of the Stetler Model for research utilization: Improving bereavement care. Oncol Nurs Forum 21:720, 1994.

59. Duffy, M: Strengthening communication signals to build a research-based practice. Nursing and Health Care 6:238, 1985.

60. American Nurses' Association Cabinet on Nursing Research: Guidelines for the Functions of Nurses. American Nurses' Association, Kansas City, Mo, 1989.

61. McClure, M: Promoting practice based research: A critical need. J Nurs Adm 11:66, 1981.

62. Oberst, M: Integrating research and clinical practice roles. Topics in Clinical Nursing 7:45, 1985.

63. Barnard, K: Knowledge for practice: directions for the future. Nurs Res 29:208, 1980.

64. Engstrom, J: University, agency and collaborative models for nursing research: An overview. Image J Nurs Sch 16:77, 1984.

65. Havelock, R, and Havelock, M: Training for Change Agents. University of Michigan, Ann Arbor, 1973.

66. Prichard, L, et al: The natural connection: The clinical nurse specialist and bedside nursing research. Clinical Nurse Specialist 8:307, 1994.

67. Gurka, A: Process and outcome components of clinical nurse specialist consultation. Dimensions of Critical Care Nursing 10:169, 1991.

68. Peglow, D, et al: Evaluation of clinical nurse specialist practice. Clinical Nurse Specialist 6:28, 1992.

69. Bloch, D: Evaluation of nursing care in terms of process and outcome: Issues in research and quality assurance. Nurs Res 24:256, 1975.

70. Ford, L: A nurse for all settings: The nurse practitioner. Nurs Outlook 27:520, 1979.

71. Hamric, A: Creating our future: Challenges and opportunities for the clinical nurse specialist. Oncol Nurs Forum 19:11, 1992.

72. Lengacher, C, et al: Effects of the partners in care practice model on nursing outcomes. Nursing Economics 12:300, 1994.

73. Iezzoni, LI (ed): Risk Adjustment for Measuring Health Outcomes. Health Administration Press, Ann Arbor, Mich, 1994.

74. American Nurses' Association: Nursing Care Report Card for Acute Care. American Nurses' Association, Washington, DC, 1995.

75. Crummer, M, and Carter, V: Critical pathways: The pivotal tool. J Cardiovas Nurs 7:30, 1993.

76. Lusk, S, and Kerr, M: Conducting worksite research: Methodological issues and suggested approaches. AAOHN Journal 42:117, 1994.

77. Corrigan, J, and Nielsen, D: Toward the development of uniform reporting standards for managed care organizations: The health plan employer date and information set. The Joint Commission Journal on Quality Improvement 19:566, 1993.

78. Delaney, C, et al: Standardized nursing language for healthcare information systems. J Med Syst 16:145, 1992.

79. Martin, K, Leak, G, and Aden, C: The OMAHA system: A research-based model for decision making. J Nurs Adm 22:47, 1992.

80. McCloskey, J, and Bulechek, G: Validation and coding of the NIC taxonomy structure: Iowa Intervention Project. Image J Nurs Sch 27:346, 1995.

81. Cromwell, J: Health professions substitution: A case study of anesthesia. In M Osterweis, et al (eds): The US Health Workforce: Power, Politics and Policy. Association of Academic Health Centers, Washington, DC.

82. Mead, M: Research: A professional responsibility. Midwives 108(1293) 322, October 1995.

83. Lehrman, E: A theoretical framework for nurse-midwifery practice. (The University of Arizona, doctoral dissertation, 1988). Dissertation Abstracts International, 49–173:5230

BIBLIOGRAPHY

Quantification and Measurement of Variables
Iezzoni, LI: Risk Adjustment for Measuring Health Care Outcomes. Health Administration Press, Ann Arbor, Mich, 1994.
Journal of Nursing Measurement. Springer Publishing Co, 536 Broadway, New York, NY 10012, phone 212–431–4370, FAX 212–941–7842.
Spilker, B (ed): Quality of Life Assessments in Clinical Trials. Raven Press, New York, 1990.

Waltz, CF, and Strickland, OL (eds): Measurement of Nursing Outcomes, Vols 1 through 4. Springer, New York, 1988.

Improved Discrimination in Interpreting Hospital Readmission Data

Farmer, RG, et al: Hospital readmissions: A re-evaluation of criteria. Cleve Clinic J Med 56:704, 1989.

Case Mix in Ambulatory Care Settings: Ambulatory Care Groups

Parkerson, GR, Broadhead, WE, and Tsa, C-K: Quality of life and functional health of primary care patients. J Clin Epidemiol 45:1303, 1992.

Smith, NS, and Weiner, JP: Applying population-based case mix adjustment in managed care: The Johns Hopkins Ambulatory Care Group system. Managed Care Quarterly 2(3):21, 1994.

Weiner, JP, et al: Development and application of a population-oriented measure of ambulatory care case-mix. Med Care 29:452, 1991.

Depression as a Risk Adjustment

Hays, RD, et al: Functioning and well-being outcomes of patients with depression compared with chronic general medical illnesses. Arch Gen Psychiatry 52:11, 1995.

Mulrow, CD, et al: Case-finding instruments for depression in primary care settings. Arch Intern Med 122:913, 1995.

Simon, GE, VonKorff, M, and Barlow, W: Health care costs of primary care patients with recognized depression. Arch Gen Psychiatry 52:850, 1995.

Sturm, R, and Wells, KB: How can care for depression become more cost effective? JAMA 273:51, 1995.

Short Forms 12 and 36

McHorney, CA, Kosinski, M, and Ware, JE: Comparisons of the costs and quality of norms for the SF-36 health survey collected by mail versus telephone interview: Results from a national study. Med Care 32:551, 1994.

McHorney, CA, Ware, JE, and Raczek, AE: The MOS 36-item short-form health survey (SF-36): Psychometric and clinical tests of validity in measuring physical and mental health constructs. Med Care 31:247, 1993.

Ware, JE, and Sherbourne, CD: The MOS 36-item short-form health survey (SF-36): Conceptual framework and item selection. Med Care 30:473, 1992.

Medical Outcomes Trust, 20 Park Plaza, Suite 1014, Boston, MA 02116–4313, phone 617–426–4046, fax 617–426–4131, e-mail motrust@delphi.com.

Measurement of Home Health Outcomes

Adams, CE, Kramer, S, and Wilson, M: Home health quality outcomes: Fee-for-service versus health maintenance organization enrollees. J Nurs Adm 25:39, 1995.

Ellenbecker, CH: Profit and non-profit home health care agency outcomes: A study of one state's experience. Home Health Care Services Quarterly 15(3):47, 1995.

Harris, MD: Clinical and financial outcomes in patient care in a home health care agency. Journal of Nursing Quality Assurance 5(2):41, 1991.

Martin, KS, Scheet, NJ, and Stegman, MR: Home health clients: Characteristics, outcomes of care, and nursing interventions. Am J Public Health 83:1730, 1995.

Williams, JK: Measuring outcomes in home care: Current research and practice. Home Health Care Services Quarterly 15(3):3, 1995.

General Chapter Support

Phillips, LRF: A clinician's guide to the critique and utilization of nursing research. Appleton-Century-Crofts, Norwalk, Conn, 1986. (**Note:** The author uses the term *consumer.*)

Titler, MG, and Goode, CJ (Guest eds): Research utilization. Nurs Clinics North Am 30:I-581, xv, 1995.

Publishing Scholarly Works

SUZANNE HALL JOHNSON, MN, RNC, CNS

Suzanne Hall Johnson, MN, RNC, CNS, is the editor of *Nurse Author & Editor; Dimensions of Critical Care Nursing;* and *Recruitment, Retention, & Restructuring Report.* She is the director of Hall Johnson Communications, where she presents seminars and provides audiotaped courses on professional development topics such as publishing, presenting, consulting, and entrepreneurship for advanced practice nurses. You may e-mail her at SuzanneHJ@aol.com.

11

OBJECTIVES

After completing this chapter, the reader will be able to:

1. Differentiate elements of style typically used in papers written to meet academic requirements from those elements of style characteristic of papers composed for publication.

2. Examine qualitative and quantitative research work for opportunities to publish using different formats, including clinical accomplishments or interesting procedural steps.

3. Appropriately target and plan an article for publication.

Nurses in advanced practice roles are the clinical leaders who are developing new nursing strategies and knowledge through their clinical research and practice. Chapter 10 emphasized the importance of conducting research on clinical questions and the effectiveness of the advanced practice nurse (APN). However, answers to clinical questions and visions of the valuable aspects of the APN role could remain a secret if the nurse does not publish these results.

In addition to publishing research findings, the APN can publish other types of manuscripts based on clinical practice. Even though quantitative studies are needed to develop nursing theory, qualitative studies have a place in scholarly writing as well. Dr. Kathleen Dracup, the editor of the *American Journal of Critical Care*, mentioned that "a case study can be considered a study with an 'n' size of one"[1] (p. 2). Indeed, even case-study reports can be valuable scholarly work because clinical observations often lead to researchable questions.

Nurse practitioners (NPs), clinical nurse specialists (CNSs), certified nurse midwives (CNMs), and certified registered nurse anesthetists (CRNAs) should consider writing for advanced practice journals as well as for specialty journals. As I edited the "Interviews with Editors" column for *Nurse Author & Editor* last year, I noticed a proliferation of new journals targeted to APNs. All of these journals will be vying for authors.

Also, many specialty journals are looking for articles on the new roles for APNs. For example, *Dimensions of Critical Care Nursing* has a new "Advanced Practice" column that covers expanded APN roles, such as NPs in intensive care units, CRNAs in postanesthesia units, and CNSs in nurse-run clinics for recently discharged acute-care patients. Similarly, the *Journal of Perinatal & Neonatal Nursing* has requested articles on advanced practice roles that might interest CNMs. APNs who have developed new roles, like those in Chapter 8, could publish these accomplishments in one of many different journals.

All APNs have the same publishing challenge: how to develop a manuscript that will be accepted by the publication. Whether the APN is interested in publishing clinical observations or research, there are two main problems to avoid:

1. Using a school-paper style
2. Sending in a thesis

Dr. Florence Downs, the editor of *Nursing Research*, mentioned the latter when she advises, "Use the journal style; do not assume the editor will rewrite your thesis to their [*sic*] style"[2] (p. 160).

These are common problems for APNs that cause rejections. You can avoid these two common problems and improve your manuscript's chance of acceptance by:

1. Recognizing the difference between the style for a school paper and the style for publication
2. Adapting a thesis report to a more concise manuscript style before submitting it

The following sections of this chapter describe specific strategies on what the APN can do to make this transition from school to professional writing. The sections include tips to help the APN make the transition from being a graduate student to a published author. APNs in several roles can use these guidelines for scholarly publication:

- Graduate students can use the publication guidelines to negotiate the style with a course instructor for their next paper. This way, they will gain experience in this style even during their graduate work.

- Faculty members can use the guidelines to teach APN students the publication format, so these students will be able to make the transition to professional publication after graduation.

- APNs in clinical practice can use the guidelines to develop their manuscripts for publication.

Avoiding the "School-Paper" Style Rejection*

Papers written in a "school-paper" style are frequently rejected. As a matter of fact, this is probably the most common reason for rejection when a manuscript is received in the editorial office. Because the school-paper problem is obvious on a quick review by the editor, many manuscripts with this problem are rejected outright by the editor. Worse yet, some potential manuscripts are declined at the query-letter stage, because it is obvious that the paper will be a school-paper type.

The problem is not that the paper comes from school work; rather, it is the style in which it is written. Many papers rejected for school-paper style problems were not written for a class; they were written for publication by a nurse who uses the last-known style—that of school work. New authors are not the only ones who encounter this problem; even experienced authors revert to this past style on occasion.

The school-paper style rejection is more serious than it might appear at first. School-paper style problems cause frustration for both the author and the editor. It is a major cause of wasted time for the author and of author-editor interpersonal problems. Because a school-paper style is very different from most publication styles, the author of a rejected manuscript must take considerable time for a major revision. In addition, when the author does not understand the difference in the publication styles and believes the work is good because of good grades in school, the author can resent the rejection or request for revision.

There are good reasons for the style differences between a school paper and a professional manuscript. One is that the purpose of the school paper is different from that of the professional publication. The purpose of the school paper is for the students to demonstrate their knowledge of theories and work done by previous nursing leaders. This is appropriate for the classroom because part of becoming a professional is to build your ideas on the nursing theory base and to quote professionals' ideas. In more advanced school papers, the students are encouraged to develop their own ideas; still, the paper usually starts with a summary of basic information on that topic.

*Adapted and reprinted with permission from Johnson, SH: Avoiding the "school-paper style" rejection, Nurse Author & Editor 1(3)1–6, Summer 1991. Copyright 1991 Hall Johnson Communications, 9737 West Ohio Avenue, Lakewood, CO 80226. All rights reserved. (The Web page is at http://members.aol.com/suzannehj/hello.htm, and the e-mail address is SuzanneHJ@aol.com.)

Another reason for the style differences between the school paper and professional manuscript is that in the school paper, the author is the student, whereas in the professional publication, the author is the expert. The author's goal in a professional publication is to communicate something new (an idea, technique, theory, or research project) that the nurse reader can use. For a clinical paper on "an effective way to secure an endotracheal tube," the expert is the clinical nurse who developed this technique. For a paper on "qualitative research on the experience of family members of patients with Alzheimer's disease," the nurse investigator is the expert. This switch in perspective from student to expert is what makes this style change difficult for most authors.

I often wonder exactly how many new nurse authors with excellent ideas and potential that we lose each year because they get a rejection due to this problem and never write again. My intuition tells me we may be losing many new ideas and reports of innovative nursing techniques because experienced clinical nurses write once using the familiar paper style and never write again if this first try is rejected. My experience with CNSs and graduate students shows me that we are losing reports of excellent research because the investigators are not certain how to adapt their theses into articles.

If you have experienced any of the following, you probably had a problem because of a school style:

- A "please-do-not-send it" response (or no response) to a query letter where you mentioned a school paper or a project that you did as a student.

- A quick rejection where you suspected the manuscript did not get through the first review.

- A rejection response with a notation that the paper looked like it was a school paper.

- An acceptance with suggestions for revision that included taking out basic information, omitting long quotations, shortening the extensive literature search, reducing the number of references, or editing the style of the references.

- An acceptance, but a surprise at page-proof stage that the editor added a new introduction, took out some material, edited the literature review, changed sentence structure, or rearranged sections.

- A rejected book proposal where the sample of the author's writing was in a school-paper style.

If you have had one or more of these experiences, you are in good company. Since all of us learned this paper style first in nursing school, all successful authors have learned how to adapt this style to that used by the professional publications. Most of us learned the hard way, and I was no exception.

Fortunately, I was one of the lucky ones. My first lesson about the difference between school and publication styles came from the fifth experience. My paper was accepted and revised by the editor. I was fortunate the editor was willing to put in this time to help convert the paper from school to publication style. My paper was from graduate work on the "premature infant's reflex behaviors: effect on the mother-infant relationship."[3]

Although I knew to adapt the paper to publication style, some school-paper style still remained, and it needed editing. My original 15 pages of literature summary on bonding theory, which I had already shortened to 3 pages for the manuscript, was edited to one paragraph.

From that experience, I was determined to learn how to write better, so the editor would not have to edit heavily the next time. I knew if the editor revised the paper, it was because I did not write it to the publisher's style in the first place. After the initial shock, I went back and asked myself, Did the editing make my paper better? The answer was, Yes, it did. The paper was more concise, focused on my points better, and to my surprise, I really was the expert on this topic.

Unfortunately most authors are still learning the hard way, because most editors and experienced authors have not clarified what makes the professional style different. See Table 11–1 for a comparison of school and professional styles.

Every journal and book publisher's style is different, and it is important to follow each one's format. If you have questions about whether an article or book project is appropriate for a particular publication, query the editor about your article or book and suggest how it would fit into their publication program. You can even query the editors directly from a new Web site sponsored by *Nurse Author & Editor*. The Web page (http://members.aol.com/suzannehj/hello.htm) will guide you to the ONLINE Nursing Editors page, where with one click, you can query many nursing editors.

However, some general components of professional writing are similar among all professional nursing publications. These basic similarities apply for clinical or research articles, as well as for book or journal formats. Following these eight steps can help convert your paper from school-writing style to professional-publications style.

ELIMINATE BASIC MATERIAL

School papers usually start with a review of basic information. In a professional publication, you do not need to review basic material before you present your

TABLE 11–1
Comparison of School-Paper and Professional-Publication Styles

School-Paper Style	Professional-Publication Style
• This style covers basic material first.	• Content is specific to the level of reader.
• It includes many long quotations.	• Quotations are rare and, when used, are short.
• Long literature search is presented in summary form in one section.	• References are spaced throughout to highlight author's ideas.
• Subject of sentence is the name of a person.	• Subject of sentence is a key point.
• Reference list is exhaustive.	• Reference list is selective.
• Reference list is in the school's style.	• Reference list is in the publication's style.
• Research format is used regardless of method.	• Research format is used only if author has reliable, valid research.
• Main idea is stated for the first time at the end.	• Main idea is stated clearly in the first paragraphs.

key point. A good policy is to omit all material that the target reader already knows. For example, if your target audience is clinical specialists, do not start your paper describing a new independent study course with a discussion about independent study; this audience already knows what it is. Instead, start with the uniqueness of your project because these readers want to know about the new independent study project you completed. Or in an article on an ethical dilemma, do not start with a definition of ethics; start with the dilemma. Writing at the audience's level is true for both books and articles. For research articles, include key definitions critical to your project or sample selection, but avoid the tendency to include definitions of common terms not specific to your research.

AVOID LONG QUOTATIONS

Avoid using long quotations in your paper. Although teachers want to make sure you know and can quote authorities, readers want to know what you think. Remember, your readers are busy, experienced nurses who are clinicians, educators, managers, or researchers, depending on the journal you pick. They probably have already read the primary sources from which you want to quote. Quotes rarely fit into your point anyway and take the reader off in another direction. Quoting others makes them the expert and takes away from your expertise.

Yes, in professional publications, do build on the work of others and do give credit to nursing leaders for their initial ideas and material. However, rather than quote them, put your ideas in your own words and then reference the authorities who agree. Remember, *you* are the expert and the readers want to know what *you* think. If they want more detail on what the other nursing leaders said about your topic, they can refer to that person's work in your reference list.

Of course, exceptions to the rule do exist, and sometimes quotations do fit nicely with your topic. For example, short quotations of actual clinical incidents or cases described in literature would fit well in an article on humor in nursing. However, avoid the tendency to spend the first half of your paper quoting others.

USE SELECTED REFERENCES

School papers frequently have long reference lists. It is important for the student to research and read all of the publications in their topical area, but you do not need to put them all in your paper. Some APN graduate students figure, because they did that much work, they can at least let their teachers know. Fortunately, faculty are starting to require more of students by requesting that they select only key references. Selecting pertinent references, deciding which are the best, and determining which ones are valid can be difficult. It is a higher level of learning than just repeating reference after reference, because it requires selection of key references.[4]

Remember, the audience for professional publications is different from that for school papers. You are writing for the readers, not a teacher. The readers are busy and want you to do some of the work for them; therefore, they are relying on you to refer them to the *best* references. Authors want guidance for finding the best references when they are seeking additional information on your topic. Even readers of research articles want help in finding the most relevant articles on the problem, instrument, or methods. A list of 150 references after an article is not as helpful as a selected list of the best 50 or even the best 20 references.

One strategy for avoiding the use of too many references is to check on the average number of references used in similar articles, so you know the style of that publication. Clinical journals like *Nursing98, RN,* and the *American Journal of Nursing* frequently use only a few references per article, whereas *Image: The Journal of Nursing Scholarship, Nursing Research, Heart & Lung,* and other nursing journals that publish research reports may list 50 or more references. However, in both cases, they include fewer references than most school papers or theses.

SYNTHESIZE THE PAST LITERATURE

In addition to too many references, school papers frequently have a different style for using literature support. School papers usually have a separate literature review section where past publications are summarized one after another. However, most clinical articles and research reports do not have a separate literature section; instead, the authors weave the key concepts that support their ideas through the entire paper. In research reports, use references that support the problem, conceptual framework, research methods, and data analysis technique throughout the respective sections of the research article, rather than create a separate section for a discussion of the literature.

Analysis is the key word here. For almost all professional publications, the author analyzes the literature to show how it fits the idea or research. This subtle change from literature review to synthesis demonstrates the transformation of the author from student to expert.

USE THE REFERENCE STYLE OF THE PUBLICATION

Learning to use precise reference list styles is painful. Faculty appropriately take off points on papers for reference lists not in the school's accepted format. This is an important lesson, but sometimes the point behind this practice is unclear. The point is that you must precisely follow a particular reference format, not that you should always use that school's format, or that there is only one format.

In fact, there are many formats for references, including the formats of the American Psychological Association and of the American Medical Association. To determine which format is the right one, study past publications to determine what style they used. Then, use that style as precisely as you did in school.[2,5–7]

AVOID PEOPLE'S NAMES AS SENTENCE SUBJECTS

Because of the need in school writing to review nursing leaders' work, the subjects of many sentences in school papers are the names of past nursing leaders. For example, one manuscript I recently read had a style similar to this:

> Knudson suggests that nurse participation is a key retention factor. VanClosen believes that nurses who participate in decision-making are more likely to stay. Yocer found that 9 out of 10 nurses wanted more decision making. . . .

In this example, the subjects are "Knudson," "VanClosen," and "Yocer." This is appropriate in a literature section of a research report, but not in a clinical article. The main problem is that the writer's idea never surfaced, so the reader is uncertain of the writer's point of view.

In a clinical article, write so that the main point is the subject of the sentence. For example, this sample paragraph is trying to express some very important (but hidden) points that might be clearer by using "participation" and "nurses" as the subjects.

> Nurse participation is a key retention factor. Because 9 out of 10 nurses want more decision making, nurses are more likely to stay when given more decisions. . . .

People who support these points can be referenced after the statement.

Yet, there are rare exceptions when you want to focus on the person, not the concept. For example, if the person is the main point, then focus on the person by making him or her the subject; otherwise, use the key word from your idea as the subject.

SELECT THE RESEARCH FORMAT CAREFULLY

School papers, which are intended to teach the research format, are written with research headings. However, sometimes the research is not reliable or valid; and the student mistakenly tries to publish it in the same research format. Use the research format when the research is reliable and valid, but select a clinical format when it is not.

For example, if an NP interviewed 10 family members of sudden death patients in the Emergency Department, selected the family members while working, and had no consistent interviewing tool, then the author should not write the report in a research format. However, this could still be valuable information, and the author might consider selecting one significant case and using a case-study format. Research is a strong format and is essential to building the practice and theory base of nursing, but it should not be used when your project will not meet acceptable research criteria.

I still remember that the first article I rejected as a journal reviewer was because of this problem. I empathized with the author because I knew the author had done an interesting project, but she used the wrong format for the paper. I suggested revising using a case-study approach, but as commonly happens when a school-paper error occurs, the revision was major and the paper was never revised.

MAKE YOUR IDEA CLEAR

Making your idea clear from the start is probably the hardest step in converting to professional writing. Most of us remember writing graduate papers Sunday evening before the Monday class when it was due. Usually, I wrote and wrote and wrote. When it was about long enough, I ended with the main point as the conclusion. I know it is still being done, because I still see these papers submitted for publication. They are often rejected because the nurse reader does not want to, nor has time to, wander around the subject before getting to the point.

In professional writing, make the point clear from the start. Make sure all paragraphs relate back to that same point. If they do not, omit those paragraphs. The reader should feel they have a good grasp of the main point and that it builds throughout the paper. Avoid the tendency to put some new point in a conclusion at the end; instead, reinforce the same key point you opened with at the end. The end should reinforce for the reader that he or she did indeed understand the main point.

Each journal and book publisher handles these aspects of style slightly differently, so investigate how they are handled in your target publication. By following these steps and the advice of the target journal's editor, APNs can develop a professional style that communicates their professional ideas as the experts that they are.

Adapting the Thesis Style for Publication†

Many APN authors are uncertain what to do with all the information they uncover in their research projects. Some try to put all the information into one manuscript, thus making the manuscript 50 or more pages long with over 200 references and more than 10 illustrations. These thesis-style articles are usually rejected or, at best, returned for revision.

Probably the reason APNs use thesis style is that it is the most common research style taught to them in graduate school. Although this style is excellent for developing a thesis, it is not the style of most research articles published in nursing journals.

Editors and editorial board members can quickly tell when authors have tried to put everything about their project into one publication. In addition to length, some typing items are a sure sign: very narrow margins, single spacing, and small typeface. When struggling with the problem of getting a 100-page thesis into a publication, some authors try to "squeeze" as much text into as small a space as possible. Those manuscripts are usually rejected.

An even greater problem for the nursing profession is the number of good research projects that are never published. I find more researchers who admit they did not write a manuscript after their project because of a prior rejection. These researchers tell me there are several reasons for the problem, including:

- Loss of interest, often after graduating from school and needing time "away" from the thesis topic
- Wanting to just retype the long thesis report "as is" for publication without having to reorganize the content
- Not knowing where to start to break down the voluminous information to a manageable size for publication
- Failing to plan manuscript development time during the research project

---

†Adapted and reprinted with permission from Johnson, SH: Getting your research published: Adapting the thesis style. Nurse Author & Editor 2(1):1–4, Winter 1992. Copyright 1992 Hall Johnson Communications, 9737 West Ohio Avenue, Lakewood, CO 80226. All rights reserved. (The Web page is at http://members.aol.com/suzannehj/hello.htm, and the e-mail address is SuzanneHJ @aol.com.)

If you are one of these researchers who finds it hard to convert your research project into a publication, the following advice can help: By dividing your topic into sections of manageable size and selecting the right research-based article style for your topic, you will find it easier to write the article and will have a greater chance of acceptance.

AVOID THE "ALL-IN-ONE" SYNDROME

First, avoid the feeling that you need to put everything about your project into one manuscript. Most research projects take considerable time to complete, often years. They go through many phases from developing the concept through collecting data, determining results, and considering implications. By the time the researcher is finished she or he knows so much about the topic, it is very difficult to put all of the information into an article.

Although journals vary in the lengths of articles, the range is 10 to 20 double-spaced manuscript pages for most research-based articles. The guideline sheet for the American Association of Critical Care Nurses' journal, *American Journal of Critical Care*, recommends 1500 to 4000 words for clinical and basic research studies. That corresponds to approximately 8 to 20 pages at 200 words per page.[8]

When you have accumulated important information such as a new conceptual framework from your literature review, a valuable research instrument developed in data collection, or significant results in a comparative study, these items need to be communicated. However, instead of putting them all into one article, develop each one of these slants into separate articles. The best way to take 100 pages of valuable information about a project and develop a 20-page manuscript is to break it apart into significant topics. Fig. 11–1 shows you how to divide a long thesis into parts.

This does not mean you "milk" the project for multiple publications by publishing the same research report multiple times or by splitting three hypotheses from one project into three separate articles. These tactics are unacceptable in

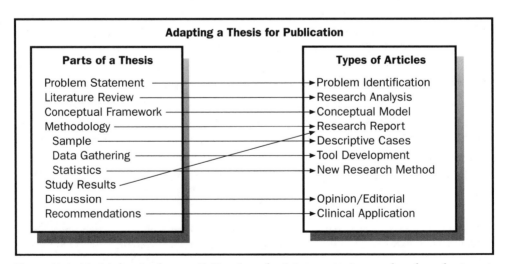

Figure 11–1 Model showing how to divide a long thesis into parts. Arrows show how thesis parts can be developed into several different types of articles (copyright 1996 SH Johnson).

nursing publication. However, it does mean that you write different articles from various *steps* in your research project.

IDENTIFY VALUABLE ASPECTS

Identify the truly valuable aspects of your research. Some research projects have several key parts; unfortunately, others have none. A project that included in-depth validity and reliability testing of an instrument plus a descriptive study using that instrument could be developed into two articles: one on the research tool and one on the descriptive study. A project using an already available research instrument on a sample size that is too small or a questionable methodology should not be submitted for publication at all.

CONSIDER MANY ARTICLE FORMATS

There are many different types of articles you can write. Review the current journals for articles based on research projects to identify examples of the many different formats. The most common types of articles written from research projects are listed below along with examples from current literature.

Problem Identification

Some projects do an excellent job of identifying a problem that was not previously recognized or understood. If your research project highlighted a new problem, consider writing a descriptive report about it. For example, the article "Nurses' Knowledge of the Code for Nurses" in the *Journal of Continuing Education in Nursing* described an interesting research project showing that a relatively small percentage of nurses had a copy of the professional code for nurses.[9]

Conceptual Framework and Theory Development

Some early steps in research projects result in new theoretical frameworks. If you analyzed the literature and developed or adapted a new conceptual framework or theory, write an article about it. For example, in the article "Empirical Development of a Middle Range Theory of Caring" in *Nursing Research,* the authors described and validated a new theory of caring.[10] If you applied a theory like one of those in Chapter 4 in a new way, consider writing about this theory application.

Research Analysis

Unique synthesis and analysis of past research are valuable. If you analyzed other research reports on a specific topic in the literature review step of your research, consider writing an article that analyzes that body of research. The article "Continuous S_vO_2 Monitoring" in *Dimensions of Critical Care Nursing* is one of several in the ongoing research-analysis section that includes charts comparing the methods and results of published research reports.[11]

Reliable and Valid Instrument

Articles on tool development can be even more valuable than studies using the instrument, because they provide tools for future research. If you demonstrated or confirmed the reliability and validity of a new or classic research tool, write an article on this part of your project. The articles "An Evaluation of Validity, Reliability, and Readability of the Critical Care Family Needs Inventory" in *Heart & Lung* and "Construct and Empirical Validity of the Self-As-Career Inventory" in *Nursing Research* show how amenable these articles are to publication.[12,13]

Descriptive Cases

Qualitative studies are a valuable addition to the literature because they add descriptive details about a situation and help to identify new research questions. If you have significant descriptive cases, develop an article that includes these case reports. Quotations regarding the difficulties in making lifestyle changes from case reports of patients in a cardiac rehabilitation program were used very effectively in the *Nursing Research* article "Empowering Potential: A Theory of Wellness Motivation."[14]

Research Method

When you have refined a research method, write an article on that procedure. For example, Regina Lederman described how to develop a coding procedure for content analysis in the article "Content Analysis: Steps to a More Precise Coding Procedure" in *MCN*.[15]

Research Report

One of the most important types of article for the nursing profession and for building your credibility as a researcher is the research report. The research report describes your research methods and results. If your research project uses credible research methods, write the research report. Usual headings include the introduction, theoretical background and/or literature review, hypotheses, methods, results, and discussion and/or implications.

Although these headings are similar to those used in a thesis, the article covers a different amount of detail in each section. Most articles include extensive details in the methods and results sections but use summaries in the other sections and fewer tables than a thesis.

To adapt your research report to a specific journal's style, check the headings and the length of each section in the journal for which you would like to write. Avoid the common misconception that it is best to include all details and tables because the editor can pick what he or she wants; most likely the editor will reject it instead. If you conducted the research in a partnership[16] and you are coauthoring a report, discuss the research format guidelines with your partner.

Research Implications and Clinical Applications

Research projects that have significant implications for nursing practice can result in publications in clinical, education, administration, and research journals.

If you have completed a research project similar to those described in Chapter 10, write a detailed article describing the clinical recommendations based on your study. After writing the research report article, consider expanding your recommendations in an article written specifically for the practicing nurse. Research application articles are printed in most nursing journals.

Research application articles usually include an abstract of the research, but primarily they emphasize what the practicing nurse can do differently based on the research. For example, in *Dimensions in Critical Care Nursing* the research methods are highlighted in a table, and the article focuses on the ways in which the critical care nurse can implement the recommendations. If you conducted the original study with a thesis advisor, be sure to negotiate in advance if this application article is a joint venture.[17]

WRITE AS YOUR PROJECT DEVELOPS

One of the mistakes of many nurse researchers is to wait until their projects are finished to start thinking about communicating the project. Plan your publications as the project evolves. This way, you will avoid the major problems of being "too tired" of your project to publish it later or seeing it as an "after-the-fact" step in your project. Even request time and support for writing in project proposals. I was granted funding for extra secretarial time for manuscript development in several projects. Many funding sponsors want you to disseminate the information, so they see the publication step as a legitimate part of the project.

In fact, many articles need to be developed as the project unfolds. For example, if you were doing a project on retention of NPs, you could write an article after each major step in the project. Here are some of the articles:

- After you developed a new model of various NP retention factors based on the literature, you could write the new concept article describing this innovative model.

- When you have analyzed 15 published research studies to determine significant NP retention factors identified in past projects, you could write the research analysis article.

- After testing the validity and reliability of an employee satisfaction tool used in other industries that you applied to NPs, you could write the research instrument article.

- After completing the study showing increased satisfaction of NPs who run their own clinics, you could write the research methods article.

- Finally, after refining your strategy further, you could write a detailed application article for an advanced nursing practice journal.

WRITE A RESEARCH-BASED BOOK

If you still cannot bring yourself to divide your research into parts because you think many sections of the project are valuable, consider writing a book. The popular book *Coping with Reality Shock* by Claudia Schmalenberg and Marlene Kramer was based on experiences from a research project.

When I wanted to publish a new family assessment tool, detailed case examples, and multiple strategies for working with high-risk families from experiences in a research project, I chose to combine them in the book. I had already published the research report article but wanted to share the clinical cases and intervention tools that would not fit in an article. This original sections based on research might have contributed to the book *High-Risk Parenting: Nursing Assessment and Strategies for the Family at Risk* (JB Lippincott, Philadelphia) being selected by the *American Journal of Nursing* for the Book of the Year award.

APNs have many ideas, clinical experiences, and research scenarios that might fit into a book. If you select the book format, you still need to reorganize your work, because even research-based books seldom use the thesis format.

Writing a research-based book is similar to the research experience; both processes have many distinct steps. Break your research project into parts and convert key accomplishments into chapters as you complete each milestone in the project.

Summary

Advanced practice nurses have valuable clinical experiences to share with colleagues and findings from research projects that can help build nursing theory. By distinguishing between school and publication formats and adapting the thesis style to a journal or book format, APNs can succeed in publishing their work.

Suggested Exercises

All of the following suggested exercises lend themselves to student peer review. Students can perform **blind peer review** by using the last four digits of their social security numbers rather than their names and having their papers fielded or refereed by faculty. Students review according to criteria developed for the assignment. In addition, students can be evaluated not only on their written products but also on their ability to provide constructive critique by developing criteria for the peer review process.

1. From the published theses or dissertations available in the library, select one on a topic that is of interest to you. The literature section constitutes an entire chapter.

   a. Rewrite the literature review, consolidating it into 2 to 3 double-spaced pages.

   b. Develop the focus (that is, the purpose and article title) for 2 to 3 individual articles that could be constructed from the thesis or dissertation.

2. Select multiple examples of direct quotations (preferably something in block form or a section of text that employs extensive use of direct quotations) from published source documents and paraphrase the citation, giving appropriate credit as is appropriate to your school's publication style guidelines.

> **3.** Plan a paper in the format of an article to be submitted for publication.
>
> a. Locate the World Wide Web site where nursing editor inquiries can be made.
>
> b. Select a journal to which the article would be sent, justifying why it is appropriate.
>
> c. Conduct a review of the article topics that appeared in the previous year of the journal, and draw conclusions about the "timeliness" and "fit" of your topic in comparison.
>
> d. Obtain a copy of the Guidelines for Authors. Write a cover letter, abstract, biographical sketch, or similar elements as dictated by the guidelines and develop at least a topical outline of your article.

REFERENCES

1. Johnson, SH: Strengthening your case study approach. Nurse Author & Editor 2(2):2 1992.
2. Johnson, SH: Adapting a thesis to publication style: Meeting editors' expectations. Dimensions of Critical Care Nursing 15:160, 1996.
3. Johnson, SH: Premature infant's reflex behaviors: Effect on the mother-infant relationship. J Obstet Gynecol Neonatal Nurs 4:15, 1975.
4. Brooks-Brunn, JA: Tips on writing a research-based manuscript: The review of literature. Nurse Author & Editor 1(2):1 1991.
5. American Psychological Association: Publication Manual of the American Psychological Association, ed 4. American Psychological Association, Washington, DC, 1995.
6. Iverson C, et al: American Medical Association Manual of Style, ed 8. Williams & Wilkins, Baltimore, 1989.
7. Damrosch, S, and Damrosch, GD: Avoiding common mistakes in APA style: The briefest of guidelines. Nurs Res 45:331, 1996.
8. Dracup, K, and Bryan-Brown, C (eds): Guide for Authors: American Journal of Critical Care. Aliso Viejo, Calif, 1991.
9. Miller, BK, Beck, L, and Adams, D: Nurses' knowledge of the code for nurses. Journal of Continuing Education in Nursing 22: 198, 1991.
10. Swanson, K: Empirical development of a middle range theory of caring. Nurs Res 40:161, 1991.
11. Copel, LC, and Stolarik, A: Continuous S_vO_2 monitoring. DCCN 10:202, 1991.
12. Macey, B, and Bouman, CC: An evaluation of validity, reliability, and readability of the Critical Care Family Needs Inventory. Heart Lung 20:398, 1991.
13. Geden, E, and Taylor, S: Construct and empirical validity of the Self-as-Carer Inventory. Nurs Res 40:47, 1991.
14. Fleury, JD: Empowering potential: A theory of wellness motivation. Nurs Res 40: 286, 1991.
15. Lederman, RP: Content analysis: Steps to a more precise coding procedure. MCN 16: 275, 1991.
16. Engebretson, J, and Wardell, DW: The essence of partnership in research. J Prof Nurs 13:38, 1997.
17. Giefer, C: Publication of a thesis: The relationship between graduate student and thesis advisor. Nurse Author & Editor 6:7, 1996.

Legal Aspects of Advanced Nursing Practice

LINDA CALLAHAN, PhD, CRNA
MARY JEANNETTE MANNINO, JD, CRNA

Linda Callahan, PhD, CRNA, received her nursing education at Rockingham Community College, Wentworth, North Carolina, and her anesthesia education at the Anesthesia Program for Nurses, North Carolina Baptist Hospital, Bowman Gray School of Medicine, in Winston Salem, North Carolina. Dr. Callahan received her bachelor of science in biology from Guilford College, Greensboro, North Carolina; her master of arts in education from California State University in Long Beach; and her doctorate in educational research and evaluation from Florida State University in Tallahassee. Dr. Callahan has a broad base of practice experience as an educator, clinician, administrator, and consultant. She has written numerous publications and is widely known as a continuing education lecturer in anesthesia and the sciences. She is past president of the American Association of Nurse Anesthetists. Dr. Callahan remains clinically active and teaches in the Department of Nursing, California State University.

Mary Jeannette Mannino, JD, CRNA, combines an independent anesthesia practice with medical-legal and business consulting. She is a graduate of George Washington University in Washington, D.C., with a bachelor of science in anesthesia, and Irvine University School of Law. Ms. Mannino's professional activities include serving as president of the American Association of Nurse Anesthetists in 1987–1988. She has been recognized for outstanding contributions to the profession, as the recipient of the Agatha Hodgins Award in 1996. *The Nurse Anesthetist and the Law* and *The Business of Anesthesia: Practice Options for Nurse Anesthetists* are the two books authored by Ms. Mannino. She has also been editor of several journals and publications for nurse anesthetists. Her professional career has included work as an educator, manager, and clinical anesthetist. She currently practices anesthesia in ambulatory surgery in her own corporation, The Mannino Group.

12

CHAPTER OUTLINE

NURSE-PRACTICE ACTS
PROFESSIONAL NEGLIGENCE (MALPRAC-
TICE)
Duty
Standard of care
Causation
Damages
Wrongful death
Proof of professional negligence
*Possible exceptions to expert witness re-
quirement*

MALPRACTICE INSURANCE
THE PATIENT AND THE ADVANCED PRAC-
TICE NURSE
PROFESSIONAL ETHICS
Historical perspectives
Ethical principles
Ethical theory bases
Ethical decision making and the clinician
Trends in ethical research in nursing
*Ethical concerns of the advanced practice
nurse*
SUGGESTED EXERCISES

CHAPTER OBJECTIVES

After completing this chapter, the reader will be able to:

1. Interpret components of the nurse-practice acts of his or her state, which define the legal scope of practice, need for collaboration, and prescriptive authority for a specific type of advanced practice.
2. Articulate the concepts of duty, standard of care, causation, and damage as applied to professional negligence in advanced nursing practice.
3. Demonstrate techniques for ethical decision making by application of a specific decision model as well as by analysis of the process of model application.
4. Incorporate knowledge about caring as an ethical concept into the development of personal moral agency within a managed-care setting.

As advanced nursing practice has evolved to new and exciting heights in the late twentieth century, legal issues become important to the practitioner, the state, and, of course, the patient. The expansion of nursing practice into areas once considered the exclusive domain of medicine and the independence of advanced practice nurses (APNs) lead to questions of legality, standards of practice, and the legendary "turf battles." The law, including statutory, regulatory, and case law, is on a different time frame from science; therefore, it may be years before a concept becomes law and legal rulings become precedent. With that in mind, advanced nurse practitioners should look at rulings in other related fields to better understand the legality of their practices.

Nurse anesthesia has set some legal trends for other APNs. Although obvious differences exist between nurse anesthetist, nurse midwife, and nurse practitioners who practice in ambulatory-care settings, most of the case law that sets precedent has been from the anesthesia portion of advanced nursing practice. The legal aspects of nurse anesthesia practice have been an area of discussion, myths, political activity, and clinical concerns for as long as the profession has existed. The legal definition of nonphysician anesthesia practitioners, the role of advanced nursing practice, state nurse-practice acts, and federal legislation continue to be debated in legal and political arenas. Likewise, medical malpractice concerns and the issue of vicarious liability accompany the nurse anesthetist to the operating room (OR) every day.

Even though nurses have been administering anesthesia for over 100 years, there have been constant legal challenges to the practice, for example, whether nurse anesthesia constitutes the illegal practice of medicine. These challenges continue in various formats and will be expanded to encompass all advanced nurse practitioners.

The American legal system functions at several levels, including laws enacted by the state and federal legislative branches, regulations at the executive levels, and the common-law system, based on precedent. The legal authorization for all of nursing practice is found in nurse-practice acts; state health and safety codes; other professional practice acts, including those of medicine, dentistry, and podiatry; and federal medical laws and cases that interpret those laws. Judicial decisions on vicarious liability and professional negligence are important in identifying the standards of practice of the profession and set a precedent for future decisions.

It is important for the reader to understand that each state has the constitutional right to set its own laws and legal process. The cases presented in this chapter and elsewhere should be evaluated with that understanding. However, to complicate the issue, one state's courts will review similar rulings in other states when formulating their opinions.

Nurse-Practice Acts

Each state has the obligation to protect the health and safety of its citizens. By various statutes, the state attempts to assure the public that a professional who is granted a license has met the qualifications and scope of practice as defined by the legislature. The nurse-practice act is the prevailing state law that defines the practice for registered professional nurses. In recent years, recognition has been given to APNs based on education, skills, and, frequently, certification. The majority of the states recognize advanced practice nursing, but there is no uniformity to their laws, with every state using different or unique language in framing its law. Generally, the advance practice portions of the nursing statutes contain:

- Definition of advance practice
- Legal scope of practice
- Educational requirements
- Collaboration and consultation requirements

Prescriptive authority may also be codified in this area of the nurse-practice act, but this practice varies from state to state.

Professional Negligence (Malpractice)

If a patient suffers harm from the actions of an advanced nurse practitioner or any other health-care professional, the legal theory that usually applies is the tort concept of negligence. Tort law recognizes the responsibility of an individual to act in the way an "ordinary, reasonable person" would under similar circumstances. A deviation from, or breach, of this reasonable person standard is considered actionable under the rules of negligence. The term **malpractice** has been used to encompass all liability-producing conduct by professionals.

For an action to be considered negligent, the following components must be present and established by the plaintiff:

- Duty
- Standard of care
- Causation
- Damages

DUTY

To be held liable for professional negligence, it must first be established that the nurse practitioner owed a duty to the injured party. This may be established under contract theory or, most frequently, by a professional-patient relationship. The legal issue is whether or not a nurse practitioner has a legal duty to the patient, when this duty starts, and when it ends.

In *Ascher v. Gutierrez*, the precedent was set for the time component of duty as it relates to anesthesia cases. There is not much direction from the courts on when the duty begins in anesthesia; however, it is generally considered to be when the anesthesia professional begins the continual care of the patient. When the legal duty ends has been addressed by the courts in the following case:

> The facts as reported in the court decision show that the patient was an 18-year-old female admitted to Columbia Hospital for Women in Washington, DC, for dilatation and curettage. Thiopental was administered and shortly thereafter the patient developed a laryngospasm. Attempts to relax the spasm manually and by injections were unsuccessful. An endotracheal tube was inserted, but the patient was cyanotic, hypotensive, and ultimately had severe disabling brain damage.

There was considerable dispute regarding the presence of the anesthesiologist in the operating room at the time of the incident. The anesthesiologist claimed he left the OR shortly after injecting the thiopental, but only after being relieved by another anesthesiologist. The plaintiff showed that the other anesthesiologist was administering an anesthetic in another section of the hospital when the incident occurred and could not have relieved on the case.

The court ruled that once a physician enters into a professional relationship with a patient, he is not at liberty to terminate the relationship at will. The relationship will continue until it is ended by one of the following circumstances: (1) the patient's lack of need for further care, or (2) withdrawal of the physician upon being replaced by an equally qualified physician. The court ruled that withdrawal from the case under other circumstances constitutes a wrongful abandonment of the patient and if patient suffers any injury as a proximate result of such abandonment, physician is liable.

The plaintiff was awarded $1,550,000.

Ascher v Gutierrez, 533 F2d 1235 (DC Cir), *add* 175 US 100 (1976)

STANDARD OF CARE

Negligence law, in general, presupposes some uniform standards of behavior against which a defendant's conduct is to be evaluated. Members of the health-care professions are expected to possess skill and knowledge in the practice of their profession beyond that of ordinary individuals and to act in a manner consistent with that added capability.

Formulation of the standard of care by which an advanced nurse practitioner is evaluated is complex when one considers that an identifying characteristic of any professional group is its inherent right to direct and control its activities.

The standards by which a nurse practitioner will be judged usually come from expert testimony and standards established by the profession. The judicial system recognizes that juries are composed of lay people with limited or no knowledge of medical activities. For that reason, expert witnesses who are members of the profession are asked to testify about the standard of care. The rationale is that all professionals should be held to the same level of skill as their peers.

Most professional organizations have formulated and published standards of practice for the profession. It is likely that those standards would be admitted into evidence in a negligence action and, though not conclusive of the standards of practice, would carry some authority.

Locality Rule

Historically, the defined standards of care for the medical profession were limited to a specific geographic setting. This narrow ruling was interpreted to mean that one had to practice in terms of the standard of practice in one's community. However, the strict locality rule proved to be impractical and severely limited the pool of expert witnesses. The courts considered the fact that modern communications have expanded access to information and modified the rule to include practice in the "same or a similar locality."

In more recent years, the locality rule has undergone continued scrutiny by the courts, and in most jurisdictions, the standard has been expanded from a local level to a national level. For that reason, it is imperative that advanced nurse practitioners remain current in state-of-the-art practice for the entire country, because they will be held accountable for practice consistent with a national standard.

CAUSATION

In malpractice actions, the plaintiff must establish that the alleged negligent act of the defendant caused the injury. This element of negligence, called **causation,** is an important factor in malpractice cases. Proof of causation may be based on direct testimony, usually by the use of expert witnesses.

The two most common tests to establish causation are classified as "but for" and "substantial factor." In the former, the plaintiff must prove that it was more probably true than not that the patient's injury would not have occurred but for the defendant's action. The latter test requires that the defendant's conduct was a substantial factor in producing the injury. The standard most commonly applied to causation requires that the patient's injury has been "more likely than not" the result of the defendant's conduct.

Multiple causation can present difficulties in malpractice cases. The cause of the injury frequently is not easily determined to be due to a single factor. An example of this can be seen in anesthesia cases where a patient dies from hypovolemia. Was the cause of the death due to errors in surgical technique or failure of the anesthetist to adequately monitor and replace lost fluid? A plaintiff's attorney usually will attempt to ascertain multiple causation, so that many defendants will be contributing to the damage awards.

DAMAGES

The final element necessary for actionable negligence is **damages.** This term generally refers to the loss or injury suffered. Damages are usually categorized as *special, general,* and *punitive.*

The purpose of compensatory damages is to make an appropriate, and usually counterbalancing, payment to the plaintiff for an actual loss or injury sustained through the act or default of the defendant, thereby "making the plaintiff whole" as much as possible. General damages are those that flow from the wrong complained of and are often known as "pain and suffering." As a result of tort reform legislation seen recently in many states, a cap to general damages has been set by the legislatures. This cap is generally $150,000 to $250,000. Special damages are the actual monetary value of the negligent act and are reflected in such awards as additional money for hospital bills because of anticipated custodial care for the life. Punitive or exemplary damages are awarded as punishment to the defendants for acts that the jury considers to be aggravated, willful, or wanton. Punitive damages are awarded or withheld at the discretion of the jury.

WRONGFUL DEATH

When a patient dies as the result of negligent acts of the provider, the survivors may collect for **wrongful death.** A number of states have wrongful death statutes that establish the bases for recovery and the maximum amount of damages that may be awarded.

The issue of recovery for loss of life's pleasures and a wrongful death action were addressed in this Pennsylvania involving a nurse anesthetist.

> A 5-year-old child, in excellent health, was admitted for a T & A [tonsillectomy and adenoidectomy]. A nurse anesthetist supervised by an anesthesiologist administered the anesthetic. During the procedure, the anesthesiologist was called to an emergency in another OR. When he returned, he noticed the child was cyanotic with no apparent heartbeat. The nurse anesthetist was still administering a full concentration of anesthetic agent and was not using precordial monitoring. Emergency resuscitation restored the patient's heartbeat, but because of the prolonged cardiac arrest, he suffered severe damage and died several weeks later.
>
> The child's father filed suit on behalf of his son's estate for wrongful death. The jury awarded the estate $455,199 and the hospital appealed.
>
> The Pennsylvania Supreme Court ruled on the trial judge's instructions to the jury on the amount of damages. The trial court instructed the jury that it could consider pain and suffering and compensate for loss of future earnings and loss of amenities or pleasures of life. In the higher court's ruling, they said loss of life's pleasures or amenities is one of the elements of recovery for wrongful death and survival.
>
> *Willinger v Mercy Catholic Medical Center of Southern Pennsylvania,* A2d 1188 (Pa 1978)

PROOF OF PROFESSIONAL NEGLIGENCE

Except for certain exceptions, expert testimony is required to establish the appropriate standard of care in professional negligence cases. Both the plaintiff and the defendant rely on the testimony of expert witnesses to prove or to defend their case. Experts may also be used to determine causation and damages. To qualify as an expert witness, a person must possess qualifications and be knowledgeable in the area in question. The federal rules of evidence indicate that an expert be qualified by "knowledge, skill, experience, training, and education."

POSSIBLE EXCEPTIONS TO EXPERT WITNESS REQUIREMENT

Expert testimony is the primary method for establishing the standard of care for professionals. There are, however, exceptions to this rule that have a direct application to advanced nursing practice.

Package Inserts and Manufacturer's Instructions

Whether package inserts of drugs or manufacturer's instructions regarding use of equipment should be admissible as evidence of the standard of care is an interesting and a complex question. It is often common practice to use drugs in ways that deviate from the package inserts. The clinician is well aware that package inserts and other drug information protect the manufacturer and can be interpreted as being restrictive in practical situations.

Most courts hold that manufacturer's recommendations are at least admissible as evidence of the standard of care. However, they have seldom, if ever, been considered conclusive. A number of courts have upheld the admissibility of manufacturer's instructions where they are properly validated or refuted by an expert witness. It appears that most courts would not accept a manufacturer's recommendations and package inserts as conclusive evidence of the standard of care. Although the instructions would probably be admitted into evidence, expert witnesses would be called to reinforce the standard of practice.

Medical Literature

The rules of evidence clearly regard the use of textbooks, periodicals, and other literature as hearsay; thus, medical literature is not admissible as direct evidence to prove the statements it contains. The arguments against using this literature for establishing conclusive evidence of the standard of care are many and include the following:

- The author may not be present.
- There is no opportunity for cross-examination.
- The literature may be out of date.

It has been recommended that a more sensible view would be to hold medical literature as admissible under limited circumstances. Where a conflict exists between the medical treatise and the standards established by expert witnesses, a good approach would hold both sources admissible as evidence. The jury or the judge could then determine which source was most probative.

Other methods of establishing standard of care include standards and guidelines published by a professional organization, departmental policies, and statutes. Except for nurse anesthetists, there have been few negligence cases against advanced nurse practitioners that have appellate court rulings setting legal precedents. It is hoped that the reason is that there are few negligence cases against nurse practitioners and not that the law moves at a slow pace.

Malpractice Insurance

Along with the independence of advanced nursing practice and the high level of knowledge and skill required, it follows that the responsibility and accountability of advanced practice leads to a greater risk of being sued. For that reason, APNs should be covered for professional negligence through an insurance program.

The employment status of the APN is important in determining whether to purchase an individual policy. Under the laws of agency, the employer is responsible for the acts of its employees and, as such, is responsible to defend and pay damages in a lawsuit occurring under the auspices of that employment. If the nurse practitioner is self-employed or uncertain of adequate coverage by the employer, it may be advisable to purchase an individual policy. The cost of malpractice insurance is dependent on the type of practice and its potential for liability claims. Nurse anesthesiology and nurse midwifery are the areas of highest malpractice insurance premiums.

The Patient and the Advanced Practice Nurse

We must not lose sight of the patient in all of the discussion of nursing theory, critical learning, and legal standards. Most nurse practitioners select the advanced practice model because they enjoy caring for patients and, in the end, concerns for patients' health and well-being and for delivery of high-quality care are the highest priorities. For that reason, the integration of legal and ethical principles into clinical practice is paramount and serves as the focus of this chapter.

Nurses tend to view legal issues from a paternalist rather than a practical standpoint. Frequently, they want to quote a law to justify a practice, when the law is rarely specific and is open to interpretation, modification, and reversal. It is much more practical for the individual nurse practitioner to use knowledge of applicable laws, regulations, and standards to determine how to manage their practice, to expect adequate reimbursement, and then to go about doing what they know and love: providing high-quality patient care.

Professional Ethics

The branch of philosophy called **ethics,** or moral philosophy, deals with questions of human conduct. The word *ethics* is derived from the Greek *ethos,* meaning customs, habitual usages, conduct, and character.[1] Ethics is concerned with defining the moral dimension of life in terms of duties, responsibilities, conscience, justice, and other societal concerns and issues. The stated fact that is nonethical in content is concerned with the "is" of the actions, whereas an ethical judgment concerns the "why" of the actions.[2]

Ethical thinking is shaped by our worldview, which is in turn shaped by all the other dimensions of our existence. Recently in the Western world, a greater concern has been expressed about our living environment. With the influences of Eastern culture, this has led to changes in attitudes. Campaigns to save the South American rain forests and endangered species are examples of such changes in thinking. Whatever our specific attitudes, there is no doubt that the scope of morality is affected by our general worldview. Today, the tendency is to separate ethics from traditional moral or religious beliefs. This is probably not entirely possible because every ethical system seems to raise questions about the worldview on which it is based.[3] Even though the world's great religions disagree in many ways, all attempt to point mankind to what lies *beyond.* Smart[3] stated that perhaps what is needed is "transcendental humanism." He defined this as valuing human welfare and seeing this welfare in the light of an eternal vision—that is, the sense of the beyond allowing one to see anew the sacredness of the person.

To think ethically requires defining the characteristics of an ethical problem. Rational choices are based on factual information but are always somewhat subjective; that is, they involve value judgment. This is also a necessary characteristic of an ethical problem. Of necessity, the concept of choice involves freedom, or the ability to make a choice, and responsibility for both right and wrong actions. Choice requires reasoning and decision making. The whole unity of knowing and valuing that comprises an individual is used when human beings make choices, especially when the choices are difficult.

A second characteristic of ethical problems is the presence of value conflicts and a lack of certainty regarding the amount or type of information needed to make appropriate decisions. Hence, ethical problems are inherently perplexing.[4]

Finally, reaching answers to ethical problems will have profound and far-reaching effects on one's perception of:

- The rights of human beings
- Relationships among human beings
- The relationship of human beings to society
- The relationship of human beings to the world

Though difficult, such judgments tend to establish precedent and justification for future activity. The decision serves as a model for our future behavior.[4]

Bioethics is the marriage of ethics and science. It is important for APNs to determine if a decision is a matter of clinical judgment rather than an ethical issue. Ethical reasoning, unlike scientific reasoning, cannot be supported by definitive proof about what is the right or wrong action in a given situation. McManus[2] noted that ethics serves as a guide to the development of a "well-traveled trail" that may lead to better behavior and better actions among people.

HISTORICAL PERSPECTIVES

In 1937, C. A. Aikens[5] wrote *Studies in Ethics for Nurses* and included chapters devoted to truth in nursing reports, discretion in speech, obedience, teachability, respect for authority, discipline, and loyalty. Such early works focused on the morality of the individual and on the nurse's duties, obligations, and loyalties.[6]

The American Medical Association (AMA) adopted a Code of Ethics in 1847 when the organization was formed. This was a hallmark event, because before this time, there was no regulation of professional behavior. The AMA's initial Code of Ethics dealt with the relationships of physicians to each other, to the patient, and to the public. Revisions followed with continual emphasis on professional conduct. Over time, this activity helped to solidify the idea that medicine was a dignified and honorable calling. Professional codes of ethics generally call for a covenant, or an agreement, between the client and the provider and are today viewed as a social contract.[2]

The contrast in ethical development between medicine and nursing has often been remarkable. This is due largely to the fact that nursing has historically been allied to the ideal of treating the person rather than the disease. From this belief, the notion of the superiority of prevention over cure developed. Medicine, on the other hand, has historically emphasized curing as a response to the presence of disease. The APN is often called on to combine the concerns of both perspectives. Complex technological problems, new legal issues, and new economic situations offer a challenging context for ethical thinking and behavior for today's APN.

Utilitarianism has probably been one of the most powerful and influential ethical systems in modern times. John Stuart Mill (1806 to 1873) was the chief proponent of this philosophy. From this viewpoint, moral action is perceived as *utility.* Utility is defined according to whether something helps to produce human happiness or reduce human suffering. This philosophical approach, or ethical system, has shaped much of modern political and economic policies in the democratic West. Often considered inherent to utility is the belief that the basis of all values lies in the individual human being and that the quality of human relationships is of ultimate importance.[3]

Opposed to utilitarian individualism is the collectivism of the Marxist tradition. In this philosophical approach, human behavior and economics are so closely interwoven that ethics is also seen as collective. Actions are good if they support the revolution and help move mankind toward a society in which all people live in harmony.[3]

ETHICAL PRINCIPLES

All ethical problems involve moral principles. Such principles are necessary to provide guidance for thought because universal solutions cannot be reached in those situations that can rotely be applied to another problem. Each ethical problem must be examined in the context of the particular circumstances. There are four guiding principles that are important to bioethics:

1. Self-determination
2. Nonmaleficence
3. Beneficence
4. Justice

Self-determination or **autonomy** is a basic social value. An autonomous act is an act of intention that is independent of coercion by others. The American Nurses' Association Code of Ethics supports patients' self-determination as a moral right.[7] This moral right was defined by Callahan[8] as follows:

> The right to control one's body and one's treatment and the emphasis given to self-determination, privacy, freedom, and autonomy. The emphasis on not being deceived and being given complete and truthful information, all point to an important aspect of a rights-based view, namely the role of an individual patient's will in individual decision making. (p. 19)

Those giving care must acknowledge and respect the autonomy of each client. It may be argued that the only permissible reason to remove a person's social or personal autonomy is to prevent harm to others. Respect for the client's autonomy and the opportunity for professional autonomy in medical practice involve possession of the threshold element of competence, the disclosure of information, and consent without duress. The presence of these three elements imposes an order on conflicting claims and offers finality, which is often sufficiently strong to override the law and prevailing custom.[2]

Nonmaleficence is the concern for doing no harm or evil. Generally, the reference is to physical harm, pain, disability, and death, but harm can be defined both broadly and narrowly. Actions that inflict harm may be necessary for ultimate client well-being, but such actions always require moral judgment. Doing something and doing nothing are both actions determined by personal decision. As an example, withdrawal of treatment is often deemed a nonmaleficence decision. If "letting die" seems justifiable, the withdrawal of nutrition and hydration is usually seen as justified. The literature does not support the concept that cessation of artificial feeding and hydration is associated with pain or suffering, although there may be increased stress for caregivers and family. The principle of nonmaleficence requires an interpretation of values and the consideration of risks and benefits as part of a thoughtful and careful action.[2]

Beneficence is the act of promoting or doing good. This principle is action oriented and requires the provision of benefits and the balance of harms and benefits. Ethical problems arise when benefits are conflicting. The principle of beneficence often appears at odds with the principle of veracity or truthfulness. As a professional, should one ever lie? Many believe that although truthful alternatives must always be sought, that intrinsically a lie may be a right choice if it is necessary to avoid greater evil. Specific criteria have been offered to assist the individual to determine whether or not a paternalistic lie is justified[9]:

- The lie produces positive benefits for the person lied to that outweigh any evil that might result.
- It is possible to describe the greater good that would occur.
- The individual would have wanted to be lied to.
- All participants would always be willing to allow the violation of truthfulness.

Justice requires weighing issues and responding to the facts that are present. Philosophically, no consensus exists about what constitutes justice. The nurse in advanced practice is responsible for distributing just behavior and comparable treatment to each client; therefore, justice is an active process. Retributive justice demands that if a client is harmed, reparation or a means by which to right the wrong be applied.[2]

ETHICAL THEORY BASES

Using the basic ethical principles, philosophers have constructed various theories that may form the bases for ethical analysis. Moral theories generally address compliance with rules, the consequences of action, or dispositions relative to behavior. The previous three variants are often classified into two broad approaches[10]:

1. Normative
2. Nonnormative.

The **normative** approach explores ethical obligations and duties. This approach allows investigation of what is right and wrong, what we are to be, and what we may value. A concern for reason formed the Socratic roots of ethics in the fifth century BC.[2] At present all humans live in a global village in which different cultures and worldviews interact. An optimal normative approach would call for tolerance and formation of a society in which there is genuine plurality of beliefs and values in order to breed an ethic of "social personalism." Under this ethic, each person respects the social values of the other because there is genuine respect for that person.

Nonnormative theoretical variants presuppose universally applicable principles of right and wrong and seek to systematically provide justifiable answers to moral questions. One may assess the rightness or wrongness of an act by examining the interests of the actor or by assessing the consequences of the act itself. **Deontology,** or the act of examining the interests of the actor in performing certain acts, is derived from the Greek word *deontais* (duty), which originally meant obedience to rules or binding duties. This sense of duty should consist of rational respect for fulfillment of obligations to other human beings. For example, the commanding duty for the health professional is to respect clients and colleagues and their right to autonomy (self-determination).[10] Emmanuel Kant (1724 to 1804) asserted that respect for persons is the primary test of duty.[11] Kant stated that all persons have equal moral worth, and no rule can be moral unless all people can apply it autonomously to all other human beings. The deontological approach is often applied by health professionals who work with individual clients.[2]

Teleology (utilitarianism) is a consequentialist approach that is paternalistic in application. The root *telos* comes from the Greek for "end of the consequences." All acts are evaluated as positive to the extent to which desirable results are achieved. The right action is that which leads to the best consequence and the greatest good. This is often the ethical foundation applied in the formation of health-care policy decisions. A difficulty with this approach is the problem of defining and properly weighing the greatest good, as well as deciding who should receive the act.[2]

ETHICAL DECISION MAKING AND THE CLINICIAN

Rapid advances in technology make many demands on the character, education, and abilities of the advanced nurse practitioner. Applying ethical responsibility in health care does not require the discovery of new moral principles on which to build a new theoretical system. Nor does it require one to evaluate new approaches to ethical reasoning. It does encourage professionals to lay down a proper foundation for the application of established moral rules. Society and the professions demand that practitioners be knowledgeable in the applied field of health-care ethics and the process of ethical decision making.[2]

The emphasis on scientific developments throughout the past several centuries has caused ethics to take a quantitative rather than a qualitative approach. Science has sought to separate itself from concerns about human values and value systems.[12] The changing demands of today's health-care environment make it clear that the application of science in medicine is not value-free. The study of values and their effect on human behavior is an area that requires vigorous research.

Physicians and nurses constantly make value judgments. McManus[2] stated that perhaps the study of ethics is best capsulized by the understanding that all health-care professionals should assume the responsibility of asking the "whys" of what "ought" to be. The issues may be reduced to what "is" and what "ought to be."

Providers are bombarded with reams of information each day in clinical practice. Consciously and unconsciously, they make selections from these data and draw conclusions about themselves, their clients, and their lives. All information carries equal weight until they assign value. Valued information stimulates further exploration of potential meaning. Dilemmas often occur as problems that require ethical decisions emerge. A **dilemma** is a choice between equally undesirable alternatives. The two essential components to an ethical dilemma are:

1. Existence of a real choice between possible courses of action

2. Placement of decision makers of different values on each possible action or on the outcome of that action

In clinical practice, dilemmas occur when the enforcement of the law does not appear to bring about justice, when there is no obvious right or wrong behavior, when right behavior appears to have the wrong outcome, or when personal sacrifice is the consequence of following ideals.[13] Resolutions to such ethical dilemmas can have a profound and far-reaching effect on personal perceptions of fellow human beings, society, and the relationship of human beings to the world.[11]

Decision-making models offer the nurse in advanced clinical practice an opportunity for self-examination and self-knowledge. Clinical decisions are most often of mixed character, containing moral dimensions but rarely being solely moral decisions. According to Fowler[14]:

> Clinical decisions often involve weighing moral values against political, economic, aesthetic, and prudent values. (p. 319)

Ethical decision making is consistent with critical thinking.[15] Situations must be processed by the identification of ethical dimensions within the context and by the application of principles of moral reasoning. This process offers the greatest assurance that final decisions or courses of action will be the "best." Use of the critical-reasoning process produces less chance for mistakes based on ignorance, personal bias, or strong paternalism.[15]

In an article on effective decision making for the occupational health nurse manager, Brown[16] discusses three types of decisions that are common to all nurses in advanced practice:

1. Operational decisions that must be made to regulate day-to-day activities

2. Ten-second decisions that require an immediate assessment of the situation and a response

3. Decisions that tend to be uncomfortable for those involved

The complex process of ethical decision making leads to making a decision, acting on it, and justifying the action. In some situations, providers are participants, but at other times, they function only to share a point of view. Three levels of decision making are believed to exist[2]:

1. The immediate level, which is characterized by no time for reflection

2. The intermediate level, in which there is some time for exploration and reflection

3. The deliberate level, in which adequate time exists to gather and examine information and to reach a rational decision after reflection[2]

Since the early 1970s, a number of decision-making models have been developed for use by health-care providers. Most of these models have focused on dilemmas as "triggers" for ethical analysis. An appropriate example, the Thompson and Thompson Decision Model for Nursing depicts a problem-solving process. The process allows critical review of the operant situation and assessment of all the variables, as well as highlighting pertinent ethical issues raised by the situation. Table 12–1 and Table 12–2 provide the model and an analysis of the process of model application.

TABLE 12–1
Thompson and Thompson Decision Model

1. Review the situation and identify
   a. Health problems
   b. Decisions needed
   c. Key individuals involved

2. Gather information that is available to
   a. Clarify the situation
   b. Understand the legal implications
   c. Identify the bureaucratic or loyalty issues

3. Identify the ethical issues or concerns in the situation and
   a. Explore the historical roots
   b. Explore current philosophical/religious positions on each
   c. Identify current societal views on each

4. Examine personal and professional values related to each issue, including
   a. Personal constraints raised by the issues
   b. Guidance from professional codes or standards
   c. Moral obligations to individuals

5. Identify the moral positions of key individuals by
   a. Direct questioning
   b. Consideration of advance directives
   c. Consideration of substituted judgments

6. Identify value conflicts, including
   a. Potential sources of each
   b. Possible strategies for the resolution of each

7. Determine who should make the final decision, considering
   a. Who owns the problem
   b. Whether the patient can participate in the decision process
   c. Who can speak on behalf of the patient (substituted on basis of best interest judgment) when patient cannot

8. Identify the range of possible actions and
   a. Describe the anticipated outcome for each action
   b. Identify the elements of moral justification for each action
   c. Note if the hierarchy of principles or utilitarianism is to be used

9. Decide on a course of action and carry it out
   a. Knowing the reasons for the choice of action
   b. Sharing the reasons with all involved
   c. Establishing a time frame for a review of the outcomes

10. Evaluate the result of the decision/ action and note
   a. Whether the expected outcomes occurred
   b. If a new decision process is complete
   c. Whether elements of the process can be used in similar situations

A clinician preparing to use any developed ethical decision-making model must have adequate knowledge of the topics involved in ethics, practice in developing skills needed for recognition of ethical dilemmas, the ability to develop an ethical stance, and the confidence to act from that stance. Adequate preparation includes understanding the premise of critical thinking and applied analysis. Knowledge can be enhanced by regular discussion of ethical topics with peers and at professional meetings.[2]

Dilemma situations have been labeled by some philosophers as incorrigible to moral reasoning. A dilemma may not be solvable but it is always resolvable. In some cases, lack of available time may limit gathering of sufficient relevant information and considering alternative actions. In this situation, the amount of time available has created a dilemma where none would have otherwise existed.[4] Having adequate time for data collection and reflection before a decision is required increases one's responsibility to gather extensive information, to weigh the values of all involved, and to estimate the results of each possible course of action. As noted by Curtin,[4] providers must guard against a tendency to avoid making a choice when it is necessary to do so. Procrastination used to

TABLE 12–2
Analysis of the Thompson and Thompson Decision Model

Step 1: Review the situation. The first step involves identifying significant components of the situation, as well as the individuals involved in making the decision. A clear understanding of the situation facilitates each subsequent action.

Step 2: Gather additional information. Additional information that may influence the situation is collected in this step. Demographic data, socioeconomic status, health status, prognosis, level of understanding, preferences, competence, and family members and/or significant others involved with the situation are examples of additional information that needs to be assessed.

Step 3: Identify the ethical issues. Understanding ethics and ethical principles is essential to accurately identify the issues of the situation. Another key to successful identification of the ethical issues is to gain a historical perspective on the issues.

Step 4: Identify personal and professional values. When a nurse defines his or her personal and professional moral positions as they relate to ethical issues, the nurse is better prepared to understand his or her position in a particular situation. Awareness of professional codes will help to identify professional values.

Step 5: Identify values of key individuals. The moral values of the key people involved in the situation are as important as the nurse's values and are assessed in this step.

Step 6: Identify value conflicts. Value conflicts can occur within one individual or between the persons involved in the situation. Understanding why conflicts exist and keeping track of how conflicts have been resolved in the past assist with the final decision.

Step 7: Determine who should decide. Many people are available to assist in making the final decision. The physician, nurse, social worker, patient, and patient's family are all involved in health-care ethics. At this point, it must be decided who should be responsible for the decision or action.

Step 8: Identify range of actions with expected outcomes. A clear list of alternatives helps the nurse recognize possible consequences of a decision and identify a course of action.

Step 9: Decide on the course of action and carry it out. The person must decide on the course of action.

Step 10: Evaluate results of the decision. The final step involves evaluating the decision made to determine if the outcome was the one anticipated. Evaluation also provides information that assists in future ethical decision making.

avoid responsibility should be avoided, as well as hastened judgment that precludes careful reflection. There are levels of immediacy in decision making. However, the fact that decisions must be made immediately in some situations cannot be used to excuse the lack of thoughtful action in other situations. For example, it is justifiable to give treatment in an emergency situation (i.e., when a person is in immediate danger of death) without the patient's informed consent. However, it is not justifiable to do this in situations in which some time is available. Though often avoided, the deliberate level of decision making is by far the most common in clinical practice. Making difficult ethical decisions is often avoided because such decisions are personally taxing, require the acceptance of great responsibility, and cannot be accomplished successfully without sensitivity to the human rights and values of others.[4]

Decisions, including ethical decisions, do not occur in a vacuum but are operant within a context that consists of an inner and outer environment. The sum total of an individual's experiences make up the inner environment. The outer environment consists of the actions and reaction of others, time constraints, and material resources. It is improbable that the environmental events that modify the setting of a decision will be repeated, and the operational self brought to the decision-making situation cannot be repeated. In this sense, all decisions are unique but not necessarily unrelated.[4]

TRENDS IN ETHICAL RESEARCH IN NURSING

The enormous and ongoing changes in the structure of the health-care delivery system are greatly affecting practice relationships, producing new concerns for both consumers and providers. Often, the resulting complex organizational environments produce significant changes in the cultural context of practice and provide the basis for a revised starting point for future research in health-care ethics. The communal moral experience that results may be used as a starting point for such research.[17]

Current biomedical ethics emphasizes problems of individual technical competence in the treatment of human beings,[18] but an exchange of ideas about specific ethical issues related to human beings has begun. Topics include the relationship between ethical theory and practical judgment,[19] the patient rights model,[20] the ideal of shared decision making within physician-patient relationships,[21] the ethical negotiation model,[22] and the way cultural, religious, social, and economic diversity complicate ethical decisions.[23] Recent nursing research has centered on exploring responsiveness to others or the ethics of caring. Studies are now enriching our understanding of the pathways by which moral interaction between health-care providers, clients, and families; advances in technology; and the changing cultural context inform and shape ethical decisions.[17]

Ketefian[24] found that 36 clinical ethics studies were reported in the literature from 1983 to 1987. A review of these studies indicated that the majority dealt with common constructs, such as moral reasoning and application of ethical precepts to nursing practice. A summary of the results of the research efforts revealed that:

- There was a positive relationship among cognitive variables such as critical thinking, intelligence, and moral decision making.
- Moral reasoning did not increase with instruction.
- Educational level was unrelated to ethical practice.
- The academic levels of most nurses were adequate to facilitate patient advocacy and risk taking.
- Prior ethics courses were unrelated to application of ethical principles in current practice.
- Cultural differences played a role in ethical nursing practice.
- The perception of powerlessness by providers within the organizational work environment was negatively related to ethical practice.

Recently, researchers have looked to practice itself as the operant domain for nursing ethics-grounded theory because ethical decision-making applications from formal or utilitarian philosophical frameworks have not always provided adequate answers to ethical dilemmas in practice. For example, a qualitative field study by Carpenter[25] revealed that ethical decision making in the clinical setting appears to be a 10-step process beginning with an emotional response to an event affecting clinical practice and ending with feelings that affect the nurse's view of self and the profession. Ethical dilemmas in practice appear to have a direct impact on whether a nurse remains in the profession. Value differences between the members of the health-care team and clients and the significance of the clinical context in the making of ethical choices are extremely important. Aroskar[26] emphasized that the ethical interaction between the nurse and physician is the starting place from which to achieve patient safety goals. This premise exemplifies the emergence of the morality of care and responsibility as a dominant force in nursing ethics during the mid-1980s. Roach[27] noted that caring is the human mode of being. The concept of caring can be conceptually "unpacked" to reveal the following components:

- The capacity or power to care
- The calling forth of this capacity
- The responsibility of being called to someone who, or something which, matters
- The actualization of the capacity or power to care
- The activity or performance of caring as manifested in specific caring behaviors

Attributes of caring include *compassion, competence, confidence, conscience,* and *commitment.*

Watson[28] defined caring as the moral ideal in nursing where protection, preservation, and enhancement of human dignity are mandates for the clinician. Leiniger[29] explored caring in nursing from a transcultural perspective and described culture as the missing link in our greater understanding of the ethical and moral dimensions of human care.

The nursing philosopher Gadow[30] more than any other has emphasized the moral position of advocacy in nursing. According to Gadow, the nurse must enter into and experience as far as possible the subjective world of the client to be an advocate through a caring presence with and for the client. Gadow further emphasized that truth telling in clinical judgment is critical and is the place where both client and nurse must be involved in disclosing information and personal values. The importance of community dynamics in ethical behavior by health-care providers has been used to link caring to public policy.[31] Benner[32] corroborated the idea of community and the importance of a community of practitioners where the "good" can be expressed and lived out. It was noted that the physician's ability to remain technically expert and humane depended, in large part, on the substance of arrangements worked out with other professionals, especially nurses. The community of practice should be the arena in which individual providers can exercise moral and practical reasoning built on values that have been collectively shaped. In this sense, community becomes an experience of shared meaning about thinking and acting, an ongoing event in which moral virtues, values, and principles guide the behavior of all within the community toward responsible decision making for the good of the whole.[17]

Experiences of moral caring with clients by nurses and physicians in responsible communal interaction create useful patterns of meaning for future application. The patterns of meaning that emerge are informed and influenced by the inner experience of values, virtues, and principles, the cultural context, and the interaction with each individual in the clinical caring context. This approach places the focus of ethical research and practice on the experience of human be- ings themselves rather than on the problems of technical competence in the treatment of human beings. It has been suggested that a phenomenologic ethical inquiry into the experiences of virtues, values, and principles of the entire com- munity of health-care providers would clarify the foundations of choice making and guide growing understanding of a new ethic of shared responsibility. The process would offer a vision to decision makers who, by virtue of their activity in the practice of clinical ethics, act as cocreators of our communal moral life.[17]

ETHICAL CONCERNS OF THE ADVANCED PRACTICE NURSE

Nurses in advanced practice today experience numerous ethical concerns, but the concept of futility as applied in decisions of patient care and the impact of managed care on practice settings are examples indicative of the changing expe- riential dynamic for clients and providers. Ethics and the law give primacy to patient autonomy, which is defined as the right to be a fully informed partici- pant in all aspects of medical decision making and the right to refuse unwanted, even recommended and life-saving, medical care. In spite of the power of this concept, it should be remembered that futile treatments are not obligatory. No ethical principle or law has ever required physicians to offer or accede to de- mands for treatment that are futile. **Futility** refers to an expectation of success that is either predictably or empirically so unlikely that its exact probability is of- ten incalculable. Futility should be distinguished from hopelessness. Hopeless- ness is a subjective attitude, whereas futility refers to an objective quality of an action. Hope and hopelessness are related more to desire, faith, denial, and other psychological responses than to the objective probability that some contem- plated action will be successful.[33]

The futility of a treatment may be evident in either quantitative or qualita- tive terms. Futility may refer to the improbability of an event happening as a re- sult of treatment or to the quality of the event that such treatment might pro- duce. The process of determining futility resembles decision analysis with one important distinction. In decision analysis, the decision to use a procedure is based on considerations of both the probability of success and the quality or util- ity of the outcome. A very low probability of success may be balanced by very high utility. However, when determining futility, the quantitative and qualita- tive aspects are treated as independent thresholds or minimum cutoff levels, either of which frees the physician from the obligation to offer a medical treat- ment.[34]

In keeping with the quantitative approach to futility, it has been suggested that when physicians conclude, through personal experience, experiences shared with colleagues, or consideration of reported empirical data, that in the last 100 cases a medical treatment has been useless, that treatment should be re- garded as futile.[33] Truog, Brett, and Frader[34] wondered how similar patients must be to apply these criteria and raise the question of stratification according to age, debility, etiologic organism, and coexisting disease. Lantes et al.[35] pro- posed that any treatment that merely preserves permanent unconsciousness or that fails to end total dependence on intensive medial care should be regarded as nonbeneficial and therefore futile. Futility is a substantive concept but may ap- pear illusive when effects on patients are confused with benefits to the patient or when the "symbolic" representation to society of treating handicapped new-borns or patients in persistent vegetative states is allowed to take precedence over patient-centered decision making. Substantive objective application of futility is suggested to be a professional judgment that takes precedence over patient autonomy and permits physicians to withhold or withdraw care deemed to be inappropriate without patient approval. Decisions of this variety are believed to be representative of the ordinary duties of physicians, duties that are applicable where there is medical agreement that the described standard of futility has been met. Appropriate resource allocation arguments for limiting treatment, although currently under intense discussion in both corporate and public arenas, are generally looked on unfavorably in our present open system of medical care. This is true because no universally shared and accepted societal value system for appropriate allocation exists and because there are no guarantees that any limit of care that a physician imposes on the client will be equally applied by other physicians under the same circumstances. Because futility is almost always a matter of probability, objective reason asks, What statistical cutoff point should be chosen as the threshold for determining futility? Certainly no answer has been derived from current discussions. However, there are some general statements of responsibility available, such as the Statement of the Council on Ethical and Judicial Affairs of the AMA, which concludes that physicians are under no obligation to provide futile cardiopulmonary resuscitation. The statement fails to specify any level of statistical certainty at which that judgment is supported. Even a decision on such statistical points would likely have limited usefulness, because studies have corroborated the limitations of clinical assessment in correctly estimating both prognosis and diagnosis.[36]

Growing pressure has been placed on all providers to control health-care costs by more rigorously controlling medical options. This produces a tension between the value of autonomy, exercised in the form of consent to use or omit various interventions, and the necessity of better control of medical resource expenditures. No consensus exists about what constitutes a just method of balancing the desires of individual patients against the diverse needs of society.[36]

When providers believe that the requested treatment would not be in the patient's best interest, even from the patient's perspective, or that persistent requests by the patient or the patient's surrogate for further interventions are based on faulty reasoning, unrealistic expectations, or psychological factors, such as guilt or denial, an obligation exists to make every effort to clarify exactly what the patient seeks to achieve with continued treatment. Adequate and sensitive communication between patient and provider often successfully resolves such problems.[36]

Truog, Brett, and Frader[34] recommended that most cases will benefit from sustained attempts to clarify the patient's values and the likelihood of the various relevant outcomes and to improve communication with patients or their surrogates. If this fails, physicians and APNs should carefully consider whether the care requested is consistent with their professional ethics and ideals. If inconsistency is perceived, alternative venues for care should be found or the conflict should be discussed in a more public forum, such as in the hospital's ethics committees or in the courts. Public scrutiny furthers the debate over the appropriate use of medical resources and fosters the development of consensus through legislation and public-policy development.

Managed care is not a new phenomenon. Zoloth-Dorfman and Rubin[37] noted that in the nineteenth and early twentieth centuries, groups of marginalized individuals created prepaid, capitated managed-care plans in response to the problems that they experienced in securing adequate health-care services. These attempts at prepaid care included immigrant aid societies, trade unions, and company insurance plans. Such plans developed as a response to a medical delivery system not designed to guarantee access to services for those unable to pay a fee at the time of need. The utility of such efforts is evidenced by the continuing success of the Kaiser Permanente system, Group Health of Puget Sound, and other nonprofit health-maintenance organizations (HMOs). The current upsurge of managed-care plans differs from their historical predecessors by being increasingly structured as for-profit rather than nonprofit corporate entities. Further, development is occurring in a marketplace that is largely unregulated. The older nonprofit managed-care model of medicine provides for rationalizing the provision of health care, incorporation of a system of greater accountability, and resource pooling to provide the highest quality of care in the most cost-effective manner.

Managed-care plans, particularly those with for-profit corporate structures, have been characterized by providers as threatening to weaken or displace the professional commitment to beneficence and nonmaleficence that form the foundation of the therapeutic relationship and, hence, quality care. The popular press has responded by raising public concern that the incentive structures built into managed care will lead to the sacrifice of quality and safety for profit.[37]

Managed care does generate concern about who will make actual treatment decisions, how decision-making authority will be established, and on which criteria clinical decisions will be made.

Clients who are ill are in an inherently unequal power relationship with providers and health plans. As buyers of health care, they are rarely in a position to effectively evaluate the practice and standards of care promoted by managed-care organizations. At present, there are few regulations by which to control policy decisions that might not be in the best interest of the patient.[37] Advanced nurse practitioners should assume a role in the evaluation of these situations. Strong individual moral agency is developed by reflection on personal goals and aspirations as well as by an understanding of the limits of one's personal and professional commitments. To develop true moral agency, the nurse in advanced practice needs to take risks in preventing all plans that call for a gag order on health-care providers or suppress healthy debate on appropriate treatment modalities. Such risk taking requires courage because of both threatened and real loss of position and status.

Advanced practice nurses must learn to accurately manage information, effectively work in teams, integrate guidelines and clinical judgment, and manage outcomes. Both nurses and consumers need to assume an activist role and seek positions on the boards of directors of large managed-care organizations. APNs must develop as expert reviewers of practice guidelines and encourage the release of such guidelines for consumers' review. Areas for future activism include striving to obtain open review of staffing patterns and reasonable compensation for providers and administrators and to secure the consumer's right to a cost rebate for improved health status or nonutilization of resources. This type of activism, properly carried out, becomes a defining opportunity for professional growth and personal advocacy of the client's right to ethical care.

Suggested Exercises

1. A major problem with access to health care exists in a remote rural area. The county commissioners are considering a clinic staffed by a family nurse practitioner and a certified nurse midwife. The county attorney obtained all of the necessary permits and documents; however, one of the commissioners still has concern regarding legality of the nurses' practicing without the immediate presence of a physician. You, a family nurse practitioner, and your spouse, a certified nurse midwife, have been accepted to fill those positions, pending final approval of the county commissioners. They have asked you to prepare policies and procedures that would adhere to the national standards of such a practice. Prepare a model document that is realistic and practical. Assume that the state allows full prescriptive authority and physician collaboration (off site).

2. You are an experienced certified registered nurse anesthetist (CRNA) who has been asked to provide anesthesia services for a plastic surgeon in his office. You will be an independent practitioner and will be paid by the patient per case. In your state, CRNAs are not required to follow protocols or standardized procedures, and your standards of practice are determined by the profession. Prepare a document delineating the clinical policies of your practice, including preanesthesia evaluation and testing, selection of patients for elective ambulatory surgery, minimum equipment and supplies, and recovery discharge criteria and responsibility.

3. Prepare documents to conduct an annual legal audit of your practice. Include clinical policies, procedures, emergency situations, transfer of patients to another level of care, medical record documentation, and review of state laws and regulations. Also include your plan for keeping current in the clinical components of your practice.

4. Form two groups. One group will represent the ethics committee of a large HMO. The other group is made up of those who have survived cancer for more than 5 years. Collaboratively seek to set down criteria for appropriate withdrawal of medical nutrition and hydration from terminal cancer patients. Provide written rationales for your decisions.

REFERENCES

1. Davis, AJ, and Aroskar, MD: Ethical Dilemmas and Nursing Practice, ed 2. Appleton-Century-Crofts, Norwalk, Conn, 1983.
2. McManus, R: Ethical decision making in anesthesia. In Foster, S, and Jordan, L (eds): Professional Aspects of Nurse Anesthesia Practice. FA Davis, Philadelphia, 1994.
3. Smart, N: Worldviews: Cross Cultural Explorations of Human Beliefs, ed 2. Prentice-Hall, Englewood Cliffs, NJ, 1995.
4. Curtin, L: Human problems, human beings. Nursing Management 25(5):35, May 1994.
5. Aikens, CA: Studies in Ethics for Nurses, ed 4. WB Saunders, Philadelphia, 1937.
6. DeLoughery, GL, and Gebbie, KM: Political Dynamics: Impact on Nurses and Nursing. CV Mosby, St. Louis, 1975.
7. Churchill, L: Ethical issues of a profession in transition. Am J Nurs 77:874, 1987.

8. Callahan, D: Minimalist ethics. Hastings Cent Rep 11(5):19, 1981.
9. Gert, B, and Culver, C: The justification of paternalism. Ethics 89(2):199, 1979.
10. Monagle, JF, and Thomasma, DC: Medical Ethics. Aspen Publishers, Rockville, Md, 1988.
11. Curtin, L, and Flaherty, MJ: Nursing Ethics: Theories and Pragmatics. Robert J. Brady, Bowie, Md, 1982.
12. Rollins, BE (ed): The Experimental Animal in Biomedical Research : A Survey of Scientific and Ethical Issues for Investigators, Vol 1. Boca Raton, Fla, 1990.
13. Flight, MR: Medical ethics: Reach out and touch everyone. The Professional Medical Assistant, p 21, Nov/Dec 1987.
14. Fowler, MD: The role of the clinical ethicist. Heart Lung 15(3):318, 1986.
15. Thompson, JE, and Thompson, HO: Ethical decision making: Process and models. Neonatal Network 9(1):69, 1990.
16. Brown, KC: Effective decision making. American Association of Occupational Nurses Journal 38(3):139, 1990.
17. Ray, MA: Communal moral experiences as the starting point for research in health care ethics. Nurs Outlook 42:104, 1994.
18. Wiggins, OP, and Schwartz, MA: Techniques and persons: Habermasian reflections on medical ethics. Human Studies 9:365, 1986.
19. Jonsen, A: Of balloons and bicycles, or the relationship between ethical theory and practical judgment. Hastings Cent Rep 21: 14, 1991.
20. Agich, G, and Younger, S: For experts only? Access to hospital ethics committees. Hastings Cent Rep 21:17, 1991.
21. Brock, D: The ideal of shared decision making between physicians and patients. Kennedy Institute of Ethics Journal 1:28, 1991.
22. Engelhardt, HT: Negotiation: The key to making ethical decisions. In Cross, R, and Nobel, M (eds): The Value of Many Voices. University of Colorado Center for Health Ethics and Policy, Denver, 1987.
23. Cross, R, and Nobel, M (eds): The Value of Many Voices. University of Colorado Center for Health Ethics and Policy, Denver, 1987.
24. Ketefian, S: Ethics and Nursing Practice: Research Perspectives. Paper presented at the 1990 Second Annual Health Care Ethics Conference, Baltimore, May 1990.
25. Carpenter, MA: Clinical Psychiatric Nurses' Ethical Decision Making Process. Paper presented at the 1990 Second Annual Health Care Ethics Conference, Baltimore, May 1990.
26. Aroskar, M: Using ethical reasoning to guide clinical decision making. Perioperative Nursing Quarterly 2:20, 1986.
27. Roach, S: Caring, the Human Mode of Being, Implications for Nursing. Perspectives for Caring Monograph I. Faculty of Nursing, University of Toronto, Toronto, Canada, 1984.
28. Watson, J: Nursing: Human Science and Human Care. Appleton-Century-Crofts, Norwalk, Conn, 1985.
29. Leininger, M: Culture: The conspicuous missing link to understanding ethical and moral dimensions in human care. In Leininger, MM (ed): Ethical and Moral Dimensions of Care. Wayne State University Press, Detroit, 1990.
30. Gadow, S: Truth-telling revisited: Two approaches to the disclosing dilemma. In Leininger, MM (ed): Ethical and Moral Dimensions of Care. Wayne State University Press, Detroit, 1990.
31. Schultz, P, and Schultz, R: Nodding's caring and public policy: A linkage and its nursing implications. In Leininger, MM (ed): Ethical and Moral Dimensions of Care. Wayne State University Press, Detroit, 1990.
32. Benner, P: Experience, narrative, and community. Advances in Nursing Science 14(2): 1, 1991.
33. Schneiderman, LJ, Jecker, NS, and Jonsen, AR: Medical futility: Its meaning and ethical implications. Ann Intern Med 112(12):949, 1990.
34. Truog, RD, Brett, AS, and Frader, J: Sounding board: The problem with futility. N Engl J Med 326:1560, 1992.
35. Lantes, JD, et al: The illusion of futility in clinical practice. Am J Med 87:81, 1989.
36. Emery, DD, and Schneiderman, LJ: Cost effectiveness analysis in health care. Hastings Cent Rep 19:8, 1989.
37. Zoloth-Dorfman, L, and Rubin, S: The patient as commodity: Managed care and the question of ethics. J Clin Ethics 6:339, 1995.

CHAPTER 13

Creating Excellence in Practice

Creating Excellence in Practice

MARLA J. WESTON, MS, RN
VICKI L. BUCHDA, MS, RN
DEBRA BERGSTROM, MS, RN, CCRN, FNP

Marla J. Weston, MS, RN, who is currently a resident of Phoenix, Arizona, received her master of science in nursing from Arizona State University in Tempe and her bachelor of science in nursing from Indiana University of Pennsylvania in Indiana, Pennsylvania. Weston is the acute care administrator for Columbia Paradise Valley Hospital in Phoenix, Arizona. She has also served as an adjunct faculty member at Arizona State University and a mentor to advanced practice nurses (APNs) experiencing the role transition to their first position and facilitated the growth and development of experienced advanced practice nurses. Ms. Weston is affiliated with the American Nurses' Association, the American Organization of Nurse Executives, and the American Association of Critical Care Nurses. She is a member of Sigma Theta Tau National Honor Society.

Vicki L. Buchda, MS, RN, received her master of science from Arizona State University in Tempe in 1987 and her bachelor of science in nursing from Marian College of Fond du Lac in Wisconsin in 1979. She is currently nurse manager for critical care and telemetry units at Del E. Webb Memorial Hospital in Sun City West, Arizona. Ms. Buchda is actively involved in several organizations, including Sigma Theta Tau, where she recently completed a term as president of Beta Upsilon Chapter. She is also a member of the American Nurses' Association, American Association of Critical Care Nurses, and Society for Critical Care Medicine.

Debra Bergstrom, MS, RN, CCRN, FNP, received her master of science in critical care nursing from Arizona State University in 1992 and her bachelor of science in nursing in 1985 from the University of Texas at El Paso. She has served in staff roles in a variety of clinical areas, including postpartum care, cardiovascular intensive care, cardiac care and neurosurgery, and cardiac catheterization laboratory. In 1995, she completed a postgraduate certification program as a family nurse practitioner. Currently, she is establishing a nurse practitioner role in an established internal medicine practice. She is the first nurse practitioner in private practice to obtain hospital privileges at Mercy Integrated Health in Phoenix, Arizona.

13

CHAPTER OUTLINE

ATTRIBUTES OF EXCELLENCE
Values
Vision
Passion

Mastery
Action
Balance
SUMMARY
SUGGESTED EXERCISES

CHAPTER OBJECTIVES

After completing this chapter, the reader will be able to:

1. Incorporate knowledge about concepts of excellence into a personal definition of excellence.
2. Apply principles of excellence to an advanced practice role.
3. Articulate strategies for creating and maintaining excellence.

dvanced practice nurses are expected to exceed the basic standards of nursing practice. Nursing's Social Policy Statement1 describes APNs as master's-prepared clinicians who:

- Practice within an area of specialization and with greater autonomy than nurses in other roles
- Function at the expanding boundaries of nursing's scope of practice
- Acquire ever-increasing levels of knowledge and skills
- Integrate advanced theoretical concepts and research-based knowledge into clinical practice

Given these already high expectations, how can one distinguish excellence in those engaged in advanced practice?

Attributes of Excellence

Badness you can get easily, in quantity: the road is smooth, and it lies close by. But in front of excellence the immortal gods have put sweat. . . .
  HESIOD, 700 BC

How does the condition or quality of being excellent arise? Webster defines the word **excellent** as "superior, very good of its kind, eminently good." Synonyms for *excellent* include *superior, premium, superb, distinct,* and *admirable.* Two other words expand on this definition. The verb *exceed* is derived from the Latin *ex cedere,* meaning "to go more." The verb *excel* is from the Latin *ex cellere,* which means "to rise above or project." The concepts of going beyond and of rising above are inherent in the word *excellent.* Pinkerton[2] wrote that

> Professional excellence implies competence and a striving for high standards in every aspect of life. (p. 280)

Excellence involves an ongoing comparison to a standard or that which is generally accepted, as well as an unceasing attempt to achieve more and to improve one's performance. Thus, excellence is a dynamic condition that is continually redefined and reinterpreted.

Although the state of excellence is dynamic, excellent organizations and individuals have been repeatedly associated with the following attributes:

- Values
- Vision
- Passion
- Mastery
- Action
- Balance

In this chapter, these attributes establish a framework for exploring excellence in advanced practice nursing. Examples of excellence in organizations and individuals are provided, and strategies for fostering excellence in advanced practice nursing are proposed.

VALUES

There is no such thing as a minor lapse of integrity.
TOM PETERS

There is always one true inner voice. Trust it.
GLORIA STEINEM

A review of the literature on values demonstrates that excellence is characterized by behaviors consistent with certain universally held values, as well as the values of one's profession, the values of one's organization, and one's own personally held values. Certain values, such as *integrity, honesty, respect for others,* and *fairness,* are universally held and are not based on any particular religion, social philosophy, or ethical system.[3] They are part of all enduring societies. Behaviors consistent with universally held values are necessary for excellence. As Henderson[4] maintained, the personal integrity of the individual [and, we add, organization] is inseparable from the quality of the service given. Integrity requires being honest and authentic with oneself and others, as well as taking substantial responsibility for agreements to which one has committed oneself.[5] Behaving with integrity and in a manner consistent with universally held values also creates *energy* for oneself and others.

When individuals, organizations, or societies fail to act according to universal principles, distrust and fear ensue, power imbalances arise, and ultimately, excellence is inhibited. Conversely, individuals and organizations that embody universal values promote harmonious relationships and excellence. When Bob Galvin, then chairman of Motorola, was negotiating a lucrative contract with a South American country, he was asked by the country's leaders to write the contract for an extra $1 million, with the understanding that the officials would skim this from the project. Because this request was clearly in violation of the principle of honesty, Motorola turned down the contract and refused further business with the country. Galvin noted that country's leaders are long deposed, whereas Motorola is still considered an organization of excellence.[5]

However, it has been suggested that there is little economic reason to justify honesty and integrity in business and minimal consequences for failure to tell the truth. In fact, some equate dishonesty with *business success.*[6] Davidhizar[7] analyzed honesty in nursing practice and found that when nurses were dishonest, they acted this way for reasons including self-protection, protection of other health-care providers, and protection of patients. She acknowledged that while paybacks for honesty are few, some important rewards include increased self-respect, peace with oneself, greater trust by others, and a reputation of integrity. Trust and honesty are the cornerstones for relationships between clients and providers and among professional colleagues.

Excellent professionals embody the core values of their professions. *Caring, advocacy, accountability, accessibility,* and *collaboration* with other health and community professionals have been articulated as values to which APNs subscribe.[8] In addition, professionals are expected to realize a "higher morality and a greater commitment to the good of others"[9] because of the special nature of the interpersonal relationship entered into with clients. The uniqueness of the relationship is based on the particular vulnerability of clients, which creates an inequality of power in the relationship. The expectation of professionals is that this vulnerability will be the source of trust and obligation, not profit or exploitation.

Excellence, whether in a company or an individual, requires clearly delineating core values. In the early 1980s, after researching attributes of excellent corporations, Peters and Waterman[10] proposed that solid commitment to the values of the organization is linked to the success of a company. Their "one all-purpose bit of advice for management" was to identify, communicate, and base actions on these values. For example, the success of Nordstrom Department Stores can be traced to clearly profiling, communicating. and enacting the value of "customer above company." The working culture of Nordstrom is filled with anecdotes of salespeople meeting the customer's needs in creative and unconventional ways. One Nordstrom saleswoman went to a rival department store for a customer to purchase a dress that Nordstrom did not carry. She then sold it to the astonished customer for less than the retail price.[11] The saleswoman's behavior was based squarely on her interpretation of the customer-above-company value and was endorsed as such. Whatever the values ascribed, successful companies are resolutely committed. Motorola, for example, strongly values honesty. As a result, discussions in Motorola often involve open disagreement and critique of ideas, even to the point of embarrassing and confronting individuals. Outsiders sometimes describe this as disrespectful or barbaric. Employees of Motorola say anything less is dishonest, and "backroom politics" and "roundabout decision making" is not tolerated.[5]

Peak performance is obtained when the values of the organization, the profession, and the person are aligned.[12] Excellent professionals are knowledgeable about the values of an organization and weigh them in comparison to the core values and traditions of the profession. In situations where the values are aligned, APNs experience a sense of participation and achievement, as well as potential for learning and growth. Koerner[13] found that for APNs, the values and job description were congruent. These values reflected initiative, decision making, accountability, and internal locus of control behaviors. Most APNs prefer to work in organizations with a participative management style.[14] Involvement in goal setting and decision making is associated with increased job satisfaction. Performing interesting and challenging work, assuming responsibility, experiencing achievement, having potential for growth, and receiving recognition as professionals add to their satisfaction.[15]

In the current health-care climate, many professional values seem to collide with those of the business environment. If an individual's values are not congruent with those of the organization, several outcomes are possible. Some professionals might continue to perform the job, ignoring the conflict and suppressing personal and/or professional values. Others may be tenacious, continuing to do the job while trying to reconcile the differences. However, excellence in practice is difficult, if not impossible, when professional or universal values are undermined by an individual or an environment.[16] Excellent APNs strive to create or find organizations and practice environments with more compatible value systems, even when the consequences can be considerable, such as making a job change. Initially, for example, the drive for increased efficiency, productivity, and profit can seem diametrically opposed to the APN's core values. To create excellence, the APN must reconcile the desire to provide caring, personalized attention to each client with the demand for ensuring cost-effective outcomes. In right-fit organizations, where individual, professional, and organizational values are aligned, APNs can excel and realize opportunities to improve the quality of care while controlling cost.[17]

At times, ethical predicaments occur when there is no option but to choose between equally unsatisfactory alternatives in which there is no "clearly best" solution. Drucker[18] advised that to obtain excellence, one has to start with what is right rather than with what is acceptable, because compromise is inevitable. In these difficult situations, basing decisions on professional and personal values can lead to excellence. In a study of nurse practitioners, Viens[19] found that strong personal and professional values guided and shaped the resolution of moral dilemmas in clinical practice. Values formed the bases for their rationales, actions, and choices. All of the values identified centered on APNs' relationship to the client. Understanding one's motives, acting for the good of the whole and not solely for oneself, caring about the values of the organization, and having concern for others are crucial to the ultimate resolution of the internal battle between the tendency toward self-interest and the obligation to serve.

VISION

If you can dream it, you can do it.
    WALT DISNEY

Reality is something you rise above.
    LIZA MINNELLI

A clear vision of what is *possible* is necessary for excellence. Creating a *new reality* occurs by first imagining that possibility. Visions may arise from speculation about the future or by posing these questions: Why are things being done in a certain way? What is missing in this situation? What is the desired state? Visions arise from what should be and require rising above "the tyranny of what is." Garfield[12] described the culture at the NASA during the Apollo 11 project. The excitement of the mission, the challenge of the task, and the vision of putting a man on the moon all combined to create a culture where otherwise unremarkable people became peak performers.

Making the vision a reality becomes the raison d'être. In all excellent organizations, decisions are made and priorities are set according to the vision. Work that does not support the vision is considered extraneous and consequently aborted.[10] Vision, based on core values, allows a powerful focus toward a future desired state or destination. Organizations and individuals characterized as excellent not only set priorities according to their vision, they concentrate on the highest priorities; that is, they do first things first.[5,18]

Successful APNs have a vision and know where they want to go. Creating a vision involves knowing what outcomes are desired and can occur on various levels, including personal, clinical, and organizational levels. Having a clear image of the future allows APNs to avoid getting caught in the inefficiency of engaging in activities that may not be vital or productive. On a basic level, creating and maintaining excellence requires the ability to discipline meeting schedules and in-boxes.[20] Moreover, excellent APNs outline long-term agendas, establish priorities, and serve as agents for constructive change. Excellent APNs guard against confusing activity with accomplishment. Bustling activity is not, in and of itself, equated with productivity and organizational imperatives, nor does it necessarily mean that one is moving toward a vision.

Unfortunately, a vision rarely provides a detailed map for a journey, but rather acts as a beacon, providing direction. A prescribed journey with much structure would likely extinguish the opportunities for chance and intuition. As evidenced by hundreds of scientists, including Jonas Salk and Albert Einstein, chance and intuition are very useful in achieving one's vision.[5] The excellent visionary is skillful in integrating reasoning, chance, and intuition.

Garfield[12] described this integrating process as "course correction," an adjustment of the critical pathway whenever cues indicate that desired results are not occurring. Setbacks and mistakes may be valuable signs that it is time to correct course. Course correction employs three skills:

1. Mental agility, which is the ability to change perspective when challenges occur

2. Concentration, which includes stamina, adaptability to changes, and hardiness

3. Learning from mistakes

The ability to correct course enhances the achievement of vision and propels one's movement further in the right direction, despite seeming setbacks.

PASSION

People can smell emotional commitment from a mile away.

Remember, passion is contagious.
TOM PETERS

Commitment to excellence is required for its *achievement*, and *passion* is essential to *sustain* excellence. Peters and Austin[21] described it as

> hanging in there long after others have gotten bored or given up; it's refusing to leave well enough alone. (p. 415)

Just as consistency between values and behavior produces energy and passion, it also enables *energy* to create excellence. Passion involves ardently striving for the best, even when repeated efforts seem tedious or appear exceedingly strenuous. Passion motivates via a clear sense of purpose and devotion to high standards.[5] The president of Racing Strollers described her turmoil, speculating about whether she was too demanding when she required that something be done over and over until it was perfect: a seam sewn straighter, a color redyed to be purer. She eventually recognized that because she cared so intensely, she was able to see more, to analyze better, and to insist that there be continuous improvement in the product. This ability to recognize the "just-noticeable difference" is a result of passion. She wrote, "Someone has to be slightly crazed, obsessive, and willing to set a high standard"[22] (p. 20).

The APN who cares a little more will encourage colleagues to become involved and will facilitate independent thinking and judgment. The APN with passion will not be satisfied with providing less than optimal care and will pursue the latest research, the most up-to-date procedures, and the most effective therapies to produce the best outcomes for patients.

A caution should be noted in the enactment of passion. One may be criticized for being unduly emotional, excessively driven, overly involved, or having unrealistic standards. Many passionate individuals experience a tension between excellence and balance in personal life.[21] Being passionate about creating excellence requires energy, time, and commitment. It may demand late nights and the sacrifice of an occasional weekend. Thus, "the adventure of excellence is not for the faint of heart"[21] (p. 414). Passion requires courage and high self-esteem and should be looked on as a gift. Yet passion must be disciplined in order to prevent inflexibility and loss of perspective. The APN can compare self-perceptions with those of colleagues to assess the degree to which passion is creating excellence. Colleagues can often assist an APN to channel passion to achieve envisioned outcomes while developing and preserving relationships.

MASTERY

People with high levels of personal mastery are continually expanding their ability to create the results in life they truly seek.
PETER SENGE

The cornerstone of mastery is expertise. The Dreyfus model[22a] of skill acquisition and development defines five levels of proficiency:

1. Novice
2. Advanced beginner
3. Competent
4. Proficient
5. Expert

As individuals evolve from novice to expert, they:

- Decrease reliance on abstract principles and increase application of past experience
- Move from viewing situations as comprising equally relevant bits of information to perceiving the whole, in which some parts have greater importance
- Diminish the detached observer orientation in favor of fuller involvement as a performer

When encountering that which has not been experienced before, or when events are unfolding in an unexpected manner, experts rely on abstract principles. However, in familiar circumstances, experts apply both theoretical and practical knowledge to actual situations. Benner[23] described expert nurses as having gestalt or holistic understanding. Because of their enormous background of experience, expert nurses perceive patterns of events in an ongoing process of contrasting and comparing scenarios. As a result, experts can sense the wholeness of a situation while recognizing separate components and are able to focus on the nature of the problem without wastefully exploring irrelevant or implausible alternatives.

Mastery is the ability to channel one's values, vision, and passion via the *milieu of expertise* to create superlative outcomes. Florence Nightingale demonstrated mastery in nursing not only through innovations in care of the sick but also by exerting her influence on powerful individuals to assist her in instituting changes to the practice of nursing. Mastery combines expert professional skills with *leadership, interpersonal,* and *organizational* proficiency. Technical and professional skills are not necessarily sufficient to make one successful within an organization. The ability to translate vision into action, clarify values, use intuition, negotiate, create consensus, implement change, and work through others is essential to progress to the master level. Masters enact these skills because they want to engage *others* in making a vision a reality.[24] Masters simultaneously hold an engaging image of a distant vision while dealing with current reality.

Mastery compels a lifelong pursuit of learning. Interestingly, although masters are confident of their competence, paradoxically they are acutely aware of what they do not know. Mastery involves approaching situations with the *inquisitiveness* of an amateur and a *willingness* to learn from mistakes. Even the master APN may feel unprepared and inadequate in certain situations. Some believe it is necessary to be perfect at everything they do, lest they be "discovered" as an impostor. Many nurses in advanced practice roles suffer from this "impostor phenomenon."[25] The impostor phenomenon denotes healthy, successful, high-achieving individuals who hide an inner feeling of inadequacy, intellectual phoniness, and a belief that they have fooled everyone. Certain situations, such as starting a new job, moving into a new role, and interacting with authority figures may escalate feelings of being an impostor, including depression, generalized anxiety, lack of self-confidence, frustration, and an overall feeling of ignorance. The risk with the impostor phenomenon is that the APN will settle for the safe and certain to avoid these uncomfortable emotions. Recognizing that many other successful individuals experience the impostor phenomenon can help the APN to celebrate achievements and continue to strive for excellence.

Candor concerning one's personal and professional strengths and weaknesses is essential to mastery. Seeking feedback and peer review for self-improvement is one of the most effective avenues for building mastery. APNs who work arduously to get feedback from many sources are more likely to achieve mastery. Peer review provides a forum for sharing information, offering guidance, contributing constructive criticism and direction to other clinical nurses and other advanced practitioners, and getting the same in return. Additional approaches to nurture mastery include ongoing dialogue, education and training, and demonstration of competence by certification. Information obtained from continuing education meetings or conferences, as well as from discussions with colleagues are the most frequent sources of practice changes for APNs.[26,27] Masters ensure they have budgeted time for ongoing learning and creative thinking.

In addition to these strategies, today's rapidly changing health-care environment demands that one be able to unlearn old ways of doing things when they no longer apply in order to relearn new methods.[24] Unlearning involves challenging the ways of thinking that worked well in the past but are no longer appropriate for the future.[28] Home Depot, a warehouse hardware store, is a good example of effective unlearning. Home Depot "forgot" that its customers were male home builders or owners; they learned to provide decorating services and a bridal registry.[29]

Perhaps the most expansive and promising mastery trajectory is that of mentorship. Mentorship is an informal, intense personal relationship in which a senior person offers the wisdom of experience to guide and influence the career of a novice. A mentor is a teacher, coach, taskmaster, confidant, counselor, and friend. Chapter 8 describes the roles and contributions of mentors in developing excellence in APNs.

ACTION

We are what we repeatedly do. Excellence, then, is not an act, but a habit.
ARISTOTLE

I think one's feelings waste themselves in words, they ought all to be distilled into actions and into actions which bring results.
FLORENCE NIGHTINGALE

Values, vision, passion, and mastery form a foundation for excellence, but action enables it. Action is what gives credibility to the values, vision, passion, and mastery of the APN.

Peters and Waterman[10] described one of eight attributes of America's best-run companies as "a bias for action." These companies are analytic when making decisions, but are not plagued by the pursuit of perfection and do not suffer from "paralysis by analysis." Experimentation and a sense of urgency reign in these companies. Standard operating procedure is "Do it, fix it, try it." For example, Bell and Howell proposed the idea of selling movie cameras by direct mail. Realizing that it would take an investment of only $10,000 to try the idea, they decided to act—a decision that ultimately spared them $100,000 worth of time to study the idea.[10]

A bias for action encompasses a focus on results. Activity is performed with a clear sense of contribution.[18] Clearly identifying and measuring contributions assist in creating excellence. Evaluations of APNs' contributions have historically been limited to documentation of time spent on various activities, number of patients seen, or amount of revenue generated. For a novice APN, an assessment and documentation of time involvement may assist in learning to effectively prioritize and organize time.[30] However, time documentation alone will not demonstrate the impact of an APN. APNs can focus on results and demonstrate their impact on cost and quality outcomes in any of the following areas[31–33]:

- Reduction of use of costly technology and inpatient care
- Reduction of inpatient lengths of stay
- Improvements in patients' levels of functioning
- Enhanced patient satisfaction
- Improvements in the quality of care provided

Combining process and outcome measurements through research, evaluative studies, or quality-improvement activities will further assist the APN in demonstrating the impact of advanced practice. For example, a clinical nurse specialist developed a comprehensive educational plan for families and children who were newly diagnosed with insulin-dependent diabetes. As an outcome, in a 2-year period, none of the children who participated in the program had been readmitted to the hospital with hypoglycemia or ketoacidosis.[34]

Excellence requires action taken with a focus on results rather than with concern for who gets credit. Actions carried out in a self-serving manner or solely directed to gain the recognition of others will not result in excellence. Block[35] presented this as the concept of "stewardship":

the willingness to be accountable for the well-being of the larger organization by operating in service, rather than control, of those around us. (p. xx)

Stewardship is based on the value of service: service to clients, the public, colleagues, and the organization. The excellent APN acts as a steward in action.

Stewardship and the pursuit of excellence also entail "giving back" to one's profession. As Curtin[36] described:

> One of the most effective ways to promote excellence in nursing practice and to disseminate new information is for nurses to offer information, support, guidance, criticism and direction to one another. (p. 28)

Mentoring others is imperative for sustaining excellence in the profession. Serving as a mentor supports the socialization of novices to the profession's values and standards as well as the development of others to take risks, to reach their full potential, and to make substantial contributions to the profession.[37]

Involvement in professional organizations also furnishes APNs with an opportunity to use their knowledge, skills, and talents to create excellence both in practice and in patient care. Involving oneself with professional organizations, both on a community and a national level, not only provides the chance to stimulate the thinking of other nurse colleagues but also stimulates the APN's thinking. In addition, most APNs find that political advocacy is most expedient through professional organizations.[38] Professional organizations often monitor health-care legislation and provide that information to their members. Professional organizations have the pooled resources of all member to influence political decisions through contributions, lobbying activities, or voting drives. Health care is becoming increasingly shaped by political decisions. Historically, nurses have not been any more active in the political process than other citizens.[39] APNs can be instrumental in working toward political consensus and cohesion with professional groups, as well as in using their visibility to influence members of the community on political issues.

Sharing clinical expertise and research results through scholarly presentations and publications provides another way for the excellent APN to give back to the profession. Poster presentations, joint presentation, or authorship with a more experienced colleague; review of an area of clinical literature; or descriptions of innovations in clinical practices provide relatively easy ways to begin presenting and publishing.

Excellence in action necessitates reasonable risk taking. Reasonable risk taking involves encouraging meritorious attempts while supporting mistakes. For example, knowing that only 1 trial in 10 results in a successful product, excellent companies encourage exploration of all possible trials, rapidly abandoning ideas that show no promise and actively pursuing those that show the potential of success.[10] McDonald's has more experimental menu items, store formats, and pricing plans than its competitors. Although most experimental menu items fail, within 2 years of experimenting with breakfast menus in a few rural franchises, breakfast accounted for 35 percent of McDonald's revenues.[10] Risk taking allows and accepts the potential for failure, minimizes control, and "steps outside of the box." While risk can sometimes be minimized by gaining additional information, time, or control,[40] the optimum direction for action is often unclear. Excellent individuals react to this ambiguity with elegance by making the best decision possible with the information available, then acting on it.

"Optimizing," that is, making the most effective use of all available and potential resources, has been shown to promote excellence.[41] Optimizing involves three phases:

- **Surviving:** making effective use of available resource to sustain current performance
- **Investing:** developing potential resources and investing in the future
- **Transforming:** reversing negative situations and creating additional resources for change and advancement

Failure to optimize results in floundering, inability to cope or to meet demands of the role. The most relevant characteristics of nursing leaders who transformed their organizations from mediocrity to excellence included:

- Total commitment guided by values
- Determination and persistence
- Courage
- Strong power base
- Political acumen
- An ability to be articulate
- A global perspective

Thus, a bias for action, reasonable risk taking, and optimizing enable excellence.

BALANCE

Balance isn't either/or; it's and.
STEVEN COVEY, ROGER MERRILL, AND REBECCA MERRILL

Move like a beam of light,

Fly like lightning,

Strike like thunder,

Whirl in circles around a stable center.
MORIHEI UESHIBA

Balance provides flexibility and stability. Being balanced is similar to having two feet on the ground: A strong wind will cause some sway but not a fall. Being unbalanced is like being tipped so that one foot is off the ground: Even a small wind can result in being toppled. Excellence requires that one balance several potentially conflicting areas: logic and emotion, home and work, urgency and importance, production and renewal. Balancing these potential incongruities makes them complementary and creates a stable base or enhances the effectiveness of a person's established base. Creating excellence requires that one be balanced. The challenge to the APN who feels pulled in multiple directions is to develop strategies for maintaining balance. Balance requires actively managing time, carefully selecting renewal activities, and becoming a well-rounded individual.

Effective time management starts with clear values and vision. Balance necessitates that time is spent on activities consistent with the identified values and vision. Balance also entails both prioritizing activities and disciplining passion to spend on only selected goals, instead of every goal. It involves resisting getting caught up in the unimportant even though it feels urgent. Saying no to seemingly urgent but lower-priority demands allows time to accomplish the truly important. One of the most effective strategies is to plan your time by *first* scheduling the most important activities.[42]

Excellence cannot be created in one area of life at the expense of all others. Working to the detriment of health or playing to the detriment of work does not maintain excellence in either category. Balance requires a holistic focus: attention to creating well-rounded, complementary skills and to spending time on renewal activities that reenergize.

However, it is unrealistic to expect that the meticulous use of even the best time management strategies will prevent periods of imbalance. Almost anything of excellence requires a short-term burst of intense time and energy. Completing a major project, starting a new job, or finishing graduate school all can require a spurt of concentrated time and attention if excellence is the goal. Short-term periods of imbalance in the use of time do not necessarily result in imbalance in the person. If the period is time limited, consistent with the overall vision, and accompanied by renewal activities, the individual can remain balanced.

Renewal activities can assist in creating excellence both during times of intense activities and during normal daily existence. Renewal activities restore energy through rest or recreation and can be physical, spiritual, mental, and social and/or emotional.[3] Renewal activities should be carefully selected to reenergize, not merely to become additions to an already lengthy "to-do" list. Purposefully selecting renewal activities that complement work activities assists in creating balance and can even enhance productivity. For example, the professional with a mentally demanding job may select renewal activities that are physical. Similarly, taking breaks every 2 hours can improve the efficiency of writing an article. Even stopping to take 10 slow deep breaths in the midst of a hectic day can assist in providing balance.

Balance also includes cultivating and applying synergistic and holistic aspects of the personality. As Henderson[4] stated, "Excellence, to me, suggests the well-rounded, or complete, person." The more complementary skills individuals possess, the more balanced they are. Integrating reason and intuition, combining the technical and the creative, and linking emotion and rationality assist in creating excellence.

Summary

How do you create excellence? Tom Watson of IBM would answer that you decide, as of this second, to quit doing less than excellent work.[43] Excellence comes from an inner core: the desire and commitment to be excellent, in other words, valuing excellence, having a vision of excellence, and being passionate about creating and maintaining excellence. APNs must arm themselves with the necessary tools to create excellence, including mastery of clinical, leadership, interpersonal, and organizational skills; the willingness and ability to translate that mastery into action; and the ability to balance conflicting demands to remain centered on achieving excellence.

Suggested Exercises

1. Admiral H. G. Rickover[44] stated, "If a profession is to have its proper place in the further development of society, it must be increasingly dissatisfied with things as they are" (p. 12). Identify an area of dissatisfaction within health care or the nursing profession. Using a variety of professional approaches, detail strategies that can be used to create excellence in this area.

2. Develop your own definition of excellence in advanced practice nursing. Identify an APN colleague who embodies excellence as you have defined it. Analyze the attributes of excellence demonstrated by this individual. What strategies did this colleague use to create excellence in advanced practice?

3. Consider whether individuals can be excellent in isolation or whether synergy is required to create excellence. What role have colleagues and mentors played in shaping your vision and achievement of excellence?

4. Evaluate how you are spending your time. Is the way you are spending your time helping or impeding you from achieving your personal and professional goals for excellence?

REFERENCES

1. American Nurses' Association: Nursing's Social Policy Statement. American Nurses Publishing, Washington, DC, 1995.
2. Pinkerton, S: Summary. In Pinkerton, S, and Schroeder, P (eds): Commitment to Excellence: Developing a Professional Nursing Staff. Aspen, Rockville, Md, 1988.
3. Covey, SR: The Seven Habits of Highly Effective People: Powerful Lessons in Personal Change. Simon and Schuster, New York, 1989.
4. Henderson, V: Excellence in nursing. Am J Nurs 90:76, 1990.
5. Hendricks, G, and Ludeman, K: The Corporate Mystic: A Guidebook for Visionaries with Their Feet on the Ground. Bantam Books, New York, 1996.
6. Bhide, A, and Stevenson, H: Why be honest if honesty doesn't pay? Harvard Business Review 68:121, 1990.
7. Davidhizar, R: Honesty: The best policy in nursing practice. Today's OR Nurse, 14(1): 30, 1992.
8. National Council of State Boards of Nursing: Position Paper on the Licensure of Advanced Practice Nursing. Unpublished material, 1992.
9. Pellegrino, ED: What is a profession? J Allied Health 12:168, 1983.
10. Peters, TJ, and Waterman, RH: In Search of Excellence: Lessons from America's Best-Run Companies. Warner Books, New York, 1982.
11. Spector, R, and McCarthy, PD: The Nordstrom Way: The Inside Story of America's #1 Customer Service Company. John Wiley & Sons, New York, 1995.
12. Garfield, C: Peak Performers: The New Heroes of American Business. William Morrow and Co, New York, 1986.
13. Koerner, JG: Congruency between nurses' values and job requirements: A call for integrity. Holistic Nurse Practitioner 10(2):69, 1996.
14. Katims, I: Nursing as aesthetic experience and the notion of practice. Sch Inq Nurs Pract 7:26, 1993.
15. Lucas, MD: Organizational management style and clinical nurse specialists' job satisfaction. Clinical Nurse Specialist 2:70, 1988.
16. Koelbel, PW, Fuller, SG, and Misener, TR: Job satisfaction of nurse practitioners: An analysis using Herzberg's theory. Nurs Pract 16:43, 1991.
17. Parr, MBE: The changing role of advanced practice nursing in a managed care environment. AACN Clin Issues 7:300, 1996.
18. Drucker, PF: The Effective Executive. HarperBusiness, New York, 1966.
19. Viens, DC: Moral dilemmas experienced by nurse practitioners. Nurse Pract Forum 5: 209, 1994.
20. Smith, PM: Blazing flashes of the obvious. Executive Excellence 10:4, 1993.

21. Peters, T, and Austin, N: A Passion for Excellence: The Leadership Difference. Random House, New York, 1985.

22. Baechler, M: Loves me, loves me not. Inc 17: 19, 1995.

22a. Dreyfus, HL, and Dreyfus, SE: Mind over Machine. Free Press, New York, 1986.

23. Benner, P: From Novice to Expert: Excellence and Power in Clinical Nursing Practice. Addison-Wesley, Menlo Park, Calif, 1984.

24. Senge, PM: The Fifth Discipline: The Art & Practice of the Learning Organization. Doubleday, New York, 1990.

25. Arena, DM, and Page, NE: The impostor phenomenon in the clinical nurse specialist role. Image J Nurs Sch 24:121, 1992.

26. Flowers, JS, et al: How obstetric/gynecologic nurse practitioners make practice changes: A national study. Journal of the American Academy of Nurse Practitioners 1: 132, 1989.

27. Johnson, TP: Continuing education survey of certified registered nurse anesthetists. AANA Journal 58:423, 1990.

28. Hamel, G, and Prahalad, CK: Competing for the Future: Breakthrough Strategies for Seizing Control of Your Industry and Creating the Markets of Tomorrow. Harvard Business School Press, Boston, 1994.

29. McGill, ME, and Slocum, JW Jr: Unlearning the organization. Organizational Dynamics 22(2):67, 1993.

30. Hamric, AB: A model for CNS evaluation. In Hamric, AB, and Spross, J: The Clinical Nurse Specialist in Theory and Practice, ed 2. WB Saunders, Philadelphia, 1989.

31. Gibson, SJ, et al: CNS-directed case management: Cost and quality in harmony. J Nurs Adm 24(6):45, 1994.

32. Cronin, CJ, and Maklebust, J: Case-managed care: Capitalizing on the CNS. Nursing Management 20(3):38, 1989.

33. Werner, JS, Bumann, RM, and O'Brien, JA: Clinical nurse specialization: An annotated bibliography: Evaluation and impact. Clinical Nurse Specialist 3:20, 1989.

34. Peglow, DM, et al: Evaluation of clinical nurse specialist practice. Clinical Nurse Specialist 6:28, 1992.

35. Block, P: Stewardship: Choosing Service over Self-Interest. Berrett-Koehler, San Francisco, 1993.

36. Curtin, L: Collegial ethics of a caring profession. Nursing Management 25(8):28, 1994.

37. Vance C: Mentoring for career success and satisfaction. J Adv Nurs 11:3, 1994.

38. Nelson, ML: Client Advocacy. In Snyder, M, and Mirr, MP: Advanced Practice Nursing: A Guide to Professional Development. Springer, New York, 1995.

39. Maraldo, PJ: Politics and Policy in Primary Care. In Mezey, MD, and McGivern, DO: Nurse Pract: Evolution to Advanced Practice. Springer, New York, 1993.

40. MacCrimmon, KR, and Wehrung, DA: Taking Risks: The Management of Uncertainty. Free Press, New York, 1986.

41. Irurita, V: Transforming mediocrity to excellence: A challenge for nurse leaders. Australian J Adv Nurs 9(4):15, 1992.

42. Covey, SR, Merrill, AR, and Merrill, RR: First Things First. Simon and Schuster, New York, 1994.

43. Peters, T: The Pursuit of WOW!: Every Person's Guide to Topsy-Turvy Times. Vintage, New York, 1994.

44. Rickover, HG: Thoughts on Man's Purpose in Life. Paper presented to the Rotary Club of San Diego, 1977.

Index